Nausea and Vomiting in Pregnancy
An Integrated Approach to Care

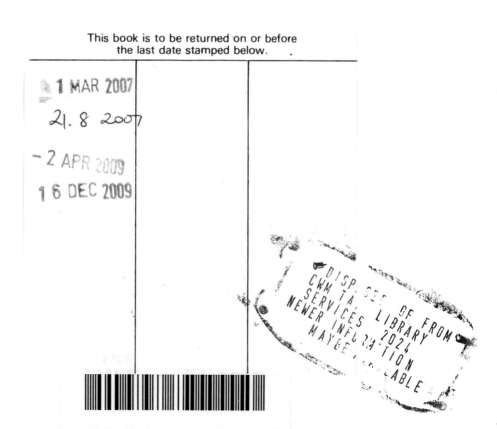

For Churchill Livingstone:

Commissioning Editor: Mary Seager
Development Editor: Catharine Steers
Project Manager: Joannah Duncan
Designer: George Ajayi

Nausea and Vomiting in Pregnancy

An Integrated Approach to Care

Denise Tiran MSc RM RGN PGCEA MTD
Principal Lecturer Complementary Medicine/Maternity Care, University of Greenwich, London, UK

Foreword by

Julian Woolfson LLM FRCOG
Consultant Obstetrician and Gynaecologist, Queen Mary's Sidcup NHS Trust, UK

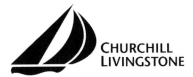

CHURCHILL
LIVINGSTONE

EDINBURGH LONDON NEW YORK OXFORD PHILADELPHIA ST LOUIS SYDNEY TORONTO 2004

Churchill Livingstone
An imprint of Elsevier Science Limited

ISBN 0 443 07392 9

British Library Cataloguing in Publication Data
A catalogue record for this book is available from the British Library

Library of Congress Cataloguing in Publication Data
A catalog record for this book is available from the Library of
Congress

Notice
Medical knowledge is constantly changing. Standard safety
precautions must be followed, but as new research and clinical
experience broaden our knowledge, changes in treatment and drug
therapy may become necessary or appropriate. Readers are advised to
check the most current product information provided by the
manufacturer of each drug to be administered to verify the
recommended dose, the method and duration of administration, and
contraindications. It is the responsibility of the practitioner, relying on
experience and knowledge of the patient, to determine dosages and
the best treatment for each individual patient. Neither the Publisher
nor the author assumes any liability for any injury and/or damage to
persons or property arising from this publication.

The Publisher

 your source for books,
journals and multimedia
in the health sciences

www.elsevierhealth.com

The
publisher's
policy is to use
**paper manufactured
from sustainable forests**

Printed in China

Contents

Foreword

To write a comprehensive book about one subject is hard enough but when it comes to writing a single book about two complementary, but in many ways divergent, subjects the potential for confusion and misinformation is great. In this book, however, Denise Tiran has not only succeeded in producing a scholarly, incisive and detailed work but has also provided the long-missing rational link between traditional and complementary medical care.

Her subject is relatively narrow but its relevance to pregnant women and their carers is enormous. At last there is a book which considers the unpleasant side-effects of pregnancy from a scientific basis and advances treatments, both traditional and complementary, based on best available evidence rather than conjecture. It is by its nature not a simple book to read but it is sufficiently fascinating to want to keep reading and reading again.

Paradoxically, its real value is not so much in its subject matter but in its approach. No idea or therapy is discarded and all are properly researched and analysed, with no preconceived ideas or artificial categorisation applied. This approach is long overdue when comparing traditional and complementary therapies and it is to be hoped that there will be more books along these lines. In the idiom of the day, coverage of these subjects in this way will provide long-overdue light rather than heat.

Julian Woolfson LLM FRCOG
Consultant Obstetrician and Gynaecologist
Queen Mary's Sidcup NHS Trust, UK 2004

Acknowledgements

I would like to thank Julian Woolfson, Consultant Obstetrician at Queen Mary's Hospital, Sidcup in Kent, for his unstinting support and friendship over many years. With reference to this book, I am particularly indebted to him for agreeing to write the Foreword and for reading the manuscript for accuracy, especially the chapter on The Conventional Approach to pregnancy sickness.

Other colleagues at the University of Greenwich and at Queen Mary's Hospital have, as always, provided moral and practical support and a sounding board for ideas.

Editors and staff at Elsevier Science have been brilliant, and I specifically wish to thank Mary Seager for her help with this project, and Inta Ozols, whom I have known for many years, who always encourages me to take up another writing challenge.

Most of all I would like to give my love to my son, Adam, now 13, the joy of my life, who has endured hours of not being able to use the computer while I worked. Without Adam, there would have been no personal experience of persistent pregnancy sickness to fuel my professional interest in the subject. Without him, there would have been no book.

Denise Tiran
London 2004

1

The conventional approach

This chapter considers the incidence, predisposing factors to and causes of nausea and vomiting in pregnancy, from a conventional perspective. Diagnosis of the condition is debated, with hyperemesis gravidarum being viewed as one end of the spectrum of severity. Issues of management, care and advice given by obstetricians, general practitioners and midwives are explored.

INTRODUCTION

Nausea and vomiting is one of the earliest, commonest and most distressing of symptoms associated with pregnancy. However, as obstetricians and general practitioners (GPs) view it merely as a physiological symptom, and one with which they frequently feel powerless to help, it is often dismissed as a normal consequence of early pregnancy without acknowledging the immense impact it can have on women and their families.

Women have stressed that part of their satisfaction with early pregnancy care is related to their perception that healthcare professionals *believe* their accounts of sickness, neither dismissing them nor over-reacting. As with pain, nausea is what the patient says it is – and if the symptom is causing her distress, then she deserves to be given the best possible means of dealing with it. The results of undervaluing women's accounts of gestational nausea and vomiting are seen as contributing to increased emotional strain, psychological stress and unnecessary delays in instigating the appropriate treatment, particularly when the condition becomes pathological (Munch 2000). Traditional professional education regarding nausea and vomiting in pregnancy has been contradicted by the findings of Lacroix et al (2000), who suggest that women's perception of pregnancy nausea may be similar to that of oncology patients undergoing chemotherapy.

INCIDENCE

Koren (2000) describes nausea and vomiting as the most common medical disorder during pregnancy. Power et al (2001) recorded an average of 51.4% of women with nausea and 9.2% who experienced vomiting. Glick and Dick (1999) assume an approximate 50% of women experience symptoms. Emelianova et al (1999) found a 67% rate of nausea and a 22% incidence of vomiting in a group of 193 women, while O'Brien and Naber (1992) suggest that 70% suffer nausea and 28% vomit. Gadsby et al (1993) reported an 80% incidence, with 28% having nausea alone and 52% experiencing both nausea and vomiting. Jewell and Young's systematic review (2000) identified a nausea rate of between 70% and 85%, with approximately half of these suffering vomiting.

Broussard and Richter (1998) suggest that up to 90% of women suffer some form of nausea and vomiting during pregnancy, which may range from the typical mild to moderate, self-limiting nausea, with or without vomiting, to the severe condition of hyperemesis gravidarum with associated weight loss, electrolyte and metabolic disturbances and the possibility of long-term sequelae. An earlier investigation by Tierson et al (1986) showed that 89.4% of women questioned in New York experienced nausea, and about 55% actually vomited. It is therefore fair to state that, contrary to popular medical opinion, some form of gestational sickness is much more prevalent than the 50% quoted in textbooks.

The pathological extreme of hyperemesis gravidarum is much less frequent than physio-logical nausea and vomiting, with Kelly (1996:306) estimating that it occurs in 1:500 pregnancies, and Walters (1999) suggesting an incidence of between three and ten per thousand pregnancies. Kuscu and Koyuncu (2002) believe the rate to be between one and twenty per thousand pregnancies. In Power et al's study (2001), approximately 2.4% of the women who suffered nausea and vomiting required hospitalisation for hyperemesis gravidarum.

TIMING AND DURATION

The term 'morning sickness' is incorrect, dismissive and inappropriate, for in many women the symptoms may last all day, or may not be present at all on rising. A prospective study of 160 women by Lacroix et al (2000) found that 74% reported nausea although a mere 1.8% experienced this as morning-only symptoms; in 80% of sufferers the nausea was continuous throughout the day. 76% of women were shown to be nauseous in a study by Vellacott et al (1988). In this survey, it was also discovered that, despite the traditional practice of informing women that pregnancy sickness is usually relieved or improved by the end of the first trimester, only 27% reported a resolution of symptoms by the twelfth week, although most were better by the 22nd week of gestation. Lacroix et al (2000) found that episodes of nausea and/or vomiting lasted an average of 34 days, from onset to resolution.

Some women experience a return to the nausea and vomiting in the last few weeks before delivery, presumably partly in response to fluctuating hormone levels in preparation for labour. This is rarely reported in professional textbooks or consumer manuals, and can be an

---

Practice point

Healthcare professionals should recognise that, although nausea and vomiting is physiological it is *not* a 'minor' disorder for sufferers; it may occur in as many as 85% of expectant women, may last all day and may persist throughout the pregnancy.

unpleasant shock to women at a stage when they are already suffering other third trimester symptoms, including tiredness, heartburn, backache, carpal tunnel syndrome, oedema and perhaps anticipatory anxiety regarding the birth.

CAUSES AND PREDISPOSING FACTORS

Physiopathology

Nausea and vomiting of pregnancy are usually attributed to changes in the endocrine system which occur during pregnancy, primarily the high fluctuating levels of *human chorionic gonadotrophin* (hCG), particularly as the most common period for gestational sickness is the first 12-16 weeks, during which time hCG is at its highest level. hCG is similar to luteinising hormone and is secreted by the trophoblast cells of the blastocyst. It bypasses pituitary-ovarian controls and prompts the corpus luteum to continue the production of oestrogen and progesterone, a function later taken over by the chorionic layer of the placenta. hCG is detectable in the woman's blood from about three weeks' gestation (i.e. one week after fertilisation), a fact which forms the basis of most pregnancy tests.

The hCG theory appears to be supported by the fact that hydatidiform mole is accompanied by excessive vomiting in approximately 26% of cases, thought to be due to increased levels of serum beta-hCG (Glick & Dick 1999). An increased amount of placental tissue in these cases is shown to increase the total hours of nausea in early pregnancy (Gadsby et al 1997).

Human chorionic gonadotrophin appears to be responsible for a decrease in *thyroid stimulating hormone* (TSH) and a rise in the amount of free thyroxine (T4) between 10 and 12 weeks' gestation (Hershman 1999; Tareen et al 1995; Goodwin et al 1992; Lao et al 1988). Many women with hyperemesis gravidarum are shown to have increased thyroid function, with a small proportion developing gestational thyrotoxicosis, in which the serum hCG exceeds 200 IU/ml (Hershman 1999). Similar findings occur where a tro-

phoblastic tumour, hydatidiform mole or choriocarcinoma is present, with the hyperthyroidism responding to treatment involving removal of the causative tumour and/or chemotherapy. However, Panesar et al (2001) suggest that hCG is not independently involved in the aetiology of hyperemesis gravidarum, but that it may be indirectly responsible by stimulating thyroid activity. Goodwin et al (1992) likewise attribute increased oestradiol concentrations in women with hyperemesis gravidarum to the effects of hCG on steroidogenesis.

Jordan et al (1999) pursue the debate about the controversial role of hCG in the aetiology of hyperemesis gravidarum and suggest that certain acidic isoforms of hCG may be a determining factor in both this and gestational thyrotoxicosis. Whilst the authors acknowledge that the mechanism by which these isoforms stimulate nausea and vomiting is still unclear, they believe oestradiol (E2) to be uninvolved in the process, but propose the theory that the longer half-life of acidic hCG isoforms may lead to thyrotrophic effects, although other theories have also been put forward. For example Mestman (1999) reported the transient hyperthyroidism of hyperemesis gravidarum to be due not to high plasma levels of hCG, but secondary to a mutation in the thyrotrophin-releasing hormone receptor. Kopp (2001) identified somatic activating mutations of the TSH receptor as being responsible for toxic adenomas, whereas mutations in the germline may give rise to congenital or non-autoimmune familial hyperthyroidism. However, Tan et al (2002) found that, in women with transient hyperthyroidism of pregnancy, free T4 levels normalised by 15 weeks' gestation and TSH levels by 19 weeks, without anti-thyroid medication, and suggest that routine assessment of thyroid function in hyperemetic women is unnecessary in the absence of any clinical features of hyperthyroidism.

Conversely, Chong and Johnston (1997) report on three cases of women whose hyperemesis gravidarum was attributed to previously undiagnosed preconceptional thyrotoxicosis. The vomiting was uncontrolled with antiemetics but resolved as the thyroid balance was re-established with anti-thyroid medication. Two cases discussed by Kort et al (1999) in which hyperemesis gravidarum presented, were found to be due to excess parathyroid activity; both were successfully treated in the second trimester with surgery.

Asakura et al (2000) demonstrated a correlation between higher levels of thyroid hormones, non-esterified fatty acids and weight loss in women with hyperemesis gravidarum than in those with mild to moderate pregnancy sickness. There appears to be a shift from T3 to reverse T3, the latter being physiologically inactive, and the authors postulate that a mechanism to minimise T3 production must occur in women with hyperemesis gravidarum, so that weight loss and lipolysis are reduced.

A possible association with the *sympathetic nervous system and gestational immunological state* has also been explored by Minagawa et al (1999), who suggest that, whilst activation of granulocytes, free thyroid cells and natural killer (NK) cells is essential for the maintenance of pregnancy, overactivation may be responsible for the development of pregnancy disorders. Leylek et al (1999) also found a correlation between higher levels of hCG, thyroid hormones and immunoglobulins in women with hyperemesis gravidarum than in controls, and a sigificantly higher level of each parameter in hyperemetics with accompanying thyroxinaemia. They concluded that immunological activity during pregnancy may have a role to play, or trigger an effect in the stimulatory mechanism of hCG in women with hyperemesis gravidarum, with or without thyrotoxicosis.

Oestrogen and progesterone have long been implicated in the aetiology of nausea and vomiting, although this theory is not entirely consistent with the first trimester incidence of symptoms in the majority of women, since levels of these hormones continue to rise past the first three months. Vellacott et al (1988) found that women who had previously experienced nausea whilst taking the contraceptive pill or during the premenstrual phase were more susceptible to gestational sickness, although this may be due to other factors, such as deficiency of vitamin B6

and zinc, the metabolism and excretion of which may be affected by the stressors of the premenstrual period or by the contraceptive pill (see also Chapter 3). There is also a higher incidence of nausea and vomiting in women with multiple pregnancies, in which both hormones are present in greater levels than in singleton pregnancies, which supports the influence of oestrogen and progesterone in the cause. However, Jarnfelt-Samsioe et al (1986) demonstrated that emetic women had significantly lower levels of progesterone, as well as cortisol, in the first trimester, while the same women had raised third trimester levels of dehydroepiandrosterone (DHEA-S) and lowered testosterone. Gadsby et al (2000) have shown a positive correlation between early emesis and levels of maternal serum *prostaglandin E2*. Goodwin (2002) suggests that the woman's response to the primary hormonal stimulus which initiates sickness is dependent on susceptibility mediated by a combination of gastrointestinal, olfactory, vestibular and behavioural factors.

Changes in *carbohydrate and lipid metabolism* are responsible for hypoglycaemia, especially on waking, giving rise to the popular, but largely incorrect term of 'morning sickness', although hypoglycaemia does not seem to be related to adverse perinatal outcome (Calfee et al 1999). Food cravings and aversions appear to be more marked in women with more severe vomiting (Crystal et al 1999), perhaps in an attempt to replace nutrients which are either lacking preconceptionally or lost due to vomiting. Flaxman and Sherman (2000) reviewed a range of related literature and found that sickness is at its worst when organogenesis of the embryo is most vulnerable to chemical disruption; the rate of spontaneous abortion is less in women who suffer these symptoms and vomiting appears to be a stronger protection against miscarrying than nausea alone. The most common food aversions appear to be alcoholic and caffeinated drinks and strong tasting vegetables, although the authors did highlight their finding that the most pronounced aversions were to meat, fish, poultry and eggs, which it would be assumed are needed for organogenesis (see also Chapter 3).

Vomiting is initiated by stimulation of the medullary vomiting centre, which controls smooth muscle in the stomach wall as well as skeletal muscle in the abdomen and respiratory system, and the chemoreceptor trigger zone on the base of the fourth ventricle, in close proximity to the vagal nerve. As the chemoreceptor trigger zone is outside the blood-brain barrier, it responds to chemical stimuli from drugs and toxins produced in certain pathological conditions; it is also responsible for motion sickness. Stimuli in the chemoreceptor trigger zone are relayed to the vomiting centre which causes muscles in the gastrointestinal and respiratory tracts to initiate the action of vomiting.

Effects on the *vestibular apparatus*, as occur in motion sickness, also play a part, with many women reporting that any sensory stimulation, especially motion, may provoke vomiting (O'Brien et al 1997). The sense of equilibrium responds to various head movements and is dependent on input from the inner ear, visual stimuli and from stretch receptors to muscles and tendons. Under normal circumstances the equilibrium receptors in the semicircular canals and vestibule of the ear (the vestibular apparatus) send signals to the brain that initiate reflexes required to adjust position, although, in the case of damage, some adaptation takes place, enabling the person to function without this process. Receptors in the vestibule monitor static equilibrium, while those in the semicircular canals monitor dynamic equilibrium.

Static equilibrium is controlled by sensory receptors called maculae which assess the position of the head in space and respond to linear acceleration forces, i.e. changes in speed and direction occurring in straight lines, but not to rotation. The maculae are flat epithelial patches containing supporting cells and hair cells which are affected by gravitational pull, causing receptor cells to release neurotransmitters in varying amounts, depending on the movement, and thereby increasing or decreasing the rate of impulse generated by the vestibular nerve endings. Dynamic equilibrium is controlled by the crista ampullaris, a minute elevation of the ampulla in each semicircular canal, and is more responsive to rotational movements, but will also be affected by acceleration and deceleration. However the vestibular apparatus does not automatically compensate for forces acting on the body, but merely sends warning signals to the central nervous system which then initiates the appropriate compensations (see also Chapter 7). Black (2002), however, suggests that, as there is currently insufficient comprehension regarding the underlying neurochemical processes, it is not yet possible to determine conclusively the role of the vestibular apparatus in the aetiology of gestational sickness.

Serotonin (5-HT), which works both on the gastrointestinal tract and the chemoreceptor trigger zone, as well as acetylcholine, dopamine, noradrenaline, histamine and endorphins, are involved in the normal vomiting reflex. Serotonin is secreted by the central nervous system, especially the midbrain, hypothalamus, limbic system, cerebellum, pineal gland and spinal cord, as well as being synthesised from tryptophan and secreted by the stomach wall in response to food, where it causes contractions of the stomach wall during digestion. It is thought that serotonin plays a part in the physiology of sleep, appetite, migraine and headache, and regulation of mood, as well as nausea of various aetiologies, although Borgeat et al (1997) failed to implicate serotonin in the aetiology of hyperemesis gravidarum. Histamine is secreted by the hypothalamus and acts as a powerful vasodilator, and by the stomach mucosa where it is synthesised from histidine and activates parietal cells to release hydrochloric acid. Dopamine is secreted by the hypothalamus, the substantia nigra of the midbrain, and is the principal neurotransmitter of the extrapyramidal system. It is synthesised from tyrosine in a shared pathway with norepinephrine and essentially acts as a 'feel good' factor. Where medication is prescribed to suppress the vomiting these will usually be acetylcholine or histamine antagonists, although Hasler (1999) suggests that 5-T3 antagonists may be effective pharmacological agents against hyperemesis gravidarum.

Physiological changes in the gastrointestinal tract, mainly due to the action of progesterone, may contribute to the problem, including relaxation of the cardiac sphincter leading to oesophageal reflux and heartburn, and reduced peristalsis resulting in constipation. Symptomatic gastro-oesophageal reflux appears to be strongly associated with nausea and vomiting. In one study, (Ho et al 1998), almost 79% of women with heartburn and/or reflux reported daily nausea and vomiting, with both symptoms commonly commencing in the first trimester and resolving by the second trimester. The results led the authors to question whether there is a common mechanism or a cause and effect relationship between the two sets of symptoms. Knudsen et al (1995) considered heartburn and oesophageal reflux in the more commonly expected third trimester and found that 60% of women experienced these symptoms, with associated nausea in 16% of sufferers and vomiting in 7%. Excessive salivation (ptyalism) also occurs in some women and can be as troublesome as, or accompanied by, nausea and vomiting. This author's experience indicates that a high proportion of women with hypersalivation are from West Africa, although no evidence regarding a racial link could be found in the literature. However, Maes et al (1999) demonstrated that, in women recovering from hyperemesis gravidarum, the rate of gastric emptying of solids was increased, appearing to correlate well with thyroid function abnormalities. These findings led the authors to postulate that gestational nausea and vomiting are unlikely to be due to disorders of the upper gastrointestinal tract. Koch (2002) also advises the exclusion of incidental gastrointestinal problems such as peptic ulcer and cholecystitis.

Jacoby and Porter (1999) considered a controversial link between hyperemesis gravidarum persisting into the second trimester and peptic ulcer due to infection with *Helicobacter pylori*, a Gram negative bacteria found in the stomach, which can cause damage to the prostaglandins protecting the mucosal cells in the stomach wall. They debated the treatment of two women whose hyperemesis gravidarum was unresponsive to standard treatment and whose persistent symptoms into the second trimester caused them to test for *Helicobacter pylori*. Positive results and appropriate antibiotic therapy resolved the nausea and vomiting, and led them to suggest the need to include active peptic ulcer disease in the differential diagnoses. Hayakawa et al (2000) found the genome of *Helicobacter pylori* present in the saliva of women with hyperemesis gravidarum and suggested that chronic *Helicobacter pylori* infection is an important factor in its pathogenesis, although it may not be the single cause of the disorder. A review by Eliakim et al (2000) also debated this possibility but evidence to confirm it is limited to date. However, Erdem et al (2002) and Wu et al (2000) found that, although the seropositivity rate for *Helicobacter pylori* was greater in the pregnant than non-pregnant population, no significant correlation between infection and gastrointestinal symptoms in pregnancy was revealed.

The theory that pregnancy sickness may be *nature's way of protecting the fetus* by discouraging the mother from eating harmful foods has also been put forward (Sherman and Flaxman 2002; Brown et al 1997), with the woman becoming nauseated at the sight, smell or taste of foods which may potentially affect the fetus, and, if the food is eaten, causing her to vomit in order to expel it. Women with hCG levels below the normal range more commonly have a poor pregnancy outcome, including miscarriage, preterm delivery or intrauterine growth retardation. Furneaux et al (2001) suggested that nutritional restriction at critical phases of organogenesis may ensure optimal production and maintenance of hCG levels, as well as facilitating placental development and optimising nutritional partitioning between the tissues of the mother and fetus. Huxley (2000) also discusses the possible protective role of nausea and vomiting in stimulating early placental growth and reducing maternal energy intake in order to ensure that nutrient partitioning favours the placenta. However, Zhou et al (1999) found that when vomiting was severe in early pregnancy it was likely to continue for longer than nausea alone, and appeared to be related to lower infant birthweights. There may also be a correlation between the severity of sickness and preconceptional Body Mass Index

---

Box 1.1 Physiopathological factors which result in vomiting

Carbohydrate and lipid metabolism changes
Corpus luteum situation
Genetic factors
Gastrointestinal tract adaptations
Helicobacter pylori infection
Human chorionic gonadotrophin
Hypotension and reduced cerebral circulation
Immunological factors
Impact on olfaction or sight
Migraine and headache

Oestrogen and progesterone
Pharyngeal vagal nerve stimulation
Protective mechanism
Sensory nerve stimulation in the stomach and duodenum
Serotonin
Thyroid hormone alterations
Uterine, bladder or renal pelvis distension, trauma or infection
Vestibular apparatus disturbance

Box 1.2 Predisposing factors to more severe nausea and vomiting

Fatigue
Female fetus
Gastro-oesophageal reflux
Nausea and vomiting in previous pregnancies
Preconceptional use of contraceptive pill
Premenstrual nausea

Smoking
Stress, anxiety and fear
Socio-economic problems
Relationship difficulties
Women with mothers who experienced nausea and vomiting in pregnancy

---

(BMI), with underweight women experiencing less nausea and vomiting than those with normal or excess BMIs (Huxley 2000) (see also Chapter 3).

Genetic incompatibility between the mother and the fetus has been propounded as a causative factor (Lindsay 1997) although this is more likely to result in spontaneous abortion, often with very few physiological symptoms of pregnancy (Flaxman & Sherman 2000; Tierson et al 1986). Klebanoff and Mills (1986) investigated whether or not vomiting was teratogenic but concluded that any increased incidence of fetal abnormality was more likely to be due to medication than to the vomiting itself. A genetic link may also be pertinent as there is an increased incidence of nausea and vomiting in women whose mothers experienced symptoms during their own pregnancies (Gadsby et al 1997), although whether this is partly due to 'nurture' as well as 'nature' has not been confirmed.

Other, less commonly acknowledged factors may be responsible for nausea and vomiting of pregnancy or hyperemesis gravidarum. It is thought that the position of the *right-sided corpus luteum* results in high levels of steroid hormones in the hepatic portal system (Lindsay 1997) but if this was the case, all women would experience nausea and vomiting. However, undue strain on the right side of the body, for example as a result of accident, injury or disease, may exacerbate this factor, leading some to be more prone than others (see also Chapter 7). Van Calenbergh et al (2001) identified a cerebral tumour presenting as hyperemesis gravidarum and advise awareness of unrelated factors when assessing emetic women.

Psychosocial factors

Psychological issues may predispose some women to nausea and vomiting in pregnancy, or to an exacerbation of existing symptoms or a reduced capacity to cope with 'normal' symptoms. A pregnancy seen as unplanned, inconvenient or unwanted, or as an occupational or financial burden will cause anguish, ambivalence and conflict. Anxieties based on previous childbearing experiences, especially anticipatory anxiety of impending hyperemesis gravidarum or pre-eclampsia, may worsen the sense of wellbeing. Women experiencing relationship difficulties may be especially vulnerable to the problem, with emotional distress adding to physical discomfort (Iatrakis et al 1988). The shock and necessary adaptation required if the pregnancy is discovered to be multiple, or pregnancies occur close together, can also be emotional factors contributing to more severe nausea and vomiting, quite apart from the physical impact such as possible anaemia (see also Chapter 8).

Raphael-Leff (1991) identified two types of women during pregnancy. The 'facilitators' who have planned for and looked forward to becoming pregnant, view it as part of the 'growing up' process of adulthood, and enjoy relinquishing themselves to the pregnant state. The 'regulators' view pregnancy as a hurdle to be overcome, a means to an end, and try to resist the loss of control which it brings. For most women there is, in any case, an element of internal conflict as they attempt to reconcile their changing roles, between lover and mother, daughter and mother, employee and career-woman, and between independence and dependence. Media portrayal of pregnant women does nothing to help those whose physiopathological or psycho-emotional state is suboptimal, and many women fail to acknowledge, perhaps even to themselves, that they are not enjoying being pregnant, seeing it, in the eyes of society, as a failure of their womanhood.

Leeners et al (2000) suggest that psychosocial factors are strongly involved in the aetiology of hyperemesis gravidarum and affect not only the duration and severity of symptoms but also the resistance (and therefore the success) of treatment strategies. Mazotta, Maltepe, Navioz et al (2000) concur with this and recognise that more severe vomiting may be linked to women's decisions to commence anti-emetic medication, but also hypothesise that the severity of nausea and vomiting does not appear adequately to reflect the degree of distress experienced by the women. Buckwalter and Simpson (2002) also suggest a psychological component in exacerbation of moderate nausea and vomiting and the development of hyperemesis gravidarum.

Feelings of guilt, anger, self pity or fear can add to physical symptoms. Women may feel guilty about the impact of the pregnancy on the family financial situation, especially if it is unplanned. Many women reveal a sense of guilt that the sickness prevents them from eating what they consider to be the 'best' and most nourishing food for the baby. They may also experience anxiety and guilt when they are unable to care adequately for other children. Anger often goes unrecognised but may manifest itself as irritability and mood swings, regarded as 'normal' emotions for women with high hormone levels. The anger may be directed towards the partner, either because he has contributed to the conception and is thus deemed responsible for the sickness, or because he is perceived as being unsympathetic (even if this is not entirely the case). The woman may feel angry about the impact of the pregnancy on her life, particularly if she is a 'regulator' (Raphael-Leff 1991), or the emotion may be directed internally, although this might more readily be viewed as self pity. In a few cases, the symptoms may be used as a means of attracting attention, or as a 'call for help' with other problems in the woman's life. Lack of knowledge, information and poor communication between the woman and her caregivers can contribute to her perception of the severity of symptoms (Iatrakis et al 1988). It may partly explain why primigravid women appear to require hospitalisation more frequently than multigravid mothers (Atanackovic, Wolpin & Koren 2001), although women in subsequent pregnancies may be preoccupied with other children and simply unable to succumb to hospitalisation. Women who responded to a survey in Toronto also cited having an obstetrician as the primary caregiver as being a reason why they were more likely to require hospitalisation, or perhaps to agree to the suggestion by obstetricians that they be admitted. Whether this is due to the increased pathological emphasis placed on the condition by obstetricians rather than by GPs or midwives is not clear (Atanackovic, Wolpin & Koren 2001). It may also relate to the paternalism of secondary medical care, in which practitioners are keen to be seen by patients to be 'doing something', whereas those working in primary care may better recognise the importance of advice and information, together with a 'normalising' attitude towards a physiological symptom and an acknowledgement of the potentially adverse impact of hospitalisation on the partner and family.

Occupational and economic issues

Although employers should not, by law, use a woman's pregnancy as a discriminatory factor in the workplace, in practice many can make time at work extremely difficult. This leads some women to conceal their pregnancies until it is no longer possible, but this in turn can cause them additional mental burdens. The anxiety of the current or impending financial situation may lead to added worry which makes the woman feel unwell, especially if she is intending to stop working completely after the birth.

The effort of journeying to work, perhaps rushing in the early morning without time for an adequate breakfast to overcome hypoglycaemia can trigger nausea and vomiting. To this may be added the exertion of coping with overcrowded public transport, possibly requiring the woman to stand on an overfull train surrounded by people whose odours, whether pleasant or not (perfume, aftershave, perspiration, breath, smoke or foods and drinks which they may be consuming) can influence the severity of her nausea.

Depending on the nature of the woman's work, aromas, chemicals or the environment may add to her nausea and cause her to vomit. Hyperolfaction in relation to hyperemesis gravidarum is explored by Erick (1995) who postulates that it may be a mechanism encouraging the expectant mother to find a better environment. Smoking has been shown to aggravate symptoms of nausea and vomiting (Gadsby et al 1997), but whether this is due to the olfactory or nutritional effects, or whether an assumption can be made of a relationship between habitual practices and psycho-emotional distress, is unclear. Certainly many women suffering nausea and vomiting will abhor the smell of cigarettes and tobacco smoke. Odours such as cooking, if working in a food shop or restaurant, or simply poorly ventilated offices, as well as close work, e.g.

computer work, which affects her eyes, leading to headaches, can also trigger nausea. Noxious chemicals in some jobs, such as printing inks, anaesthetic gases or cleaning fluids can also make the problem worse, both physiologically and pathologically (see also Chapter 5).

Poor posture as a result of inappropriate seating may aggravate the gastrointestinal tract by compressing the abdomen (see also Chapter 7). Infrequent visits to empty her bladder may irritate the urinary tract, distend the abdomen and increase the symptoms of nausea, particularly if this leads to a urinary tract infection.

Although nausea and vomiting of pregnancy occurs across all cultures and has been recorded for centuries, contemporary western society – and thus women themselves – places unrealistic expectations on those who are pregnant. More than ever before, most couples require two incomes in order to provide an acceptable standard of living. The emphasis on commercially viable productivity in industry does not facilitate women who may be working at less than 100% of their normal efficiency and effectiveness. Fatigue, already a physiological problem for many women, may be worsened by long hours of work and travel to and from the place of employment, and a positive correlation between the severity of nausea and vomiting and the intensity of tiredness has been shown to aggravate the situation (van der Lier et al 1993).

Colleagues may be jealous or appear unsympathetic when they become aware of the pregnancy, seeing it as placing more of a burden on them. Women often seem to be even less facilitative than male colleagues. This author frequently meets expectant mothers whose colleagues are unhelpful, some of the worst cases being general practitioners, already overworked, who simply interpret a colleague's pregnancy as an increase in their own workload! This leads pregnant women to continue working, often at the expense of their health and wellbeing, with an increase in fatigue, hypoglycaemia and stress, all of which contribute to the nausea and vomiting.

Current UK maternity and sick leave allowances discourage women from taking more than an absolute minimum of absence from work in the antenatal period, and leads them to continue working until the latest possible gestation in order to prolong their maternity leave following the birth. The resulting anxiety and stress of fulfilling their obligations to the employer, their colleagues and to themselves can cause worse than normal complaints to manifest during pregnancy, including prolonged or more severe nausea and vomiting.

There is some evidence to suggest that women expecting girls are more prone to hyperemesis gravidarum than those carrying boys (del Mar Melero-Montes & Jick 2001), particularly where there is a multiple pregnancy or concomitant pre-eclamspia (Basso & Olsen 2001), although no other research has been found in the academic literature to dispute what appears to be an 'old wives' tale'. Where a woman is aware of the sex of the fetus, she may experience extremes of either positive or negative emotion, perhaps related to her desire for a particular sex of the baby; this in turn may manifest in physical symptoms such as nausea and vomiting.

DIAGNOSIS

Nausea is often the first symptom experienced by the mother, frequently occurring even before the first missed menstrual period. It is therefore self-diagnosed, and in many cases, self-managed. Vomiting is also a visual manifestation of the problem and does not require medical or midwifery assistance to make a diagnosis, although confirmation of the pregnancy may be undertaken by the health professional. If, however, the woman delays her initial appointment for booking of maternity care, the condition may have resolved itself before she meets her midwife or obstetrician, which may contribute to the low priority given by healthcare professionals to dealing with it.

Whilst midwives and general practitioners may recognise the impact of severe nausea and vomiting on the woman's day-to-day life and that of her partner and family, obstetricians do not normally witness this in the community, and are concerned only with the pathological

effects on the mother and fetus when the condition becomes more serious. A difficulty in assessment may then occur, for if the woman feels unwell enough to report her symptoms to her obstetrician, he may feel obliged to take action to deal with it, one of the few options available being to admit the mother to hospital. Various methods of assessment have been trialled, including the Rhodes Index of Nausea, Vomiting and Retching (Rhodes & McDaniel 1999), the McGill Nausea Questionnaire (Lacroix et al 2000) and the pregnancy-unique quantification of emesis and nausea (PUQE) system (Koren et al 2002; 2001), with variable success. The impact on women's quality of life has also been assessed by Magee et al (2002) and Attard et al (2002).

However, there are wide variations in the coping abilities of women experiencing nausea and vomiting during pregnancy, which will be affected by their personality and attitudes to illness, family and occupational commitments, general health and available support mechanisms. One mother may complain of untenable symptoms, although perhaps vomiting only two or three times a day, and be grateful for hospital admission and attention, while others may be carrying on their daily lives feeling constantly nauseous and frequently vomiting. It is the mother's *perception* of the severity of her symptoms which is important in the first instance, and a simple grading tool, similar to the Likert scales used to measure pain perception can be introduced to assist in the *mother's* assessment of severity (Figure 1.1)

There appears to be, as may be expected, a strong correlation between the maximal number of daily vomiting episodes and the maximal weight loss (Emelianova et al 1999). Walters (1999) advocates hospital admission only for

---

Practice point

Health professionals should endeavour to validate women's perceptions of their nausea and vomiting, rather than dismiss it simply as a normal symptom of pregnancy.

Figure 1.1 Simple grading tool to assess maternal perception of nausea and vomiting

1   5   10

The mother should be asked to identify, on a scale of 1-10, how *she* perceives the severity of her nausea and vomiting. The parameters she uses to make this assessment are irrelevant: this tool indicates the degree of distress caused by the condition. This will assist in determining whether or not *she* perceives any improvement in her symptoms in response to treatment.

Box 1.3 Differential diagnosis

Acute fatty liver	Hypercalcaemia
Gastroenteritis	Intra-abdominal conditions
Hiatus hernia	Intracranial hypertension (benign)
Helicobacter pylori infection	Pyelonephritis
Hepatitis	Reflux oesophagitis as a feature of medical problems

---

Box 1.4 Clinical assessment for hyperemesis gravidarum

Weight loss: over 3kg or 5%	Biochemical assessment for vitamin and mineral status
Appearance – face, skin	Urea and electrolytes
Pulse, blood pressure	Liver function tests
Urinalysis, specific gravity, MSU for microscopy	? endoscopy in third trimester
Fluid intake and output measurement	Fetal assessment – ultrasound scan/cardiotocograph
Full blood count	

---

those who have lost at least 3kg in weight and who require intravenous rehydration, but not necessarily for those who report frequent vomiting without weight loss. Gross et al (1989) suggest that there is an increased chance of intrauterine growth retardation if the mother loses more than 5% of her pre-pregnancy weight, as fetal growth patterns are disturbed by alterations in the maternal metabolism. Hershman (1999) also uses the 5% parameter of weight loss as an indicative feature of hyperemesis gravidarum.

Where dehydration, electrolyte disturbance, protein-calorie malnutrition and vitamin deficiency co-exist, hospitalisation is essential for the health of both mother and fetus. It is important however to exclude other causes of excessive vomiting before a diagnosis of hyperemesis gravidarum is confirmed. Women with a previous personal or maternal history of hyperemesis gravidarum are more prone to the condition, as are women with pre-existing liver disease. Walters (1999) states that caution should be exercised after 16 weeks as the cause of the vomiting is unlikely to be pregnancy related, and, indeed, in the third trimester, could herald much more serious conditions such as acute fatty liver, biliary or other disease. He suggests a flexible endoscopic investigation, which 'carries no excess risk to the pregnancy', be performed to exclude gastritis or ulcerative oesophagitis (see Box 1.3 for differential diagnosis).

Walters, an obstetrician, (1999) fails, however, to take account of the woman's appearance or temperament as the condition worsens, whereas Stables, a midwife, (1999) focuses on the clinical signs and maternal symptoms. These may include sunken eyes, dryness of the mouth and offensive-smelling breath, loss of skin elasticity and weight loss. There is likely to be bradycardia and hypotension. There will be oliguria with dark urine containing ketones, bile, sugars and protein and having a high specific gravity. A microscopy, culture and sensitivity test of a midstream specimen of urine will exclude or confirm infection such as pyelonephritis. A blood picture will reveal anaemia, disruption of vitamin B12, folic acid and vitamin C levels, and assessment of electrolyte balance will show hyponatraemia, hypochloraemia, hypokalaemia and low urea levels. There will be a raised haematocrit. Liver function tests may show abnormalities and abnormal thyroid function may be revealed.

MANAGEMENT

It is fascinating to note that medical textbooks give scant attention to the management of physiological nausea and vomiting, and, in James et al's *High Risk Pregnancy: Management Options* (1999), even hyperemesis gravidarum is awarded less than two pages of cover, in a chapter devoted to hepatic conditions in pregnancy. Even midwifery texts, normally more concerned with aspects of psychological as well as physiopathological care, offer minimal discussion of 'normal' sickness and, as in Stables' *Physiology in Childbearing with Anatomy and Related Biosciences* (1999), approximately three columns of information on hyperemesis gravidarum. This may be due to the limited priority given to the condition in clinical practice, with the attitude being that there is little that can be done for the physiological symptoms, and treatment is only offered when it becomes pathological. However, more attention to helping women to deal with the 'normal' levels of sickness may reduce the incidence and impact of hyperemesis gravidarum and its associated problems for both the individual and the service.

Advice by health professionals on physiological nausea and vomiting

The majority of women will attempt to manage their symptoms by themselves, occasionally asking for advice from their midwives, GPs or obstetricians, although Dilorio et al (1994) found that medical practitioners look to the women as the primary source of information regarding the problem. The approach of most conventional healthcare professionals is usually to include advice to eat little and often in order to maintain blood sugar levels (Power et al 2001; Stables 1999:383; Broussard & Richter 1998; Lindsay 1997; Dilorio et al 1994; Iatrakis et al 1988). This includes the ubiquitous advice to eat a dry biscuit or piece of toast before rising from bed in the morning, traditional advice related to nocturnal hypoglycaemia, yet in many cases, completely impractical and ineffective. Lindsay (1997:508) reiterates the conventional dietary advice to be issued by midwives, such as avoiding fatty, spicy or strong-smelling or flavoured foods and suggests that fresh fruit and savoury foods are 'usually acceptable'. Milky drinks before retiring are also advocated, but as any nauseated person will know, milk is quite often the last beverage desired. Jednak et al (1999) suggest that protein-dominant meals assist in reducing nausea and dysfunction in gastric emptying. For some, citrus fruits may be helpful, whereas others may find that they exacerbate the condition.

In practice, women should be advised to try everything and anything that they feel able to eat or drink – at this time, good nutrition is almost irrelevant. Many expectant mothers possibly contribute to their symptoms because of their anxiety about fetal nourishment and much can be done by health professionals to lessen their concerns. Adding feelings of guilt to the physical and emotional distress already experienced as a result of this debilitating condition is unrealistic, inappropriate and unkind. This author's personal experience of severe nausea and vomiting until 20 weeks' gestation involved living for several weeks on nothing more than muesli and Coca-Cola, with no adverse effects on mother or baby! Most essentially, women should be encouraged to maintain adequate fluid intake, especially when they are vomiting frequently.

Rest and sleep are important to reduce the impact of fatigue; indeed, many women spontaneously resort to 'napping' (O'Brien et al 1997),

Box 1.5 Complementary therapies for relaxation	
Aromatherapy	Reiki
Bach flower remedies	Relaxation classes
Hypnotherapy	Shiatsu
Massage	Swimming
Reflexology	Yoga

although it is unclear whether any improvement is the result of renewed physical energy or simply the facilitation of a period of unconscious mental relief. Any means of alleviating associated stress should be advised, including time off work where possible, manageable recreation and relaxation and complementary therapies (see Box 1.5). A recognition that health professionals empathise and appreciate the effects of the problem will go a long way towards influencing the mother's perception of her condition, even though the amount of nausea and the frequency of vomiting may be very little different from before.

It is also necessary to ensure that partners and family members appreciate the nature of the problem. Partners seem to have one of two possible responses to the mother's vomiting: either they become over-solicitous, or they disregard the intensity of the woman's feelings, both physical and psychological. Diplomatic advice could help to ensure that, as far as possible, they understand the problem and suggestions could be made for them to participate in essential domestic chores, as well as, in some cases, advising the woman herself to prioritise aspects of the housework. If there are children old enough to understand they can also play their part in helping the mother to cope.

Practice point

When mothers wish to use complementary therapies for relaxation they should be encouraged to find practitioners who are experienced in treating pregnant women, who fully understand pregnancy physiopathology and who appreciate their relationship with conventional maternity professionals.

MEDICAL MANAGEMENT OF HYPEREMESIS GRAVIDARUM

Medical management of hyperemesis gravidarum, where the mother is hospitalised, aims to rehydrate her, correct electrolyte and other haematological disturbances, prevent complications and transfer the mother home as soon as possible, although many women have a high readmission rate. It is necessary to determine the cause of the excessive vomiting, not merely to make a differential diagnosis, but also to consider other factors such as psychological issues, which may be adding to the severity of the mother's condition. Somewhat presumptuously, Edmonds (1999:239) suggests that the first action to be taken in the event of a mother becoming pathologically unwell is that she 'should be *removed* from her stressful home environment' (this author's italics). It is, however, vital to assess the impact of hospitalisation on the mother and her family and to weigh this against the implications of treating her condition either as an inpatient or an outpatient. For some, the distress and domestic upheaval caused by insisting on admission to the antenatal ward may be counter-productive to the benefits of medical management.

Almost half of American obstetricians surveyed by Power et al (2001) would admit women who showed signs of dehydration and weight loss to hospital. There needs to be a balance between a reactionary medicalisation of care for women whose nausea and vomiting could be managed at home, and avoiding unnecessary delays in instigating appropriate treatment when the condition becomes pathological (Lee at al 2000). Wagner et al (2000) postulate that it is an increased comprehension of the condition together with a more aggressive approach to dealing with the metabolic upheaval which has contributed to a decline in maternal deaths from hyperemesis gravidarum.

Fluid and electrolyte replacement is usually achieved through the intravenous administration of a solution such as Hartmann's. Fluid intake and output, including measurement of vomitus, should be undertaken and vital signs of pulse, blood pressure and temperature recorded regularly. Any signs of disorientation, drowsiness, ataxia or abnormal eye movements should be noted and action taken to prevent further complications. Ditto et al (1999) found that intravenous normal saline, glucose and vitamins with the addition of diazepam was significantly more effective in reducing nausea, vomiting, length of hospital stay and rate of readmission than infusions without diazepam. Intravenous fluid replacement has also been carried out successfully, safely and cost effectively in the home and could be considered for women without additional complications (Naef et al 1995).

The mother should not be given anything to eat or drink other than ice to suck, and attention to oral and personal hygiene should be maintained. Undue disturbance should be minimised, by nursing the woman in a single room if possible. It is generally considered appropriate to introduce oral fluids and foods gradually when vomiting has ceased for 24 hours.

Total parenteral nutrition (TPN) or slow drip enteral feeding may be implemented in order to maintain maternal nutrition. Zibell Frisk et al (1990) suggest that TPN is safe, when individually tailored to each woman's needs, despite the inclusion of lipids, the safety of which in pregnancy has been questioned. However the use of both TPN and enteral feeding is not without risk. Aspiration pneumonia may occur if persistent vomiting occurs during enteral feeding, or cardiac tamponade may develop in association with TPN (Greenspoon et al 1989). Russo-Stieglitz et al (1999) found a higher rate of complications from centrally inserted TPN catheters (50%) than from peripherally inserted catheters (9%) with incidents of infection, thrombosis, occlusion, pneumothorax and catheter dislodgement, and recommended the insertion of peripheral catheters. Katz et al (2000) reported the case of a woman in whom the catheter tip became infected with *Mycobacterium chelonae* after prolonged use and suggested the judicious removal of catheters as soon as possible. In another case, TPN without multivitamin therapy resulted in increased lactate levels and acute beri-beri due to lack of thiamine pyrophosphate supplementation. Hsu et al (1996) favour nasogastric enteral feeding, having demonstrated success in treating seven women, first in hospital and then at home.

Antiemetics, initially intramuscularly and later orally, are given primarily to prevent the complications of further fluid loss. Phenothiazines, which are dopamine antagonists and act by blocking the chemoreceptor trigger zone, include prochlorperazine, which has the advantage of being available in the more easily administered suppository form. Metoclopramide is an effective antiemetic which works similarly to the phenothiazines but also has a peripheral action on the gut. Subcutaneous metoclopramide on an outpatient basis has been found to be a safe and clinically- and cost-effective means of dealing with the problem (Buttino et al 2000). Walters (1999) suggests that intradermal scopolamine may be appropriate, although the British National Formulary (BNF) (September 2001:205) lists pregnancy as a precaution.

The use of steroids such as intravenous hydrocortisone and oral prednisolone or dexamethasone may also be effective and safe (Safari et al 1998; Nelson-Piercy 1998; Taylor 1996). Nelson-Piercy et al (2001) randomly allocated 25 women to receive either oral prednisolone or a placebo, changed after three days to intravenous hydrocortisone or normal saline (placebo) if women were still vomiting. When compared to placebo, steroid therapy resulted in an increase in the sense of wellbeing, appetite and weight. The research team therefore supported the use of steroids in the management of severe hyperemesis gravidarum, although it was not felt that they led to a rapid or a complete resolution of symptoms.

The Committee on the Safety of Medicines has recently reviewed steroid use in pregnancy

---

Box 1.6 Recommendations for the management of enteral or total parenteral nutrition in pregnancy

Individually tailored to each woman's needs
Monitor blood levels for nutritional deficiencies
Consider nasogastric feeding before TPN

Peripherally inserted TPN catheters have lower risks
Remove catheters as soon as possible

---

and concluded that dexamethasone will readily cross the placenta, whereas 88% of prednisolone is inactivated as it crosses the placenta, however there is no convincing evidence of an increase in the incidence of congenital abnormalities such as cleft lip and palate. Prolonged use may lead to intrauterine growth retardation but adrenal effects in the infant will resolve spontaneously and are rarely of clinical significance (BNF 2001:342).

The teratogenicity of antiemetic pharmacological preparations is of concern to both health professionals and to expectant women, although, where drug therapy is prescribed, counselling regarding its safety appears to reduce parental concern (Mazotta et al 1999). Concern is more marked where medication is prescribed in response to unresolved nausea and vomiting secondary to advice about adaptations to diet and lifestyle, whereas women whose obstetricians' first line of management is drug therapy appear to be less worried about the teratogenicity (Mazotta et al 1999). Antihistamines such as promethazine or meclozine act centrally but do not appear to be the usual drug of choice, although Kallen (2002) suggests that there is no clear indication of any teratogenic effect.

In the USA no FDA-approved antiemetic drug for use in pregnancy has been available since the voluntary withdrawal of Bendectin (Debendox) in 1983 by the manufacturers, Merrel Dow, pending many product liability suits. A generic form, Diclectin, a combination of doxylamine and pyridoxine, continues to be used in Canada. Bishai et al (2000) have reviewed the evidence for the use of Diclectin and concluded that it is an effective antiemetic whilst refuting the claims made against its safety in pregnancy. Indeed, Boneva et al (1999) found a lower risk of congenital heart defects in the infants of women with severe nausea and vomiting who had taken

---

Practice point

'Nausea in the first trimester of pregnancy does **not** require drug therapy. On rare occasions if vomiting is severe, an antihistamine (e.g. promethazine) or a phenothiazine may be required. If symptoms have not settled in 24 to 48 hours then a specialist opinion should be sought.'
(British National Formulary 2001:200)

---

doxylamine and pyridoxine, and suggest that this may be due either to endocrine factors or a component of the drug, deemed most probably to be the pyridoxine.

However, the cost to the health services of the removal of Bendectin has been estimated at $73 million in the USA and $16 million in Canada, between 1983 and 1987 (Neutel & Johnson 1995), and by 1984 hospital admissions for hyperemesis gravidarum in both countries had risen by approximately 50%. These estimates do not take account of the increased cost to society of obstetricians' time, additional absenteeism from work and the psychosocial impact on women and their families. The authors conclude that, without any perceived decline in the rates of congential abnormalities, there appears to be no real justification for the withdrawal of a drug which was effective and relatively safe. A meta-analysis of 16 cohort and 11 case-control studies which reported birth defects in women exposed to Bendectin also failed to show any significant difference in risk for congenital abnormalities between women who had taken Bendectin in the first trimester and those who had not. The authors therefore refuted the role of the drug in the prevalence of defects (McKeigue et al 1994). More recently, Brent (2002) addressed the medical, social and legal implications of treatments for pregnancy sickness, confirming that studies investigating Bendectin have shown no evidence that therapeutic doses of the drug cause adverse effects in either mother or fetus, a fact which has been supported by the re-publication of these conclusions by the US Food and Drug Administration, thus possibly setting the scene for its re-introduction. Similarly, analysis of controlled studies into the safety of pharmacological preparations for pregnancy sickness was undertaken by Magee et al (2002), who found more evidence of safety for Bendectin, H1-antagonists and phenothiazines than for metoclopramide, droperidol, ondansetron or corticosteroids.

Mazotta, Stewart and Atanakovic et al (2000) compared contemporary attitudes to antiemetic medication for pregnancy sickness of American and Canadian women and found that Americans were more wary of the potential teratogenic effects of the drugs, whereas Canadian mothers, for whom medication is available, considered the effects of severe nausea and vomiting to be more likely to pose considerable risk to the fetus. Atanackovic, Navioz, Moretti et al (2001) investigated the incidence of adverse maternal and fetal effects and pregnancy outcomes in women taking the recommended four tablets of Diclectin daily, and those taking a higher than recommended dose. 33.6% of women reported tiredness, sleepiness or drowsiness whilst taking the medication, but there did not appear to be a dose-per-kg of maternal body weight-related effect. Pregnancy outcome and infant birthweight were not found to be associated with a higher than recommended dose of the drug and it was concluded that it was safe to administer more than four tablets daily.

Van Stuijvenberg et al (1995) expressed concern regarding the risk of malnutrition of hyperemetic women. They found that there was a statistically significant difference, when compared to controls, in the levels of thiamine, riboflavin, pyridoxine, vitamin A and retinol-binding protein, whereas there were higher levels of vitamin C, calcium, albumin, haematocrit and haemoglobin, suggestive of dehydration. Correction of the biochemical profile was associated with cessation of vomiting.

Vitamin supplementation, including thiamin (vitamin B1), is especially necessary, in an attempt to prevent the rare complication of Wernicke's encephalopathy from developing; should this develop, thiamin injections are usually effective in treating the condition. Wernicke's encephalopathy is characterised by small petechial haemorrhages in the hypothalamus and upper brain stem, leading to disturbed consciousness, impaired memory, ataxia, abnormal eye movements and polyneuropathy. Lesions around the hypothalamus may trigger hypothermia as a result of an inability to control the temperature. Coma and death may follow. Correct diagnosis is important to enable prompt treatment; magnetic resonance imaging will confirm encephalopathic changes and differentiate the condition from an acute thyroid storm of Graves' disease (Ohmori et al 1999).

Ohkoshi et al (1994) reported the case of an 18-year-old woman whose Wernicke's encephalopathy was induced by hyperemesis gravidarum, initially treated with antiemetic therapy, intravenous glucose and low dose insulin, but without thiamin. As a result she developed polyneuropathy, nystagmus, ataxia and became comatose. Computed tomography and magnetic resonance imaging revealed symmetrical periventricular lesions of the thalamus and hypothalamus, as well as bilateral caudate lesions, which occur only rarely. In another case, Gardian et al (1999) found, on MR imaging, lesions in the nuclei of thalami, the hypothalamus and the periaqueductal gray matter of a woman with a history of prolonged vomiting. Successful treatment involved the administration of intramuscular vitamin B1 followed by oral thiamin until term, when a healthy infant was delivered. However, their review of previous cases shows a perinatal loss rate of approximately 50%. A similar case was also reported by Togay-Isikay et al (2001).

Rotman et al (1994) also advocate parenteral thiamin supplementation in cases where severe hyperemesis gravidarum persists for more than three weeks, especially if there is associated liver dysfunction. They report on a woman who vomited for 11 weeks, and by 18 weeks' gesta-

---

Box 1.7 Potential complications of hyperemesis gravidarum

Central pontine myelinolysis
Coagulopathy
Death – maternal or fetal
Haematemesis
Hypothermia
Intrauterine growth retardation if weight loss excessive
Jaundice and hepatic failure

Malnutrition
Oesophageal lacerations
Polyneuritis and other neurological disorders
Renal failure
Thyrotoxicosis
Wernicke's encephalopathy

---

tion had lost 21kg in weight, and in whom the fetus died. Liver function was moderately disturbed; a review of other cases of hyperemetic Wernicke's encephalopathy revealed a 40% incidence of raised aspartate aminotransferase values (more than 100 U/l) and the authors suggest that hepatic abnormality contributes to the pathogenicity of Wernicke's encephalopathy.

Coagulopathy has also been reported by Robinson et al (1998) as a consequence of vitamin K deficiency induced by the malnutrition of excessive nausea and vomiting. They recommend that, where hyperemesis is protracted and severe, coagulation disorders should be considered and prophylactic vitamin K should be administered. Larrey et al (1984) described the case of a woman who suffered jaundice, caused by conjugated hyperbilirubinaemia, in three consecutive hyperemetic pregnancies. There were increased levels of alanine aminotransferase, and necrotic hepatocytes were revealed by electron microscopic examination. The jaundice resolved completely following cessation of vomiting.

Elective termination of pregnancy is only occasionally performed as a last resort in the most severe cases of hyperemesis gravidarum where the life of the mother is at risk if the pregnancy continues. Mazotta, Stewart and Koren et al (2001) surveyed 3201 callers to a healthline in Toronto and, when independent factors were excluded, found that 413 women had considered termination of pregnancy to stop the sickness and 108 had actually had a termination performed. Where the pregnancy was unplanned, there was more than one fetus, the mother was clinically depressed as a result, or the condition was profoundly affecting both the mother's and her partner's daily life or their relationship, termination was more likely to have been performed. The authors conclude that pyschosocial factors must be taken into account when women request termination of the pregnancy. However, Koren and Levichek (2002) express concern that there is a misplaced perception of the teratogenic risk of medication which may lead some women to consider termination of pregnancy in which nausea and vomiting might otherwise have been treated effectively and safely.

CONCLUSION

It can be seen from this introductory discussion that pregnancy-associated nausea and vomiting is a complex phenomenon, with multifactorial aetiology, although some of the more recent theories remain controversial. The condition ranges from a mild, short-term and self-managed inconvenience to a major complication of pregnancy with variable prognoses. Conventional management usually commences with simple dietary and lifestyle advice offered by midwives, progressing to pharmacological and intensive medical intervention for those with the most serious manifestations.

Further chapters in this book explore a range of different approaches, both to the causes and predisposing factors and to the care and management of women suffering nausea and vomiting in pregnancy. The final chapter attempts to draw the themes together in an integrated approach, which empowers women to make informed choices and increases the management options for maternity care providers.

REFERENCES

Asakura H, Watanabe S, Sekiguchi et al 2000 Severity of hypermesis gravidarum correlates with serum levels of reverse T3. Archives of Gynecology and Obstetrics 264 (2): 57-62

Atanackovic G, Wolpin J, Koren G 2001 Determinants of the need for hospital care among women with nausea and vomiting of pregnancy. Clinical Investigations in Medicine 24 (2): 90-93

Atanackovic G, Navioz Y, Moretti M E et al 2001 The safety of higher than standard dose of doxylamine-pyridoxine (Diclectin)n for nausea and vomiting of pregnancy. Journal of Clinical Pharmacology 41 (8): 842-845

Attard C L, Kohli M A, Coleman S et al 2002 The burden of illness of severe nausea and vomiting of pregnancy in the United. States American Journal of Obstetrics and Gynecology 186 (5 suppl): S220-227

Basso O, Olsen J 2001 Sex ration and twinning in women with hyperemesis or pre-eclampsia. Epidemiology 12 (6): 747-749

Bishai R, Mazzotta P, Atanackovic G et al 2000 Critical appraisal of drug therapy for nausea and vomiting of pregnancy II : efficacy and safety of diclectin (doxylamine-B6). Canadian Journal of Clinical Pharmacology 7 (3): 138-143

Black F O 2002 Maternal susceptibility to nausea and vomiting of pregnancy: is the vestibular system involved? American Journal of Obstetrics and Gynecology 186 (5 suppl): S204-209

Boneva R S, Moore C A, Botto L et al 1999 Nausea during pregnancy and congenital heart defects: a population-based case-control study. American Journal of Epidemiology 149 (8): 717-725

Borgeat A, Fathi M, Valiton A 1997 Hyperemesis gravidarum: is serotonin implicated? American Journal of Obstetrics and Gynecology 176 (2): 476-477

Brent R 2002 Medical, social and legal implications of treating nausea and vomiting of pregnancy. American Journal of Obstetrics and Gynecology 186 (5 suppl): S262-266

British Medical Association/Royal Pharmaceutical Society of Great Britain 2001 British National Formulary 42 (September) Section 4.6 Drugs used in nausea and vertigo: 200-203; 342-343 and Appendix 4 Pregnancy: 669-683

Broussard C N, Richter J E 1998 Nausea and vomiting of pregnancy. Gastroenterology Clinics of North America 2791:123-51

Brown JE Kahn ES Hartman TJ 1997 Profet, profit and proof: do nausea and vomiting of early pregnancy protect women from 'harmful vegetables'? American Journal of Obstetrics and Gynecology 176 (1 Pt 1): 179-181

Buckwalter J G, Simpson S W 2002 Psychological factors in the etiology and treatment of severe nausea and vomiting in pregnancy. American Journal of Obstetrics & Gynecology 186 (5 suppl): S210-214

Buttino L, Coleman S K, Bergauer N K et al 2000 Home subcutaneous metoclopramide therapy for hyperemesis gravidarum. Journal of Perinatology 20 (6): 359-362

Calfee E F, Rust O A, Bofill J A et al 1999 Maternal hypoglycemia: is it associated with adverse perinatal outcome? Journal of Perinatology 1995: 379-382

Chong W, Johnston C 1997 Unsuspected thyrotoxicosis and hyperemesis gravidarum in Asian women. Postgraduate Medicine 73 (858): 234-236

Crystal S R, Bowen D J, Bernstein I L 1999 Morning sickness and salt intake, food cravings and food aversions. Physiology and Behavior 67 (2): 181-187

Del Mar Melero-Montes M, Jick H 2001 Hyperemesis gravidarum and the sex of the offspring. Epidemiology 12 (1): 123-124

Dilorio C, van der Lier D, Manteuffel B 1994 Recommendations by clinicians for nausea and vomiting of pregnancy. Clinical Nursing Research 3 (3): 209-227

Ditto A, Morgante G, la Marca A et al 1999 Evaluation of treatment of hyperemsis gravidarum using parenteral fluid with or without diazepam. A randomised study. Gynecological and Obstetric Investigations 48 (4): 232-236

Edmonds D K 1999 Miscellaneous disorders in pregnancy. In: Edmonds D K (ed) Dewhurst's Textbook of Obstetrics and Gynaecology for Postgraduates , 6th edn. Blackwell Science , London

Eliakim R, Abulafia O, Sherer D M 2000 Hyperemesis gravidarum: a current review. American Journal of Perinatology 17 (4): 207-218

Emelianova S, Mazotta P, Einarson A et al 1999 Prevalence and severity of nausea and vomiting of pregnancy and effect of vitamin supplementation. Clinical Investigations in Medicine 22 (3): 106-110

Erdem A, Arslan M, Erdem M et al 2002 Detection of Helicobacter pylori seropositivity in hyperemesis gravidarum and correlation with symptoms. American Journal of Perinatology 19 (2): 87-92

Erick M 1995 Hyperolfaction and hyperemesis gravidarum: what is the relationship? Nutritional Review 53 (10): 289-295

Flaxman S M, Sherman P W 2000 Morning sickness: a mechanism for protecting mother and embryo. Quarterly Reviews in Biology 75 (2): 113-148

Furneaux E C, Langley-Evans A J, Langley-Evans S C 2001 Nausea and vomiting of pregnancy: endocrine basis and contribution to pregnancy outcome. Obstetrical and Gynecological Surveys 56 (12): 775-782

Gadsby R, Barnie-Adshead A M, Jagger C 1993 A prospective study of nausea and vomiting during pregnancy. British Journal of General Practice 43 (373): 325

Gadsby R, Barnie-Adshead A M, Jagger C 1997 Pregnancy nausea related to women's obstetric and personal histories. Gynecological and Obstetric Investigation 43 (2): 108-111

Gadsby R, Barnie-Adshead A, Grammatoppoulos D et al 2000 Nausea and vomiting in pregnancy: an association between symptoms and maternal prostaglandin E2. Gynecological and Obstetric Investigations 50 (3): 149-152

Gardian G, Voros E, Jardanhazy T et al 1999 Wernicke's encephalopathy induced by hyperemesis gravidarum. Acta Neurologica Scandinavica 99 (3): 196-198

Glick M M, Dick E L 1999 Molar pregnancy presenting with hyperemesis gravidarum. Journal of the American Osteopathic Association 99 (3): 162-164

Goodwin T M 2002 Nausea and vomiting of pregnancy: an obstetric syndrome. American Journal of Obstetrics and Gynecology 186 (5 suppl): S184-189

Goodwin T M, Montoro M, Mestman J H et al 1992 The role of chorionic gonadotrophin in transient hyperthyroidism of hyperemesis gravidarum. Journal of Clinical Endocrinology and Metabolism 75 (5): 1333-1337

Greenspoon J, Masak D, Kurz C 1989 Cardiac tamponade in pregnancy during central hyperalimentation. Obstetrics and Gynecology 73 (3): 465-466

Gross S, Librach C, Cecutti E 1989 Maternal weight loss associated with hyperemesis gravidarum: a predictor of fetal outcome. American Journal of Obstetrics and Gynaecology 160 (4): 906-909

Hasler W L 1999 Serotonin receptor physiology: relation to emesis. Digestive Diseases and Sciences 44 (8Suppl): 108S-113S

Hayakawa S, Nakajima N, Karassaki-Suzuki M et al 2000 Frequent presence of Helicobacter pylori genome in the saliva of patients with hyperemesis gravidarum. American Journal of Perinatology 17 (5): 243-247

Hershman J M 1999 Human chorionic gonadotrophin and the thyroid: hyperemesis gravidarum and trophoblastic tumours. Thyroid 9 (7): 653-657

Ho K Y, Kang J Y, Viegas O A 1998 Symptomatic gastro-oesophageal reflux in pregnancy: a prospective study among Singaporean women. Journal of Gastroenterology and Hepatology 13 (10): 1020-1026

Hsu J J, Clark Glena R, Nelson DK et al 1996 Nasogastric enteral feeding in the management of hyperemesis gravidarum. Obstetrics and Gynecology 88 (3): 343-346

Huxley R R 2000 Nausea and vomiting in early pregnancy: its role in placnetal development. Obstetrics and Gynecology 95 (5): 779-782

Iatrakis G M N, Sakellaropoulos G G, Kourkoubas A H et al 1988 Vomiting and nausea in the first 12 weeks of pregnancy. Psychotherapeutics and Psychosomatics 49 (1): 22-24

Jacoby E B, Porter K B 1999 Helicobacter pylori infection and persistent hyperemesis gravidarum. American Journal of Perinatology 16 (2): 85-88

James D K, Steer P J, Weiner C P et al 1999 High risk pregnancy: management options. Saunders, London

Jarnfelt-Samsioe A, Bremme K, Eneroth P 1986 Steroid hormones in emetic and non-emetic pregnancy. European Journal of Obstetrics, Gynecology andReproductive Biology 2192: 87-99

Jednak M A, Shadigian E M, Kim M S et al 1999 Protein meals reduce nausea and gastric slow wave dysrhythmic activity in first trimester pregnancy American Journal of Physiology 277 (4 Pt 1): G855-861

Jewell D, Young G 2000 Interventions for nausea and vomiting in early pregnancy. Cochrane Database Systematic Review (2): CD000145

Jordan V, Grebe S K, Cooke R R et al 1999 Acidic isoforms of chorionic gonadotrophin in European and Samoan women are associated with hyperemesis gravidarum and may be thyrotrophic. Clinical Endocrinology 50 (5): 619-627

Kallen B 2002 Use of antihistamine drugs in early pregnancy and delivery outcome. Journal of Maternal-Fetal and Neonatal Medicine 11 (3): 146-152

Katz V L, Farmer R, York J et al 2000 Mycobacterium chelonae sepsis associated with longterm use of an

intravenous catheter for treatment of hyperemesis gravidarum. A case report. Journal of Reproductive Medicine 45 (7): 581-584

Kelly S 1996 Disorders caused by pregnancy. In: Bennett V R, Brown L K (eds) Myles' Textbook for Midwives, 12th edn. Churchill Livingstone, Edinburgh

Klebenoff M A, Mills J L 1986 Is vomiting during pregnancy teratogenic? British Medical Journal (Clinical Research Edition) 15: 292 (6522): 724-726

Knudsen A, Lebech M, Hansen M 1995 Upper gastrointestinal symptoms in the third trimester of the normal pregnancy. European Journal of Obstetrics, Gynecology andReproductive Biology 60 (1): 29-33

Koch K L 2002 Gastrointestinal factors in nausea and vomiting of pregnancy. American Journal of Obstetrics and Gynecology 186 (5 suppl): S198-203

Kopp P 2001 The TSH receptor and its role in thyroid disease. Cellular and Molecular Life Sciences 58 (9): 1301-1302

Koren G 2000 Appraisal of drug therapy for nausea and vomiting of pregnancy: I: the placebo effect – methodological and practical considerations. Canadian Journal of Clinical Pharmacology 7 (3): 135-137

Koren G, Boskovic R, Hard M et al 2002 Motherisk – PUQE (pregnancy-unique quantification of emesis and nausea) scoring system for nausea and vomiting of pregnancy. American Journal of Obstetrics and Gynecology 186 (5suppl): S228-231

Koren G, Levicheck Z 2002 The teratogenicity of drugs for nausea and vomiting of pregnancy: perceived versus true risk. American Journal of Obstetrics and Gynecology 186 (5 suppl): S248-252

Koren G, Magee L, Attard C et al 2001 A novel method for the evaluation of the severity of nausea and vomiting of pregnancy. European Journal of Obstetrics, Gynaecology andReproductive Biology 94 (1):31-6

Kort K C, Schiller H J, Numann P J 1999 Hyper-parathyroidism and pregnancy. American Journal of Surgery 177 (1): 66-68

Kuscu N K, Koyuncu F 2002 Hyperemesis gravidarum: current concepts and management. Postgraduate Medical Journal 78 (916): 76-79

Lacroix R, Eason E, Melzack R 2000 Nausea and vomiting during pregnancy: a prospective study of its frequency, intensity and patterns of change. American Journal of Obstetrics and Gynecology 182 (4): 931-937

Lao T, Chin R, Mak Y et al 1988 Plasma zinc concentration and thyroid function in hyperemetic pregnancies. Acta Obstetrica et Gynaecologica Scandinavica 677: 599-604

Larrey D, Rueff B, Feldmann G et al 1984 Recurrent jaundice caused by recurrent hyperemesis gravidarum. Gut 25 (12): 1414-1415

Lee J, Einarson A, Gallo M et al 2000 Longitudinal change in the treatment of nausea and vomiting of pregnancy in Ontario. Canadian Journal of Clinical Pharmacology 7 (4): 205-208

Leeners B, Sauer Rath W 2000 Nausea and vomiting in early pregnancy/hyperemesis gravidarum. Current status of psychosomatic factors. Zeitschrift fur Neonatologie 204 (4):1 28-134

Leylek O A, Toyaksi M, Erselcan T et al 1999 Immunologic and biochemical factors in hyperemesis gravidarum with or without hyperthyroxinaemia. Gynecologic and Obstetric Investigation 47 (4): 229-234

Lindsay P 1997 Vomiting. In: Sweet B with Tiran D (eds)

Mayes' Midwifery, 12th edition. Bailliere Tindall, London

Maes B D, Spitz B, Ghoos Y F et al 1999 Gastric emptying in hyperemesis gravidarum and non-dyspeptic pregnancy. Alimentary Pharmacology and Therapeutics 13 (2): 237-243

Magee L A, Chandra K, Mazzotta P et al 2002 Development of a health-related quality of life instrument for nausea and vomiting of pregnancy. American Journal of Obstetrics and Gynecology 186 (5 suppl): S232-238

Magee L A, Mazotta P, Koren G 2002 Evidence-based view of safety and effectiveness of pharmacological therapy for nausea and vomiting of pregnancy (NVP). American Journal of Obstetrics and Gynecology 186 (5 suppl): S256-261

Mazotta P, Magee L A, Maltepe C et al 1999 The perception of teratogenic risk by women with nausea and vomiting of pregnancy. Reproductive Toxicology 13 (6): 573

Mazotta P, Stewart D, Atanackovic G et al 2000 Psychosocial morbidity among women with nausea and vomiting of pregnancy: prevalence and association with anti-emetic therapy. Journal of Psychosomatic Obstetrics and Gynaecology 21 (3): 129-136

Mazotta P, Maltepe C, Navioz Y et al 2000 Attitudes, management and consequences of nausea and vomiting of pregnancy in the United States and Canada. International Journal of Gynaecology and Obstetrics 70 (3): 359-360

Mazotta P, Stewart D E, Koren G et al 2001 Factors associated with elective termination of pregnancy among Canadian and American women with nausea and vomiting of pregnancy. Journal of Psychosomatic Obstetrics and Gynecology 22 (1): 7-12

McKeigue P M, Lamm S H, Linn S et al 1994 Bendectin and birth defects. I: A meta-analysis of the epidemiologic studies. Teratology 50 (1): 27-37

Mestman J H 1999 Diagnosis and management of maternal and fetal thyroid disorders. Current Opinion in Obstetrics and Gynecology 11 (2): 167-175

Minagawa M, Narita J, Tada T et al 1999 Mechanisms underlying immunologic states during pregnancy: possible association of the sympathetic nervous system. Cellular Immunology 196 (1): 1-13

Munch S 2000 Commentary. A qualitative analysis of physician humanism: women's experiences with hyperemesis gravidarum. Journal of Perinatology 20 (8 part 1): 540-547

Naef R W, Chauhan S P, Roach H 1995 Treatment for hyperemesis gravidarum in the home: an alternative to hospitalisation. Journal of Perinatology 15 (4): 289-292

Nelson-Piercy C, Fayers P, de Swiet M 2001 Randomised double-blind placebo-controlled trial of corticosteroids for the treatment of hyperemesis gravidarum. British Journal of Obstetrics and Gynaecology 108 (1): 9-15

Nelson-Piercy C 1998 Treatment of nausea and vomiting in pregnancy. When should it be treated and what can safely be taken? Drug Safety 19 (2): 155-164

Neutel C I, Johansen H L 1995 Measuring drug effectiveness by default: the case of Bendectin. Canadian Journal of Public Health 86 (1): 66-70

O'Brien B, Naber S 1992 Nausea and vomiting during pregnancy: effects on the quality of women's lives. Birth 19 (3): 138-143

O'Brien B, Relyea J, Lidstone T 1997 Diary reports of nausea and vomiting during pregnancy. Clinical Nursing Research 6 (3): 239-252

Ohkoshi N, Ishii A, Shoji S 1994 Wernicke's encephalopathy induced by hyperemesis gravidarum associated with bilateral caudate lesions on computed tomography and magnetic resonance imaging. European Neurology 34 (3): 177-180

Ohmori N, Tushima T, Sekine Y et al 1999 Gestational thyrotoxicosis with acute Wernicke encephalopathy: a case report. Endocrinology Journal 46 (6): 787-793

Panesar N S, Li C Y, Rogers M S 2001 Are thyroid hormones of hCG responsible for hyperemesis gravidarum? A matched paired study of pregnant Chinese women. Acta Obstetricia et Gynecologica Scandinavica 80 (6): 519-524

Power M L, Holzman G B, Schulkin J 2001 A survey on the management of nausea and vomiting in pregnancy by obstetricians/gynecologists. Primary Care Update in Obstetrics and Gynecology 8 (2): 69-72

Raphael-Leff J 1991 Psychological processes of childbearing. Chapman and Hall, London

Rhodes V A, McDaniel R W 1999 The index of nausea, vomiting and retching: a new format of the index of nausea and vomiting. Oncology Nursing Forum 26 (5): 889-894

Robinson J N, Bannerjee R, Thiet M P 1998 Coagulopathy secondary to vitamin K deficiency in hyperemesis gravidarum. Obstetrics and Gynecology 92 (4 pt 2): 673-675

Rotman P, Hassin D, Mouallem M et al 1994 Wernicke's encephalopathy in hyperemesis gravidarum: association with abnormal liver function. Israeli Journal of Medical Science 30 (3): 225-228

Russo-Stieglitz K E, Levie A B, Wagner B A et al 1999 Pregnancy outcome in patients requiring parenteral nutrition. Journal of Maternal and Fetal Medicine 8 (4): 164-167

Safari H R, Alsulyman O M, Gherman R B et al 1998 Experience with oral methylprednisolone in the treatment of refractory hyperemesis gravidarum. American Journal of Obstetrics and Gynecology 178 (5): 1054-1058

Sherman P W, Flaxman S M 2002 Nausea and vomiting of pregnancy in an evolutionary perspective. American Journal of Obstetrics and Gynecology 186 (5 suppl): S190-197

Stables D 1999 Physiology in childbearing with anatomy and related biosciences. Bailliere Tindall, London

Tan J Y L, Loh K C, Yeo G S H et al 2002 Transient hyper-thyroidism of hyperemesis gravidarum. British Journal of Obstetrics and Gynaecology 109 (6): 683-688

Tareen A K, Baseer A, Jaffry H F et al 1995 Thyroid hormone in hyperemesis gravidarum. Journal of Obstetrics and Gynaecology 21 (5): 497-501

Taylor R 1996 Successful management of hyperemesis gravidarum using steroid therapy. Quarterly Journal of Medicine 89: 103-107. Cited by Walters B N J 1999 Hepatic and gastrointestinal disease. In: James D K, Steer P J, Weiner C P, Gonik B (eds) High risk pregnancy management options. Bailliere Tindall, London

Tierson F D, Olsen C L, Hook E B 1986 Nausea and vomiting of pregnancy and association with pregnancy outcome. American Journal of Obstetrics and Gynecology 155 (5): 1017-1022

Togay-Isikay C, Yigit A, Mutluer N 2001 Wernicke's encephalopathy due to hyperemesis gravidarum: an under-recognised condition. Australian and New

Zealand Journal of Obstetrics and Gynaecology 41 (4): 453-456

Van Calenbergh S G K, Poppe W A J, van Calenbergh F 2001 An intracranial tumour: an uncommon cause of hyperemesis in pregnancy. European Journal of Obstetrics, Gynecology and Reproductive Biology 95 (2): 182-183

van der Lier D, Manteuffel B, Dilorio C et al 1993 Nausea and fatigue during early pregnancy. Birth 20 (4): 193-197

van Stuijvenberg M E, Schabort I, Labadarios D et al 1995 The nutritional status of patients with hyperemesis gravidarum. American Journal of Obstetrics and Gynecology 172 (5): 1585-1591

Vellacott I D, Cooke E J, James C E 1988 Nausea and vomiting in early pregnancy. International Journal of Gynecology and Obstetrics 27 (1): 57-62

Wagner B A, Worthington P, Russo-Stieglitz K E et al 2000 Nutritional management of hyperemesis gravidarum. Nutrition in Clinical Practice 15 (2): 65-76

Walters B N J 1999 Hepatic and gastrointestinal disease. In: James D K, Steer P J, Weiner C P, Gonik B (eds) High risk pregnancy management options. Bailliere Tindall London

Wu C Y, Tseng J J, Chou M et al 2000 Correlation between Helicobacter pylori infection and gastrointestinal symptoms of pregnancy. Advances in Therapy 17 (3): 152-158

Zibell Frisk D, Jen K L, Rick J 1990 Use of parenteral nutrition to maintain adequate nutritional status in hyperesis gravidarum. Journal of Perinatology 10 (4): 390-395

Zhou Q, O'Brien B, Relyea J 1999 Severity of nausea and vomiting during pregnancy: what does it predict? Birth 26 (2): 108-114

2

The complementary medical approach

This chapter examines the increase in the use of complementary and alternative medicine and the possible reasons for this. The evidence for the safety and efficacy of natural remedies and complementary therapies is debated, with specific reference to the care of pregnant and childbearing women.

INTRODUCTION

Complementary and alternative medicine (CAM) has become a hugely popular force with which orthodox medicine must now reckon. In the UK it is estimated that one person in three, two thirds of whom are women, has used some form of CAM (Thomas, Nicholl & Coleman 2001). Use of CAM amongst children appears to be approximately 18% with almost 7% having visited a CAM practitioner, although Simpson and Roman (2001) recommend that parents should be encouraged to adhere to conventional treatments where appropriate. Young healthy men are the least likely to access complementary medicine, possibly due to insufficient knowledge and a perceived lack of support from medical doctors (Jain & Astin 2001).

In Britain, in 1998, 22 million visits were made to practitioners of the six main complementary therapies, of which 10% were provided by the NHS (Thomas, Nicholl & Coleman 2001). An estimated £450 million (Thomas, Nicholl & Coleman 2001) is spent by the public on accessing CAM outside NHS provision, although private medical insurance policies will increasingly provide cover for some aspects of CAM. In the USA it is estimated that 60 million people, or between 30% and 50% of the population, use CAM (Barrett 2001; Crock et al 1999; Astin et al 1998), with many health insurance companies prepared to provide cover, notably for acupuncture, chiropractic and osteopathy (Pelletier & Astin 2002), and access in Australia is also high (Hall & Giles-Corti 2000; Pirotta et al 2000) with the annual amount spent by the general public on CAM being comparable with patient contributions to pharmaceutical drugs (Easthope et al 2000).

REASONS FOR THE INCREASING USE OF COMPLEMENTARY AND ALTERNATIVE MEDICINE

Ernst (2001) attributes the increase in the use of complementary therapies to a profound criticism of orthodox healthcare provision and a belief amongst CAM users that conventional medicine has the power to do more harm than good, although this does not seem to be entirely the case. One Boston, USA, survey of 831 adults who accessed both conventional and complementary medicine indicated that many people appreciate the synergistic effect of combined use (Eisenberg et al 2001). Patients may be dissatisfied with the conveyor-belt, profit-motivated service within conventional healthcare, but do not generally feel aggrieved about the individual professionals with whom they come into contact. They dislike the lack of time available to talk about issues of concern, a fact which may lead to a perception of doctors as dismissive and uncaring, although many consumers acknowledge that medical practitioners are themselves caught up in 'the system'. This lack of time, of necessity, means that doctors, especially general practitioners who average approximately seven minutes per patient, focus on the presenting symptoms rather than on the whole person.

Reilly (2001) postulates that it is the desire of the general public for a different, more person-centred approach to care and claims that CAM is the second biggest growth industry in Europe. Conventional healthcare is seen by users and practitioners of CAM therapies to be widely accessible and socially legitimate, but also disempowering and mechanistic, leading consumers to turn to different modalities (Barrett et al 2000). Where CAM therapies are provided by the NHS, patients feel they are either more effective or more acceptable than orthodox treatments, and practitioners are seen as caring and focusing on the therapeutic relationship (Luff & Thomas 2000a). Conventional medicine is valued for the effectiveness of its diagnosis and speed of its intervention, particularly for symptom relief, but systems such as Traditional Chinese Medicine are seen as being better at determining the root cause of illnesses and therefore better at preventing recurrence (Tang & Easthope 2000).

The emphasis of complementary medicine on the psychological and spiritual aspects of health, as well as on the physiopathological aspects of illness, is valued by users (Mitzdorf et al 1999; Hebert et al 2001) and CAM treatments appear to attain better patient satisfaction than conventional healthcare, even when the treatment outcome is not wholly successful (Freivogel & Gerhard 2001). This is especially noticeable amongst oncology patients for whom the use of CAM treatments enhances their empowerment in the decision-making process (Shumay et al 2001). Swisher et al (2002) suggest that oncologists caring for women with gynaecological cancers should initiate discussion about the safe and appropriate use of CAM, which in turn will legitimise the self-administration of natural remedies by patients who might otherwise conceal the fact from their physicians.

This concept of holism is fundamental to complementary medicine and is diametrically opposed to the reductionist approach of orthodox medicine, in which the body is artificially compartmentalised to comply with the specialisms which occur in conventional medicine. There appears to be little appreciation of the interlinking of body, mind and spirit, nor of the sociological factors which impact on health and wellbeing. Eastwood (2000) discusses the globalisation which has occurred with the onset of

Box 2.1 Reasons for increased interest in complementary medicine

Attention to more than just the symptoms: mind-body-spirit approach
Disenchantment with orthodox healthcare system (but not practitioners)
Communication difficulties/lack of time of orthodox health professionals
'Doctor-shopping' for second opinions – resort to CAM practitioners
Patient desire for control and empowerment
Perception of risks of pharmaceutical preparations
Reduced efficacy of existing medications

Environmental factors – move towards a more natural approach
Public generally more informed
Media coverage and encouragement including Internet
Multicultural society: immigrants dependent on traditional medicine
Financial: herbal, homeopathic remedies may be cheaper than OTC drugs or prescription charges

Adapted from Kayne (1997)
and Spencer and Jacobs (1999)

rapid social change. GPs have had to respond to increasing consumer demand, yet are also acting as agents of change by acknowledging the limitations of the biomedical approach of orthodox medicine and advocating alternatives, offering an artistic rather than a scientific approach to care, in the latter of which 'clinical legitimacy' overrides 'scientific legitimacy'.

The plethora of information available to the general public, particularly via the Internet, also means that people are more knowledgeable about health-related issues, often more so than their doctors, although concern has been expressed, by both conventional and complementary experts, about the health risks associated with advice offered over the Internet (Ernst & Schmidt 2002). Even within conventional healthcare, patients may discover a wider range of treatment options than is at first offered by their general practitioners or consultants, and may challenge their doctors to seek a second opinion. This extends to a consumer-driven demand for complementary and alternative medicine, although one of the issues of concern is the 'therapy shopping' which many patients seem to pursue in an attempt to find the quickest, most effective or most pleasant resolution to their problems, without giving any one therapy the chance to work efficiently.

Users of all health services ever more frequently ask for advice regarding CAM therapies, and orthodox medical professionals can no longer afford to remain ignorant or unfacilitative. Those who remain sceptical have an obli-

gation, at the very least, to facilitate patient choice by 'permitting' them to seek alternatives, should they so wish. Lack of knowledge of doctors and other healthcare professionals should also be no barrier to patient access, and their oft-quoted justification for reticence to accept CAM, that 'there is no evidence to support it', is unacceptable, since CAM research is increasingly being undertaken, often in conjunction with conventional practitioners.

People respond well to the increased focus in CAM on a partnership with their healthcare providers, rather than the traditional paternalistic approach of conventional medicine. Working in partnership is not only client-focused and desirable, but in CAM, is essential, since many aspects of care require lifestyle changes to be made by the patient. However, a Swiss survey by Messerli-Rohrbach and Schr (1999) suggests that this desire for and ability to work in partnership declines with worsening health in favour of a more directive approach for a speedy resolution to the condition. Similarly, Passalacqua et al (1999), who questioned oncology patients about an emotive Italian media campaign for an alternative cancer therapy, found that patients value the advice of a trusted doctor and would be guided by their advice rather than scientific evidence of efficacy, although many would be prepared to try even unproven treatments in the hope of a cure.

Within maternity care this is seen as a means of empowerment of women, in keeping with the philosophy of the *Changing Childbirth* (Department of Health 1993) approach, which advocated 'choice, control and continuity' of care and carers for expectant, labouring and newly-delivered mothers. The physiological aetiology of many of their symptoms can lead to a dismissive attitude of some obstetricians and GPs, for conditions such as nausea and vomiting do not normally require medical attention, yet they have a profound sociological and psychological effect for the women. When even these physiological conditions require more treatment, complementary therapies provide more choice for women who may not wish to resort to the other options, namely pharmacological drugs or conservative or no treatment. Informed choice thus gives women more control over their care, enabling them to elect whichever is the most appropriate course of action for them, given their individual circumstances.

However, despite the increasing recognition of CAM by orthodox healthcare providers, many patients fail to inform their doctors about concomitant use of natural remedies, perhaps perceiving medical practitioners as being unable to comprehend the differences between the two systems, and unable to incorporate them into their current practice (Eisenberg et al 2001). Confidence of users in their healthcare providers is comparable between conventional and complementary practitioners, but many patients feel that their doctors would disapprove of their use of CAM therapies and may refuse to continue acting as their primary care physician (Eisenberg et al 2001). Indeed, this threat of termination of conventional treatment

may be a real one, although consultants in secondary healthcare appear more likely to take this stance than family practitioners (Crock et al 1999). This can be a cause of conflict between healthcare providers and patients, and between healthcare disciplines (see Case 2.1, which, although not an obstetric case, clearly demonstrates this potential for conflict).

This failure to inform conventional medical practitioners about patients' use of CAM seems to be universal. Emergency department patients surveyed in Sacramento, USA, were knowledgeable about herbal remedies and 43% had used some form of CAM at some time. However, 16% of patients presumed that CAM therapies and remedies were safe and women generally felt that natural medicines did not interact with other pharmaceutical preparations. Only 67% would inform their doctors about their use (Weiss et al 2001). Crock et al (1999) found that an astounding 70% of CAM users fail to inform their GPs when accessing orthodox medical care. Wagner et al (1999) suggest that 425 million visits to CAM practitioners have been made in total in the USA, with, for example, users of herbal remedies such as St John's wort seeing little necessity for informing their GPs. Montbriand (2000) expressed similar concerns regarding patients' lack of communication about CAM use, especially herbal medicines, in Canada, but also highlighted the need for greater communication between doctors, nurses and pharmacists on possible drug interactions (see also Chapter 5).

Case 2.1

An elderly male patient was admitted to a medical ward following a cerebrovascular accident, caused by severe essential hypertension. Despite intravenous antihypertensive therapy his blood pressure remained extremely high for several days. On the sixth day, however, the blood pressure plummeted to below normal levels. By chance the nurses discovered that the man's wife had been surreptitiously administering Chinese herbal remedies to him, aimed at reducing the blood pressure, and it is likely that a potentiation had occurred as a result of both this and the prescribed medication. The consultant physician refused to treat the man further as he appeared to view the patient's choice of herbal remedies as a threat to his own clinical autonomy. The nursing staff were caught in the middle, attempting to act as the patient's advocate to facilitate his right to self-treat, as well as complying with the instructions of the consultant, yet bound by the Code of Conduct of their own governing body to continue to provide care. A resolution to this ethical dilemma only occurred when the wife decided to transfer her husband to a private nursing home, from where it was reported later that he had died.

ATTITUDES OF HEALTHCARE PROFESSIONALS

Although, in Britain, NHS provision remains limited, there appears to have been an increasing acceptance and interest amongst conventional healthcare professionals, not least in an attempt to respond to consumer demand. Undergraduate medical education now includes an introduction to CAM in at least 15 medical schools in Britain (FIM 2001) and there is also tremendous interest amongst nurses, midwives and physiotherapists as seen by the numerous papers in professional journals.

In the USA Einarson et al (2000) found that 86% of physicians, 74% of medical students, 66% of naturopaths and 50% of naturopathic students considered that complementary medicine should be included as standard in the conventional medical curriculum. Interest amongst medical students in Kansas was shown in Greiner et al's survey (2000), with 72% desiring its inclusion in the undergraduate curriculum and 84% viewing a knowledge of CAM as important to their future medical practice. There is a belief that more comprehensive knowledge of CAM would better prepare medical students to act as patient advocates once qualified (Chez et al 2001), and indeed would assist in the prevention of unanticipated complications from interactions between the two systems. Boucher and Lenz (1998) revealed that almost 59% of physicians advocate improved CAM education to assist them in referral and response to consumer demand. 56% of Australian trainee doctors surveyed in Melbourne had no knowledge of CAM therapies and it was shown that even a single lecture on the subject can have a positive effect on their attitudes towards the use of CAM (Hopper & Cohen 1998). Similar results regarding the value of exposure to CAM education during pre-registration training of a range of health professionals were found in Ontario by Baugniet et al (2000).

Indeed, there has been a dramatic change in the views of those working in orthodox medicine since the British Medical Association published its first report into 'alternative' medicine (BMA 1986) in which it was dismissed as a passing trend with no credibility. The 1993 report went some way further towards a greater degree of acceptance by the medical profession (BMA 1993) and made some much-needed recommendations for improvements in education, regulation and practice, with GPs retaining the 'gatekeeper' responsibility for patients' health. The Foundation for Integrated Medicine (1997) reiterated the importance of education, regulation, research and improved delivery of integrated services and called for a more integrated and accessible approach to CAM in order that the best of both orthodox and complementary medicine could be made available to patients. These issues were debated further by a Select Committee of the House of Lords, resulting in a report which classified the main therapies into three categories (HoL 2000) (see Boxes 2.2-2.4).

A 1995 survey of 1226 general practitioners in England (Thomas, Nicholl & Fall 2001) showed that an estimated 39.5% of GP partnerships in England provided access to some form of CAM for their NHS patients. 21.4% of these offered access via a member of the primary healthcare team and 6.1% employed an independent therapist, while 24.6% had made NHS referrals to external CAM practitioners. It was acknowledged, however, that fundholding practices at the time were more likely to offer CAM therapies than non-fundholding practices and the authors of the report suggested that patterns of provision of CAM may change as Primary Care Groups and Trusts become more established. A similar survey of 254 general practices in Birmingham showed approximately 50% offering in-house CAM services, usually provided by the doctors, more commonly in larger, fund-holding practices with a teaching commitment. Luff and Thomas (2000b) explored ten existing complementary therapy services within primary care in England and confirmed that there was an 'ad hoc' development of CAM provision, historically facilitated by the fundholding arrangements of the 1990s. They were keen that these services should be maintained within the Primary Care Group context and for there to be a more standardised approach to the development of further CAM services, particularly as lack of time is perceived as a serious constraint on the capability of GPs to provide CAM in their own practice (Adams 2001).

Lack of time, and lack of knowledge, are also reasons why integrating CAM into secondary care, such as intensive care units, is difficult (Hayes & Cox 1999), although Manga (2000) argues that greater integration of therapies such as chiropractic is cost-effective and could improve health outcomes. The ignorance of some primary care doctors regarding homeopathy is felt to put them at risk of failing to understand patients' expectations, and that these practitioners use a disease-focused, rather than a person-centred approach to treatment (Calderon 1998). The point here, however, is whether the CAM therapies are incorporated into the care provided by individual conventional practitioners, or whether CAM therapists are contracted to provide additional treatment alongside medical care. Many doctors are trained in and use homeopathy or acupuncture together with orthodox treatment, selecting whichever is the most appropriate for individual patients. Increasing numbers of nurses, midwives and physiotherapists use supportive therapies such as massage, aromatherapy, reflexology or hypnotherapy as adjuncts to caring for their patients. The number of CAM practitioners 'allowed' to practise in the NHS or other conventional services is probably less, and is certainly not widespread, except in clinical specialisms such as oncology and terminal care.

Medical practitioners most likely to support CAM therapies are younger, female general practitioners (Rooney et al 2001; Perry & Dowrick 2000) who have had personal experience of complementary medicine, but the socioeconomic status of the area in which they practise does not appear to influence their decisions (Perry & Dowrick 2000). Naturopaths, physiatrists (rehabilitation specialists) and physician assistants in Canada and America are more willing than medical practitioners to prescribe CAM to patients, although this is largely dependent on their level of knowledge (Einarson et al 2000; Ko & Bernrayer 2000; Houston et al 2001).

Acupuncture, primarily for the treatment of pain (Diehl et al 1997), chiropractic and osteopathy appear to be the most widely recommended and used CAM therapies in Britain, America, Canada and Australia (Perry & Dowrick 2000; Rooney et al 2001; Hall & Giles-Corti 2000; Pirotta et al 2000; Astin et al 1998) as these are seen to be the most clinically effective. There are divided opinions regarding homeopathy due to its need to individualise treatments so specifically, making controlled research studies difficult (Merrell & Shalts 2002), although the emphasis on evidence-based medicine presents conflict for some GPs, who turn to CAM in an attempt to retain clinical autonomy (Adams 2000). Hypnotherapy, medical herbalism, aromatherapy and reflexology are viewed more sceptically.

In Britain at least, this may partly be due to an unacknowledged political distinction, with those therapies in group 1 (the 'Big Five') more frequently practised by doctors than by nurses and other professions supplementary to medicine; these practitioners tend, on the whole, to incorporate therapies from group 2 into their work, since they are more supportive than diagnostic methods or discrete systems of treatment.

USE OF COMPLEMENTARY THERAPIES DURING PREGNANCY AND CHILDBIRTH

It is evident from developments in the past decade that complementary and alternative medicine has increasingly become more integrated into mainstream healthcare. The term 'integrated medicine' is now frequently used in favour of 'alternative' or 'complementary', implying a move towards combining the best from both the conventional and complementary fields. Nowhere is this more apparent than in materni-

---

Box 2.2 Group 1

Therapies which are discrete, professionally organised systems of healthcare and which have a reasonable body of evidence to support practice.
- Acupuncture (see Chapter 4)
- Medical herbalism (see Chapter 5)

- Homeopathy (see Chapter 6)
- Osteopathy (see Chapter 7)
- Chiropractic (see Chapter 7)

(House of Lords 2000)

Box 2.3 Group 2

Therapies which have only limited evidence to support practice but which provide relaxation and symptom relief to patients and are considered to be complementary to conventional healthcare.
- Nutrition (see Chapter 3)
- Shiatsu (see Chapter 4)
- Aromatherapy (see Chapter 5)
- Reflexology (see Chapter 7)

- Massage (see Chapter 7)
- Yoga, meditation (see Chapter 8)
- Bach flower remedies (see Chapter 8)
- Hypnotherapy (see Chapter 8)
- Alexander technique
- Counselling, stress management
- Healing

(House of Lords 2000)

Box 2.4 Group 3

Therapies which have little or no body of evidence to support practice.
   3a: Traditional systems of medicine: Traditional Chinese Medicine, Chinese herbal medicine, Ayurvedic medicine, Tibetan medicine, naturopathy,

anthroposophical medicine
   3b: Other, alternative therapies: kinesiology, iridology, radionics, crystal healing, dowsing.

(House of Lords 2000)

(see Glossary for definitions of terms)

ty care, for which women are already receiving conventional care. A survey by the NHS Confederation in 1997 identified that approximately 34% of British midwives had used one or more elements of CAM in their practice. An astounding 93.9% of nurse-midwives in North Carolina, USA have recommended CAM therapies to pregnant women (Allaire et al 2000) and approximately 18% of nurse-midwives across America appear to use herbal preparations to stimulate labour (McFarlin et al 1999).

GPs, obstetricians and midwives may find themselves being asked for advice about different therapies, such as homeopathic arnica for postpartum perineal bruising, raspberry leaf herbal tea to tone the uterus in preparation for labour, or the safe use of aromatherapy essential oils during pregnancy. Certainly, most gynaecologists will have had queries on natural progesterone and dietary phytoestrogens from perimenopausal women wishing to avoid hormone replacement therapy. Gordon et al (1998) found that 75% of Californian consultants in obstetrics and gynaecology were interested in recommending herbal and homeopathic medicines to women, mainly for treating the menopause and premenstrual syndrome. However enthusiasm for and interest in complementary medicine amongst doctors, nurses and midwives are often misinterpreted as 'knowledge', and care should be taken to ensure that lack of depth of knowledge and inadequate understanding does not compromise patient safety or professional accountability. Some examples of this are included in Box 2.5.

Obstetricians in Britain may be tacitly sup-

Box 2.5 Examples of inappropriate complementary medical advice to pregnant women

- Injudicious advice on the use of ginger for nausea and vomiting without appreciating why it may, on occasions, exacerbate the symptoms
- Universal advice to take raspberry leaf tea in the last trimester without checking whether or not there are contraindications such as a uterine scar
- Agreeing with a woman suffering backache that receiving massage during pregnancy is relaxing (and therefore 'harmless') without understanding that

inappropriate massage by an inadequately trained therapist can do more harm than good, including initiating preterm labour by inadvertent stimulation of acupuncture points known to trigger uterine contractions
- Facilitating a labouring woman's choice to use lavender essential oil for pain relief as a complement to epidural analgesia without acknowledging that the hypotensive effect of certain chemicals in lavender can potentiate the hypotensive effect of bupivicaine

---

Box 2.6 Access to complementary medicine by pregnant women

Self-administered prior to pregnancy
Self-administered for the first time during pregnancy
Consultation with CAM practitioner for relaxation during pregnancy
Consultation with CAM practitioner for specific condition during pregnancy

Recommended by midwife, health visitor, GP or obstetrician
Referred by midwife, health visitor, GP or obstetrician
Practised by midwife, health visitor, GP, obstetrician or other conventional healthcare professional, e.g. physiotherapist or anaesthetist

---

portive of women's wishes to use natural remedies but are possibly less likely to utilise complementary medicine themselves. This is because the role of the obstetrician in the UK is fundamentally related to dealing with *abnormal* pregnancies and labours, for which most women will be prepared to accept conventional assistance, especially in an emergency situation. British midwives, whose role focuses on caring for women with *normal* pregnancies and labours, are in a more favourable position to use complementary therapies for the relief of physiological symptoms, which come within their remit of normal practice, and as general relaxation strategies. In the United Kingdom it is illegal for anyone, other than a midwife or doctor, or one in training under supervision, to take sole responsibility for care during childbirth, except in an emergency. This means that the vast majority of pregnant women will access antenatal care in good time to prepare for the birth. Therefore, any complementary and alternative therapies used during pregnancy, labour or the puerperium must be used in addition to orthodox maternity care.

The integration of CAM therapies into maternity care is well publicised, and primarily, in

Practice point

The use of any natural remedies or alternative therapies *must* be *complementary* to conventional maternity care.

Britain, provided by midwives. Tiran (2001) reported on the use of a variety of complementary therapies to treat physiological disorders of pregnancy within an NHS clinic, and on reflexology in particular (Tiran 1996; 2002). Aromatherapy services have been described by Ager (2002); and Budd (1992) and West (1997) provide accounts of midwifery acupuncture clinics. There are also frequent reports in the professional texts of the varied applications of CAM therapies to the care of pregnant and childbearing women including chiropractic (Tellefsen 2000; Daly et al 1991; Fallon 1986), osteopathy (Conway 2000), herbal medicine (Stapleton & Tiran 2000) and homeopathy (Cummings 2000) although many of these are outside NHS provision.

Consumer interest demands, at the very least, an awareness of CAM by conventional healthcare professionals and an acknowledgement that women will use these therapies irrespective of approval from doctors, nurses and midwives. A survey of pregnant women in a Rhode Island, USA, maternity hospital showed that almost 10% self-administered herbal remedies during pregnancy (usually as a follow-on to preconceptional use) and 13.3% had accessed other complementary therapies (Gibson et al 2001). Ranzini et al (2001) suggested that almost one third of pregnant women in an area of New Jersey use potentially harmful natural remedies, of which physicians are rarely aware. Over half of women in New York have been shown to use a CAM treatment or remedy and 40% have visited a CAM practitioner (Factor-Litvak et al 2001). A Canadian survey regarding women's self-management of pregnancy sickness showed that 61% used complementary and alternative therapies, of which 21% had consulted CAM practitioners, 8% had discussed CAM with their doctor or pharmacist and 71% had spoken to family, friends or, occasionally, other allied health professionals (Hollyer et al 2002). Westfall (2001) and Pinn and Pallett (2002) believe that expectant mothers most frequently use herbal medicine as tonics and to prevent miscarriage or to induce labour at term. However, there seems to be a misplaced belief that, because they are natural, complementary therapies are also safe – or at least, safer than conventional medicine. On the one hand, women believe them to offer effective alternatives to medically prescribed drugs, yet on the other, they fail to acknowledge that any powerful tool used inappropriately has the potential to be, at best, ineffective and, at worst, harmful. It is therefore essential that those who provide orthodox maternity care should appreciate issues of efficacy and safety, even if the individual personally remains sceptical or is not in a position to provide or facilitate access to CAM therapies for pregnant and childbearing women.

Expectant mothers can usually be persuaded to be cautious about their use of complementary and alternative remedies once the possible hazards have been highlighted, in order to protect their babies, although this is dependent on adequate knowledge of their obstetricians, GPs and midwives. There is much media coverage of natural remedies to deal with women's health concerns and it is precisely because pregnancy and childbirth are essentially normal that women choose to reject pharmaceutical preparations, sometimes to their detriment. Women's magazines often carry articles about natural means of inducing labour. For example, this author is frequently contacted by journalists requesting information on 'DIY induction', who fail to recognise that induction is a medical technique performed for specific clinical reasons.

The use of complementary medicine for other phases of physiological adaptation, such as the premenstrual or perimenopausal phases, is also debated at length by the media. However, although this information may empower women to help themselves, conversely and at the very least, it may give women false hope or, in extreme circumstances be potentially dangerous. Women generally believe 'natural' to imply substances derived from plants, which are not synthesised or made with chemicals, and the majority appear to endorse the value of remedies such as natural hormone replacement to be superior to drugs, both in their effectiveness and their safety (Adams & Cannell 2001). This is despite the conflicting evidence regarding various herbal remedies. For example, black cohosh, when tested using standard clinical trial methodology, was not found to be significantly more effective in relieving menopausal symptoms such as hot flushes than placebo (Jacobson et al 2001) and Amato et al (2002) urge the cautious use of other remedies such as dong quai and ginseng which have been shown to stimulate the growth of MCF-7 cells, a human breast cancer cell line. Furthermore, protracted use of herbal remedies may not be cost-effective for the individual, for they are much more expensive than paying for prescriptions, especially when required for a number of years. More importantly, while natural remedies may relieve some of the discomforts of the perimenopausal phase, they will do little to prevent the long-term sequelae of oestrogen withdrawal.

It is interesting in clinical practice to find that women will generally be prepared to take natu-

---

Practice point
'Natural' does not automatically mean 'safe'.

ral remedies in the form of herbal and homeopathic *tablets*, yet fail to accept that any drugs prescribed antenatally by the obstetrician or GP will only be prescribed when necessary, will be appropriate for their particular needs and will be those approved as safe to use in pregnancy. They seem to reject these with an implication that they are being 'forced' to take drugs, yet fail to understand the possible dangers of not complying. An example of this might the woman with a urinary tract infection who refuses to take antibiotics, without realising the risks of preterm labour which might ensue.

On the other hand there are occasions when women will reject oral complementary medicines, even when it has been explained, for example in the case of homeopathy, that the amount of the active ingredient is negligible, because it has been impressed on them that they should avoid *all* drugs (with 'drugs' being interpreted as oral preparations only). Strangely, these same women are often more accepting of manual therapies with less scientific evidence to support them, e.g. reflexology, than of herbal remedies with a greater body of research findings and a mechanism of action akin to pharmaceutical drugs. This may be because they view manual and manipulative therapies simply as relaxation strategies rather than powerful therapeutic techniques, without realising the hazards of inappropriate use. An example of this is the mother seen for pregnancy sickness by this author, who had rejected homeopathic remedies as unsafe but who had been advised by a friend to press 'an acupuncture point' in the webbing of the thumb and forefinger, and who was actually stimulating the Large Intestine 4 point (see Chapter 4), a point which could potentially induce preterm labour or miscarriage!

CAM RESEARCH IN MATERNITY CARE

Only limited research has been carried out into the effectiveness of CAM therapies and techniques during pregnancy and childbirth, and often the numbers of subjects are small, studies lack control groups or there are other concerns regarding methodology. It is sometimes difficult to ascertain whether positive results are attributed to the CAM intervention or whether the nature of the client-therapist relationship (or, with many therapies, simply the use of human touch), has a bearing on the patient's perception of effectiveness (Kiernan 2002).

Burns et al (2000) successfully administered essential oils to over 8000 women for pain relief in labour, with less than 1% of side-effects or complications, all of them minor, and none affecting the fetus/baby. Kvorning et al (1998) found that acupuncture was an effective method of relieving labour pain and reduced the need for other analgesia, when compared to a control group. Positive results have been obtained by Cardini and Weixin (1998) and Kanakura et al (2001) with moxibustion, a Traditional Chinese Medicine technique applying heat to the Bladder 67 acupuncture point for correction of breech presentation, when com-

---

Case 2.2

A 28-year-old woman was in her second pregnancy, at 32 weeks' gestation and suffering very painful varicose veins in her legs, together with heartburn and haemorrhoids. However, when it was suggested by the complementary therapy midwife that she might try homeopathic pulsatilla, a remedy admirably suited to women suffering these three conditions concurrently, she refused on the grounds of concern about taking any medication during pregnancy. Conventional management involving supportive tights and advice to rest with her legs raised failed to improve the condition, which gradually worsened as the pregnancy progressed. Two weeks later her discomfort was so intense that she agreed, (against her beliefs), to try the pulsatilla, with almost immediate effects.

pared to external cephalic version and a control. 'Heat', in the form of a ginger paste applied to the same acupuncture point, has also been used successfully to effect cephalic version (Cai et al 1990), and hypnosis may offer an additional strategy for the management of breech presentation (Mehl 1994).

Raspberry leaf appears to shorten labour, decrease the likelihood of preterm or post-term delivery and reduce the incidence of amniotomy or operative delivery (Parsons et al 1999). Relaxation therapy in women who experience preterm labour may help to prolong pregnancy and increase infant birthweight when compared to controls (Janke 1999). Reflexology has also been shown to have a beneficial effect on the duration of labour and the woman's perception of pain (Motha & McGrath 1993; Feder et al 1993). However, the evidence for the use of homeopathic caulophyllum to induce labour is deemed to be insufficient (Smith 2001). Ripening of the cervix using acupuncture may be feasible (Rabl et al 2001), and successful induction of uterine contractions has been achieved with transcutaneous electrical nerve stimulation at specified acupuncture points (Dunn et al 1989).

Antenatal perineal massage may help to reduce the need for episiotomy and the risk of second and third degree lacerations (Shipman et al 1997). Dale and Cornwell (1994) investigated the use of lavender oil for perineal healing in over 650 postpartum mothers and although the results were inconclusive in respect of wound healing, the women reported feeling much more relaxed and experienced less perineal pain. In women with faecal incontinence after obstetric trauma, biofeedback training has been found to be superior to sensory feedback alone, with improved continence and anal musculature (Fynes et al 1999).

Although complementary therapies are likely to be used with more caution in women with complications of pregnancy, third trimester administration of garlic tablets may reduce the occurrence of hypertension, but has not been found to be effective in preventing pre-eclampsia (Zinaei et al 2001). Nutritional supplementation with calcium may also be a means of reduc-

ing the severity, but not the incidence, of pre-eclampsia (Wanchu et al 2001), although Atallah et al (2000) advocate further study to determine optimum doses. A Chinese study demonstrated a significant difference in a group of women with pregnancy induced hypertension who were given prepared rhubarb with nifederpine, compared with a group given nifederpine alone, and the authors postulated that the prepared rhubarb may reduce damage to vascular endothelial cells and alter the immune balance (Wang & Song 1999).

SAFETY OF COMPLEMENTARY AND ALTERNATIVE MEDICINE IN PREGNANCY

The interest in using complementary therapies for symptoms of pregnancy and aspects of labour is growing, but there is a dearth of knowledge about what is safe to use at this time. Pinn (2001) expresses concern that a lack of clinical trials on efficacy and safety make it almost impossible to determine which remedies are of benefit. This is echoed by Pinn and Pallett (2002), Petrie and Peck (2000) and Chez and Jonas (1997a; 1997b). A problem arises, however, for if there is insufficient evidence about effectiveness of a particular remedy, there is no reason to investigate its safety. Conversely, an ethical dilemma arises if therapies, as yet untested for safety, are used, although there may be a plethora of anecdotal reports confirming their value in reducing symptoms.

This is particularly pertinent for pregnant women, for whom the range of options within conventional medicine is often limited because of the potential teratogenicity or mutagenicity of pharmacological preparations, especially in the first trimester, the commonest period for women to experience nausea and vomiting. Where information regarding the hazards of natural remedies is available this is largely on herbal medicines. This may be because herbalism is the therapy most commonly used by expectant mothers, or because its mode of action is similar to pharmaceutical drugs and can be comprehended by medical practitioners, whereas that of therapies within the 'energy medicine' category, such as homeopathy, Reiki or acupuncture, is less well understood. Information regarding possible dangers of CAM therapies is often in the form of case reports following accidental overdose or as a result of inexperienced or poorly trained practitioners, but caution is needed to refrain from making an assumptive leap and reaching an unsupported conclusion about the generalisability of these reports. Similarly, the application of small-scale research studies on animals must be put into context for human significance.

The potential interaction of herbal medicines with medical drugs has been questioned by Miller (1998), Klepser and Klepser (1999), Cupp (1999), Izzo and Ernst (2001), and Ernst (2002), with particular emphasis on St John's wort, ginkgo biloba, ginseng and echinacea. Indeed, Ernst et al (2001) recommend refraining from using any herbal medications in pregnancy. St John's wort is contraindicated during the pre-conception phase and during pregnancy, although no longterm effects on fetal growth and maturation were found when administered to mice (Rayburn et al 2000; 2001). Some of the evidence on humans appears to suggest that echinacea is comparatively safe to take during pregnancy (Gallo & Koren 2001), and St John's wort taken during breastfeeding has not been shown to produce side-effects in either mothers or infants (Klier et al 2002). The evidence for the safety of raspberry leaf is inconclusive (Simpson et al 2001). However, there have been reports of irregular menstrual bleeding in non-pregnant women taking St John's wort (Ratz et al 2001), which poses the question of the extent to which any perceived emmenagoguic action can be related to risks of bleeding in pregnancy. A case of profound neonatal congestive heart failure was attributed to maternal consumption of blue cohosh (caulophyllum) due to its vasoactive glycosides and an alkaloid known to produce toxic effects on the myocardia of laboratory animals (Jones & Lawson 1998). Of relevance for women requiring surgery are the reports of herb/drug interactions and coagulation dysfunction following laparoscopic cholecystecto-

my and with general anaesthesia (Fessenden et al 2001; Ang-Lee et al 2001).

The safety of acupuncture has also been called into question by Wilson (2002), and a case of acute intracranial haemorrhage following acupuncture treatment is reported by Choo and Yue (2000). However, the overall percentage of adverse events appears to be small, with an incidence of fourteen per 10,000 acupuncture consultations in one prospective study (White et al 2001) and 43 adverse reactions in over 34,000 treatments in another investigation (Macpherson et al 2001), most of which involved episodes of nausea, vomiting and fainting. A Japanese survey recorded only 94 minor adverse events in 65,000 treatments, which included needles being left in situ (Yamashita et al 1999). There does not appear to be any evidence of potential hazards of acupuncture used specifically during pregnancy and childbirth. Acupressure and shiatsu seem to be less challenged in general, with no accounts of side-effects from the use of wristbands being found in the literature, although one case of shingles developing after shiatsu treatment was reported by Mumm et al (1993).

Ernst et al (2001:29) state that the first trimester of pregnancy is often quoted as an acupuncture contraindication, except for the treatment of nausea and vomiting, although no rationale is given for its avoidance for other symptoms at this time, nor for the safety of its use specifically for gestational sickness. This is typical of the unsupported theory of many complementary therapies which is passed on from one 'authority' to another. Reflexology is a particular example of a therapy which traditionally teaches a set of contraindications and precautions, including pregnancy, probably more as a protection for its practitioners than in response to any evidence against its use. O'Hara (2002) and Tiran (2002) challenge these 'rules' for reflexology practice, but Tiran (2000; 2002) also emphasises the need for 'dual knowledge' where generic complementary therapists choose to specialise, particularly in the care of pregnant women when there is also the fetus to consider.

Bensoussan et al (2000) collated data from registered and unregistered, medical and non-medical practitioners of Traditional Chinese Medicine, which includes the use of acupuncture and Chinese herbs, and found an average of one adverse event with every 633 consultations. There was an interesting difference between the mean adverse event rate of medical and non-medical practitioners with that of medical practitioners being more than twice that of non-medical practitioners, although the authors postulated that this might reflect a more conscientious reporting of adverse events by doctors.

The embryotoxicity and teratogenicity of an Ayurvedic herbal method of contraception has been considered by Chaudhury et al (2001) and concern has been expressed over traditional childbirth remedies used by Tongan women (Ostraff et al 2000) and Nigerian women (Opaneye 1998). Traditional massage used by Pacific Island women to turn breech presentations has been blamed for 47 cases of intrauterine subdural haemorrhage; subsequent medical antenatal advice about its possible risks has coincided with a reduction in the incidence of haemorrhages (Becroft & Gunn 1989).

Chiropractic and osteopathy are not without risks either, but no reports of complications in pregnant women could be found in the literature. Shvartzman and Abelson (1988) questioned the long-term effects of chiropractic and recommended that caution be exercised when treating patients with specific conditions, although those cited are considered to be generally accepted contraindications. Practitioners working within defined boundaries (as with any therapy) should, in theory, experience a low incidence of adverse events. Senstad et al (1997) and Leboeuf-Yde et al (1997) suggest that approximately half of patients may suffer short-term local discomfort immediately after chiropractic treatment, but major complications are rare and include stroke or arterial dissection resulting from upper spinal manipulation and cauda equina after lower spinal manipulation (Assendelft et al 1996; Fibio 1999). Ernst et al (2001:65) cited similar potential complications from osteopathy.

Within general healthcare, homeopathic remedies are considered to be reasonably safe,

---

Practice point
Obstetricians, GPs and midwives must develop a facilitative attitude to support women who wish to use complementary and alternative therapies to ensure safe and effective maternity care.

possibly due to the misconception that because the amount of the original substance is so diluted it can do no harm. It is interesting to note that Ernst et al (2001:55) do not consider homeopathy to be contraindicated in pregnancy, whereas they take a cautious stance with almost every other therapy discussed, yet there is no more evidence in favour of homeopathy in pregnancy than for any other system of complementary medicine. Dantas and Rampes (2000) found that any adverse effects reported by patients appear to be an aggravation of symptoms, but in homeopathic theory, this is an indication of selection of the most appropriate remedy and cannot truly be considered as a complication. Some homeopaths, however, believe that, as the remedies are developed from much-diluted substances, some of which in large doses are toxic (e.g. arsenic), it is safer in pregnancy to administer a dose which is homeopathically more potent yet chemically more dilute, for example to use the 30C potency rather than the 6C strength.

CONCLUSION

It can be seen that complementary and alternative therapies are increasingly popular with the general public and with healthcare professionals. The incidence of usage is between 30% and 50% in many countries of the developed world, varying according to knowledge, availability and acceptability within different gender, age, social and geographical groups. Expectant mothers are keen to resort to a variety of means of dealing with the symptoms of pregnancy and labour, but do not always take into account the possible risks as well as the benefits of so doing.

There are many case reports and accounts of services where complementary medicine has helped women during the antenatal period, parturition and the puerperium. However, directly related clinical research on the efficacy of different therapies is not readily available, although it is sometimes possible to apply the findings of generic studies to the physiopathology of childbearing.

There is even less evidence regarding the safety of complementary medicine for pregnant and labouring women, but it is necessary to put into context the number of adverse events as a percentage of overall usage, and to balance this with an appreciation of the percentage of adverse events resulting from conventional medical or midwifery practice. Collation of single case reports and problems arising from accidental overdose or misuse will add to the body of knowledge required to practise evidence-based complementary medicine. However, the incidence of self-administration of natural remedies by the general public is high enough to provide the foundations of statistical data on both efficacy and safety.

Pregnant women will continue to use complementary and alternative medicine, with or without the sanction of their obstetricians, GPs or midwives. Healthcare professionals providing maternity care must therefore develop a facilitative attitude and an awareness of the subject in order to assist women to cope safely with symptoms of pregnancy and childbirth. Improved education of both consumers and professionals is needed in order to enhance communication between them and so provide optimum maternity care for mothers and their infants.

REFERENCES

Adams J 2000 General practitioners, complementary therapies and evidence-based medicine: the defence of clinical autonomy. Complementary Therapies in Medicine 8 (4): 248-252

Adams J 2001 Direct integrative practice, time constraints and reactive strategy: an examination of GP therapists' perceptions of their complementary medicine. Journal of Management in Medicine 15 (4-5): 312-322

Adams C, Cannell S 2001 Women's beliefs about 'natural' hormones and natural hormone replacement therapy. Menopause 8 (6): 433-440

Ager C 2002 A complementary therapy clinic – making it work. RCM Midwives' Journal 5 (6): 198-200

Allaire A D, Moos M K, Wells S R 2000 Complementary and alternative medicine in pregnancy: a survey of North Carolina certified nurse-midwives. Obstetrics and Gynecology 95 (1): 19-23

Amato P, Christophe S, Mellon P L 2002 Estrogenic activity of herbs commonly used as remedies for menopausal symptoms. Menopause 9 (2): 145-150

Ang-Lee M K, Moss J, Yuan C S 2001 Herbal medicines and perioperative care Journal of the American Medical Association 286 (2): 208-216

Assendelft W J, Bouter L M, Knipschild P G 1996 Complications of spinal manipulation. Journal of Family Practice 42: 475-480

Astin J A, Marie A, Pelletier K R et al 1998 A review of the incorporation of complementary and alternative medicine by mainstream physicians. Archives of Internal Medicine 23,158 (21): 2303-2310

Atallah A N, Hofmeyr G J, Duley L 2000 Calcium supplementation during pregnancy for preventing hypertensive disorders and related problems. Cochrane Database Systematic Review (2): CD 001059

Barrett B, Marchand L, Schneder J et al 2000 Bridging the gap between conventional and alternative medicine. Journal of Family Practice 49 (3): 234-239

Barrett B 2001 Complementary and alternative medicine: what's it all about? Wisconsin Medical Journal 100 (7):20-26

Baugniet J, Boon H, Ostbye T 2000 Complementary/alternative medicine: comparing the view of medical students with students in other health care professions. Family Medicine 32 (3): 178-184

Becroft D M, Gunn T R 1989 Prenatal intracranial haemorrhages in 47 Pacific Islander infants: is traditional massage the cause? New Zealand Medical Journal 102 (867): 207-210

Bensoussan A, Myers S P, Carlton A L 2000 Risks associated with the practice of Traditional Chinese Medicine: an Australian study. Archives of Family Medicine 9 (10): 1071-1078

Boucher T A, Lenz S K 1998 An organizational survey of physicians' attitudes about and practice of complementary and alternative medicine. Alternative Therapies in Health and Medicine 4 (6): 59-65

British Medical Association 1986 Alternative therapy. Report of the Board of Science and Education. British Medical Association, London

British Medical Association 1993 Complementary medicine: new approaches to good practice. Oxford University Press, Oxford

Budd S 1992 Traditional Chinese Medicine in obstetrics. Midwives Chronicle and Nursing Notes 105: 140

Burns E, Blamey C, Ersser S J et al 2000 The use of aromatherapy in intrapartum midwifery practice: an observational study. Complementary Therapies in Nursing and Midwifery 6 (1): 33-34

Cai R, Zhou A, Gao H 1990 Study on the correction of abnormal fetal position by applying ginger paste at zhihying acupoint. A report of 133 cases. Zhen Ci Yan Jiu 15 (2): 89-91

Calderon C 1998 Homeopathic and primary care doctors: how they see each other and how they see their patients: results of a qualitative investigation. Aten Primaria 21 (6): 367-375

Cardini F, Weixin H 1998 Moxibustion for correction of breech presentation: a randomised controlled trial. Journal of the American Medical Association 280 (18): 1580-1584

Chaudhury M R, Chandrasekaran R, Mishra S 2001 Embryotoxicity and teratogenicity studies of an ayurvedic contraceptive – pippaliyadi vati. Journal of Ethnopharmacology 74 (2): 189-193

Chez R A, Jonas W B, Crawford C 2001 A survey of medical students' opinions about complementary and alternative medicine. American Journal of Obstetrics and Gynecology 185 (3): 754-757

Chez R A, Jonas W B 1997a Complementary and alternative medicine. Part 1: clinical studies in obstetrics. Obstetric and Gynecologic Survey 52 (11): 704-708

Chez R A, Jonas W B 1997b Complementary and alternative medicine. Part II: clinical studies in gynecology. Obstetric and Gynecologic Survey 52 (11): 709-716

Choo D C, Yue G 2000 Acute intracranial hemorrhage caused by acupuncture. Headache 40 (5): 397-398

Conway P 2000 Osteopathy during pregnancy. In: Tiran D, Mack S (eds) Complementary therapies for pregnancy and childbirth, 2nd edn. Bailliere Tindall, London

Crock R D, Jarjoura D, Polen A et al 1999 Confronting the communication gap between conventional and alternative medicine: a survey of physicians' attitudes. Journal of Alternative Therapies in Health and Medicine 5 (2): 61-66

Cummings B 2000 Homeopathy for pregnancy and childbirth. In: Tiran D, Mack S (eds) Complementary therapies for pregnancy and childbirth, Bailliere Tindall London

Cupp M J 1999 Herbal remedies: adverse effects and drug interactions. American Family Physician 59 (5): 1239-1245

Dale E, Cornwell S 1994 The role of lavender oil in relieving perineal discomfort following childbirth: a blind randomised clinical trial. Journal of Advanced Nursing 19 (1): 89-96

Daly J M, Frame S P, Rapoza P A 1991 Sacroiliac subluxation: a common treatable cause of low back pain in pregnancy. Journal of Orthopaedic Medicine 13 (3): 60-65

Dantas F, Rampes H 2000 Do homeopathic medicines provoke adverse effects? A systematic review. British Homeopathic Journal 89 (Suppl 1): S35-38

Department of Health 1993 Changing Childbirth. HMSO, London

Diehl D L, Kaplan G, Coulter I et al 1997 Use of acupuncture by American physicians. Journal of Alternative and Complementary Medicine 3 (2): 119-126

Dunn P A, Rogers D, Halford K 1989 Transcutaneous electrical nerve stimulation at acupuncture points in the induction of uterine contractions. Obstetrics and Gynecology 73 (2): 286-290

Easthope G, Tranter B, Gill G 2000 Normal medical practice of referring patients for complementary therapies amongst Australian general practitioners. Complementary Therapies in Medicine 8 (4): 266-233

Eastwood H L 2000 Complementary therapies: the appeal to general practitioners. Medical Journal of Australia 173 (2): 95-98

Einarson A, Lawrimore T, Brand P et al 2000 Attitudes and practices of physicians and naturopaths toward herbal products, including use during pregnancy and lactation. Canadian Journal of Clinical Pharmacology 7 (1): 45-49

Eisenberg D M, Kessler R C, Van Rompay M I et al 2001 Perceptions about complementary therapies relative to conventional therapies among adults who use both: results from a national survey. Annals of Internal Medicine 135 (5): 344-351

Ernst E, Pittler M, Stevinson C, White A (eds) 2001 The Desktop guide to complementary and alternative medicine: an evidence-based approach. Mosby, Edinburgh

Ernst E 2001 Rise in popularity of complementary and alternative medicine: reasons and consequences for vaccination. Vaccine Oct 15; 20 Suppl 1: S90-93

Ernst E 2002 The risk-benefit profile of commonly used herbal therapies: Ginkgo, St John's wort, Ginseng, Echinacea, Saw Palmetto and Kava. Annals of Internal Medicine 136 (1): 42-53

Ernst E, Schmidt K 2002 Health risks over the Internet: advice offered by 'medical herbalists' to pregnant women. Wiener Medizinische Wochenschrift 152 (7-8): 190-192

Factor-Litvak P, Cushman L F, Kronenberg F 2001 Use of complementary and alternative medicine among women in New York City: a pilot study. Journal of Alternative and Complementary Medicine 7 (6): 659-666

Fallon J M 1986 Chiropractic manipulation in the treatment of costovertebral joint dysfunction with resultant intercostal neuralgia during pregnancy. Journal of the Neuro-musculo-skeletal System 4 (2): 73-75

Feder E, Liisberg G B, Lenstrup C et al 1993 Zone therapy in relation to birth. Proceedings of International Confederation of Midwives 23rd International Congress 2: 651-656

Fessenden J M, Wittenborn W, Clarke L 2001 Ginkgo biloba: a case report of herbal medicine and bleeding postoperatively from a laparascopic cholecystectomy. American Surgery 67 (1): 33-35

Fibio R 1999 Manipulation of the cervical spine: risks and benefits. Physical Therapy 79: 50-65

Foundation for Integrated Medicine 1997 Complementary medicine: a way forward for the next five years? FIM, London

Foundation for Integrated Medicine 2001 Symposium on undergraduate medical familiarisation with complementary and alternative medicine. Proceedings of Conference held at the British Medical Association 23rd November 2001

Freivogel K W Gerhard I 2001 Complementary medicine and patient contentedness – a survey. Forsch Komplementarmed Klass Naturheilkd 8 (3): 137-142

Fynes M M, Marshall K, Cassidy M et al 1999 A prospective randomised study comparing the effect of augmented biofeedback with sensory biofeedback alone on fecal incontinence after obstetric trauma. Diseases of the Colon and Rectum 42 (6): 753-758

Gallo M, Koren G 2001 Can herbal products be used safely during pregnancy? Focus on echinacea. Canadian Family Physician September 47: 1727-1728

Gibson P S, Powrie R, Star J 2001 Herbal and alternative medicine use during pregnancy: a cross-sectional survey Obstetrics and Gynecology 97 (4: Suppl 1): S44-45

Gordon N P, Sobel D S, Tarazona E Z 1998 Use of and interest in alternative therapies among adult primary care clinicians and adult members in a large health maintenance organisation. Western Journal of Medicine 169 (3): 153-161

Greiner K A, Murray J L, Kallail K J 2000 Medical student interest in alternative medicine. Journal of Alternative and Complementary Medicine 6 (3): 231-234

Hall K, Giles-Corti B 2000 Complementary therapies and the general practitioner. A survey of Perth GPs. Australian Family Physician 29 (6): 602-606

Hayes J A, Cox C L 1999 Integration of complementary therapies in North and South Thames regional health authorities' critical care units. Complementary Therapies in Nursing and Midwifery 5 (4): 103-107

Hebert R S, Jenckes M W, Ford D E et al 2001 Patient perspectives on spirituality and the patient-physician relationship. Journal of General Internal Medicine 16 (10): 685-692

Hollyer T, Boon H, Georgousis A et al 2002 The use of CAM by women suffering from nausea and vomiting during pregnancy. Complementary and Alternative Medicine 2 (1): 5

Hopper I, Cohen M 1998 Complementary therapies and the medical profession: a study of medical students' attitudes. Alternative Therapies in Health and Medicine 4 (3): 68-73

House of Lords Select Committee on Science and Technology 2000 Sixth report on complementary and alternative medicine. HMSO, London

Houston E A, Bork C E, Price J H et al 2001 How physician assistants use and perceive complementary and alternative medicine. Journal of the American Association of Physician Assistants 14 (1): 29-30, 33-4, 39-40

Izzo A A, Ernst E 2001 Interactions between herbal medicines and prescribed drugs: a systematic review. Drugs 61 (15): 2163-2175

Jacobson J S, Troxel A B, Evans J et al 2001 Randomized trial of balck cohosh for the treatment of hot flashes among women with a history of breast cancer. Journal of Clinical Oncology 19 (10): 2739-2745

Jain N, Astin J A 2001 Barriers to acceptance: an exploratory study of complementary/alternative medicine disuse. Journal of Alternative and Complementary Medicine 7 (6): 689-696

Janke J 1999 Effect of relaxation therapy on preterm labour outcomes. Journal of Obstetric, Gynecologic and Neonatal Nursing 28 (3): 255-263

Jones T K, Lawson B M 1998 Profound neonatal congestive heart failure caused by maternal consumption of blue cohosh herbal medication. Journal of Paediatrics 132 (3 Pt 1): 550-552

Kanakura Y, Kometani K, Nagata T et al 2001 Moxibustion treatment of breech presentation. American Journal of Chinese Medicine 2991: 37-45

Kayne S B 1997 Homeopathic pharmacy: an introduction and handbook. Churchill Livingstone, Edinburgh

Kiernan J 2002 The experience of Therapeutic Touch in the lives of five postpartum women. American Journal of Maternal and Child Nursing 27 (1): 47-53

Klepser T B, Klepser M E 1999 Unsafe and potentially safe herbal therapies. American Journal of Health Systems and Pharmacy 56 (2): 125-138

Klier C M, Schafer M R, Scmid-Siegel B et al 2002 St John's wort (Hypericum perforatum) – is it safe during breastfeeding? Pharmacopsychiatry 35 (1): 29-30

Ko G D, Bernrayer D 2000 Complementary and alternative medicine: Canadian physiatrists' attitudes and behaviour. Archives in Physical Medicine and Rehabilitation 81 (5): 662-667

Kvorning T N et al 1998 Acupuncture for pain relief during childbirth. Acupuncture and Electro-Therapeutics Research: The International Journal 23: 19-26

Leboeuf-Yde C, Hennius B, Rudberg E et al 1997 Side effects of chiropractic treatment: a prospective study. Journal of Manipulative and Physiological Therapeutics 20: 511-515

Luff D, Thomas K J 2000a 'Getting somewhere', feeling cared for: patients' perspectives on complementary therapies in the NHS. Complementary Therapies in Medicine 8 (4): 253-259

Luff D, Thomas K J 2000b Sustaining complementary therapy provision in primary care: lessons from existing services. Complementary Therapies in Medicine 8 (3): 173-179

Macpherson H, Thomas K, Walters S et al 2001 The York acupuncture safety study: a prospective survey of 34,000 treatments by traditional acupuncturists. British Medical Journal 323: 486-487

Manga P 2000 Economic case for the integration of chiropractic services into the health care system. Journal of Manipulative and Physiological Therapeutics 23 (2): 118-122

McFarlin B L, Gibson M H, O'Rear J et al 1999 A national survey of herbal preparation use by nurse-midwives for labour stimulation. Review of the literature and recommendations for practice. Journal of Nurse Midwifery 44 (3): 205-216

Mehl L E 1994 Hypnosis and correction of the breech to the vertex presentation. Archives of Family Medicine 3 (10): 881-887

Merrell W C, Shalts E 2002 Homeopathy. Medical Clinics of North America 86 (1): 47-62

Messerli-Rohrbach V, Schr A 1999 Complementary and conventional medicine: prejudices against and demands placed on natural care and conventional doctors. Schweizerische Medizinische Wochenschrift 129 (42): 1535-1544

Miller L G 1998 Herbal medicinals: selected clinical considerations focusing on known or potential drug-herb interactions. Archives of Internal Medicine 158 (20): 2200-2211

Mitzdorf U, Beck K, Horton-Hausknecht J et al 1999 Why do patients seek treatment in hospitals of complementary medicine? Journal of Alternative and Complementary Medicine 5 (5): 463-473

Montbriand M J 2000 Alternative therapies. Health professionals' attitudes. Canadian Nurse 96 (3): 22-26

Motha G, McGrath J 1993 The effects of reflexology on labour outcome. Reflexions: Journal of the Association of Reflexologists 1: 2-4

Mumm A H, Morens D M, Elm J L et al 1993 Zoster after shiatsu massage. Lancet 341 (8842): 447

NHS Confederation 1997 Complementary medicine in the NHS: managing the issues. NHS Confederation, Birmingham

O'Hara C 2002 Challenging the 'rules'. In: Mackereth P, Tiran D (eds) Clinical reflexology: a guide for health professionals. Elsevier, London

Opaneye A A 1998 Traditional medicine in Nigeria and modern obstetric practice: need for cooperation. Central African Journal of Medicine 44 (10): 258-261

Ostraff M, Anitoni K, Nicholson A et al 2000 Traditional Tongan cures for morning sickness and their mutagenic/toxicological evaluations. Journal of Ethnopharmacology 71 (1-2): 201-209

Parsons M, Simpson M, Ponton T 1999 Raspberry leaf and its effect on labour: safety and efficacy. Journal of the Australian College of Midwives 12 (3): 20-25

Passalacqua R, Campoine F, Caminiti C et al 1999 Patients' opinions, feelings and attitudes after a campaign to promote the Di Bella therapy. Lancet 353 (9161): 1310-1314

Pelletier K R, Astin J A 2002 Integration ad reimbursement of complementary and alternative medicine by managed care and insurance providers: 2000 update and cohort analysis. Alternative Therapies in Health and Medicine 8 (1): 38-9; 42; 44

Perry R, Dowrick C F 2000 Complementary medicine and general practice: an urban perspective. Complementary Therapies in Medicine 8 (2): 71-75

Petrie K A, Peck M R 2000 Alternative medicine in maternity care. Primary Care 27 (1): 117-136

Pinn G 2001 Herbs used in obstetrics and gynaecology. Australian Family Physician 30 (4): 351-354

Pinn G, Pallett L 2002 Herbal medicine in pregnancy. Complementary Therapies in Nursing and Midwifery 8 (2): 77-80

Pirotta M V, Cohen M M, Kotsirilos V et al 2000 Complementary therapies: have they become accepted in general practice? Medical Journal of Australia 7, 172 (3): 105-109

Rabl M, Abner R, Bitschnau M et al 2001 Acupuncture for cervical ripening and induction of labour at term – a randomized controlled trial. Wiener Kliniks Wochenschrift 113 (23-24): 942-946

Ranzini A, Allen A, Lai Y 2001 Use of complementary medicines and therapies among obstetric patients. Obstetrics and Gynecology 97(Suppl 4): S46

Ratz A E, von Moos M, Drewe J 2001 St John's wort: a pharmaceutical with potentially dangerous interactions. Schweiz Rundschau-fur-Medizin undPraxis 90 (19): 843-849

Rayburn W F, Christensen H D, Gonzalez C L 2000 Effect of antenatal exposure to Saint John's wort (Hypericum) on neurobehaviour of developing mice. American Journal of Obstetrics and Gynecology 183 (5): 1225-1231

Rayburn W F, Gonzalez C L, Christensen H D et al 2001 Effect of prenatally administered hypericum (St John's wort) on growth and physical maturation of mouse offspring. American Journal of Obstetrics and Gynecology 184 (2): 191-195

Reilly D 2001 Comments on complementary and alternative medicine in Europe. Journal of Alternative and Complementary Medicine 7: Suppl 1: S23-31

Rooney B, Fiocco G, Hughes P et al 2001 Provider attitudes and use of alternative medicine in a midwestern medical practice in 2001. Wisconsin Medical Journal 100 (7): 27-31

Senstad O, Leboeuf-Yde C, Borschgrevink C 1997 Frequency and characteristics of side-effects of spinal manipulative therapy. Spine 22: 435-441

Shipman M K, Boniface D R, Tefft M E et al 1997 Antenatal perineal massage and subsequent perineal outcomes: a randomised controlled trial. British Journal of Obstetrics and Gynaecology 104 (7): 787-791

Shumay D M, Maskarinec G, Kakai H et al/Cancer Research Center of Hawaii 2001 Why some cancer patients choose complementary and alternative medicine instead of conventional treatment. Journal of Family Practice 50 (12): 1067

Shvartzman P, Abelson A 1988 Complications of chiropractic treatment for low back pain. Postgraduate Medicine 83 (7): 57-58

Simpson M, Parsons M, Greenwood J et al 2001 Raspberry leaf in pregnancy: its safety and efficacy in labor. Journal of Midwifery and Women's Health 46 (2): 51-59

Simpson N, Roman K 2001 Complementary medicine use in children: extent and reasons. A population based study. British Journal of General Practice 51 (472): 914-916

Smith C A 2001 Homeopathy for induction of labour (Cochrane Review) Cochrane Database Systematic Review 4: CD 003399

Spencer J W, Jacobs J J 1999 Complementary/alternative medicine: an evidence-based approach. Mosby, St Louis

Stapleton H, Tiran D 2000 Herbal medicine. In: Tiran D, Mack S (eds) Complementary therapies for pregnancy and childbirth, 2nd edn. Bailliere Tindall, London

Swisher E M, Cohn D E, Goff B A et al 2002 The use of complementary and alternative medicine among women with gynecologic cancers. Gynecologic Oncology 84 (3): 363-367

Tang K C, Easthope G 2000 What constitutes treatment effectiveness? The differential judgements of Chinese Australian patients and doctors. Complementary Therapies in Medicine 8 (4): 241-247

Tellefsen T 2000 The chiropractic approach to healthcare during pregnancy. In: Tiran D, Mack S (eds) Complementary therapies in pregnancy and childbirth, 2md edn. Bailliere Tindall, London

Tiran D 2001 Complementary strategies in antenatal care. Complementary Therapies in Nursing and Midwifery 7 (1): 19-24

Tiran D 2000 Clinical aromatherapy for pregnancy and childbirth. Churchill Livingstone, Edinburgh

Tiran D 1996 Complementary therapies in maternity care: a focus on reflexology. Complementary Therapies in Nursing and Midwifery 2 (1): 32-37

Tiran D 2002 Supporting women during pregnancy and childbirth. In: Mackereth P, Tiran D (eds) Clinical reflexology: a guide for health professionals. Elsevier Science, Edinburgh

Tiran D 2002 Theories on reflexology. In: Mackereth P, Tiran D (eds) Clinical reflexology: a guide for health professionals. Elsevier Science, Edinburgh

Thomas K J, Nicholl J P, Coleman P 2001 Use and expenditure on complementary medicine in England: a population based survey. Complementary Therapies in Medicine 9 (1): 2-11

Thomas K J, Nicholl J P, Fall M 2001 Access to complementary medicine via general practice. British Journal of General Practice 51 (462): 25-30

Wagner P J, Jester D, LeClair B 1999 Taking the edge off: why patients choose St John's wort. Journal of Family Practice 48 (8): 615-619

Wanchu M, Malhotra S, Khullar M 2001 Calcium supplementation in pre-eclampsia. Journal of the

Association of Physicians of India 49: 795-798

Wang Z, Song H 1999 Clinical observation on therapeutical effect of prepared rhubarb in treating pregnancy induced hypertension Zhingguo Zhong Xi Yi Jie He Za Zhi 19 (12): 725-727

Wearn A M, Greenfield S M 1998 Access to complementary medicine in general practice: survey in one UK health authority. Journal of the Royal Society of Medicine 91 (9): 465-470

Weiss S J, Takakuwa K M, Ernst A A 2001 Use, understanding and beliefs about complementary and alternative medicine among emergency department patients. Academic Emergency Medicine 8 (1): 41-47

West Z 1997 Acupuncture within the National Health Service: a personal perspective. Complementary Therapies in Nursing and Midwifery 3 (3): 83-86

Westfall R E 2001 Herbal medicine in pregnancy and childbirth. Advanced Therapy 18 (1): 47-55

White A, Hayhoe S, Hart A et al 2001 Adverse events following acupuncture: prospective survey of 32,000 consultations with doctors and physiotherapists. British Medical Journal 323: 485-486

Wilson T 2002 Safety of acupuncture. British Medical Journal 324 (7330): 170A

Yamashita H, Tsukayama H, Tanno Y et al 1999 Adverse events in acupuncture and moxibustion treatment: a six year survey at a national clinic in Japan. Journal of Alternative and Complementary Medicine 5: 229-236

Zinaei S, Hantoshzadeh S, Rezasoltani P et al 2001 The effect of garlic tablet on plasma lipids and platelet aggregation in nulliparous pregnants at high risk of preeclampsia. European Journal of Gynecology Reproduction and Biology 99 (2): 201-206

FURTHER READING

Ernst E, Pittler M, Stevinson C et al 2001 The desktop guide to complementary and alternative medicine: an evidence-based approach. Mosby, Edinburgh

Tiran D 2001 Natural remedies for morning sickness and other pregnancy problems. Quadrille, London [for consumers]

Tiran D, Mack S (eds) 2000 Complementary therapies for pregnancy and childbirth, 2nd edn. Bailliere Tindall, London

3

The nutritional approach

Complementary nutritional advice is based on an understanding that good nutrition is not only about the quality and quantity of food eaten, but also the ability of the body to absorb adequate amounts of nutrients and the factors which adversely affect absorption and utilisation of those nutrients. This chapter explores the effects of nutrition on nausea and vomiting in pregnancy, particularly the roles of vitamin B6, zinc, magnesium and copper.

INTRODUCTION

Good nutrition in pregnancy has long been acknowledged as being of importance for the development of the fetus and maintenance of the mother's health. Many authorities advocate comprehensive nutritional assessment preconceptionally and at booking in order to identify potential problems resulting from malnutrition (Pearson et al 1996; Sujitor 1994), as well as nutritional counselling between pregnancies to prevent recurrences of previous problems predisposed by poor nutrition (Fernandes 1998). Nutritional status, generally, is influenced by the quality and quantity of the food eaten, as well as the body's ability to absorb, digest and utilise nutrients, and the biochemical profile of each individual.

Food quality can be affected by nutrient deficient soil, variations in which may be due to local agricultural policy regarding crop rotation and the use of pesticides and herbicides. Manufacture and storage of food, the addition of preservatives and colourings and domestic food preparation can also impair or improve its quality. In today's fast-paced life, changes in shopping practices, storage and types of food eaten, as well as the predominance of the ingestion of highly processed and 'fast' foods, containing little of the essential nutrients, all contribute to an element of malnourishment amongst many members of the general public. Increased intake of stimulants such as tea, coffee, alcohol and cola drinks may lead to reduced absorption of essential nutrients, and increased sensitivity to certain foods, e.g. wheat or dairy products, can also result in compromised health, although this may not always be apparent. Environmental toxins and pollutants, prescribed or illicit drug use, plus individual biochemical factors may additionally cause nutritional deficiency conditions, despite adequate food intake, possibly as a result of excessive excretion or impaired utilisation.

Each individual has unique nutritional requirements but this may alter at times of growth, such as puberty and pregnancy, and is affected by age, gender, genetics and health and illness, including psychological and emotional stress. The medical profession is well informed about the severe acute and chronic conditions which arise from serious nutritional deficiencies, but may be less aware of the range of health issues caused by mild to moderate dietary problems. An example of this is the recognition of diseases such as Crohn's disease or scurvy, but scepticism about less specific conditions e.g. chronic systemic candidiasis, rather than just oral or vaginal thrush.

Attention to *nutrition*, rather than merely to *refuelling*, requires time, effort and motivation which many people do not have, although pregnancy is often a period in which women will consider more carefully the nutritional value of the family's meals. Optimum nutritional status is achieved by consuming a balance of foods from all groups, but a reduction for most people of animal fat, salt, sugar, stimulants, processed foods and those with additives, and an increase in fibre, fresh vegetables and water would be wise.

General nutrition prior to and during pregnancy, labour and breastfeeding has always been the subject of much discussion, since the health, birth weight and subsequent growth of the baby as well as the mother's future risks of obesity and associated diseases, are dependent on the quality and quantity of food eaten and the timing and amount of weight gain at these times (Stephenson & Symonds 2002; Reifsnider & Gill 2000; Harding 1999). Poor fetal nutrition may lead to long-term conditions such as lowered bone mass density in childhood (Jones et al 2000), cardiovascular disease in adulthood (Barker 1999), and may possibly affect even the next generation (Harding 1997). Nutritional inadequacies may be implicated in infertility, recurrent miscarriage and birth defects, although Stoll et al (1999) found no definitive differences in vitamin and mineral profiles between women who had delivered an abnormal infant and those who had not. Various other factors are known to influence nutritional status and pregnancy outcome, including smoking (Mathews et al 1999), caffeine (Eskenazi et al 1999), alcohol (Kesmodel et al 2002), age (Mathews et al 2000) and vitamin and mineral supplementation (Dolk et al 1999; Kulier et al 1998). Advice to women in the UK intending to conceive now routinely includes a recommendation to take folic acid (Fernandez-Ballart & Murphy 2001; Shaw et al 1999) since the original work by Smithells et al (1980) on the aetiological role of folic acid in neural tube defects, although there is some suggestion that folic acid suppresses zinc uptake (see below). Various individual vitamin and mineral deficiencies have been implicated in pregnancy-specific complications, particularly in the prevention of pre-eclampsia with calcium (Levine et al 1997) or magnesium (Hussain & Sibley 1993; Spatling et al 1989). A link between low consumption of seafood in early pregnancy (with consequent low intake of n-3 fatty acids) and increased incidence of preterm labour has been found by researchers in Scandinavia (Olsen & Secher 2002; Grandjean et al 2001), although high mercury levels found in certain fish, such as shark, marlin and swordfish, and the possible link with neurological impairment in offspring, have led the Food Standards Agency to discourage intake of these foods in pregnancy (FSA 2002; Olsen 2001). Other research has focused on the impact of what is considered to be acceptable carbohydrate, fat and protein intake in pregnancy (Cattalano et al 1999; Kramer et al 1996), the benefits of essential fatty acids (Brooks et al 2000; Satter et al 1998) and whether or not supplementation is advisable (Winkvist et al 1998; Urgell et al 1998). Selective supplementation of at risk women may reduce the incidence of congenital abnormality such as omphalocele (Botto et al 2002), although Cikot et al (2001) emphasise the importance of knowing preconceptional and postpartum concentrations of vitamins when evaluating pregnancy-induced alterations. Otto et al (2001) found that maternal plasma and erythrocyte phospholipid concentrations increased during the first trimester, which seems unlikely to be related to dietary changes alone, and is probably due to adaptations to deal with the proliferating and differentiating tissues at this stage of embryonic development. Routine supplementations for all women are unnecessary and, indeed, could lead to complications from ingesting higher than recommended levels of vitamins or minerals (Voyles et al 2000). Inter-pregnancy nutritional counselling has also been advocated, but may not always be effective in reducing dietary-related problems in future pregnancies (Doyle et al 1999).

Although Mathews and Hall (1998) suggested, in one survey, that the nutritional intake of pregnant women was very similar to non-pregnant women, this does not appear to be the case, especially amongst younger expectant mothers, usually as a result of increased appetite, an altered sense of taste, food cravings and, most significantly, concern for the baby (Pope et al 1997). However, there seems to be some correlation between decreased frequency of eating during the third trimester and risks of preterm delivery (Osendarp et al 2001). Financial, social, emotional and behavioural factors may all impact on antenatal eating habits (Reid & Adamson 1997). Cultural factors are important and differences in levels of consumption of specific food types must be considered (Siega-Riz et al 2002) as pregnancy-specific problems

may be seen in women with different dietary habits (Bronner 2000). For example, Alfaham et al (1995) expressed concern about the incidence of vitamin D deficiency amongst pregnant Asian women, while a Canadian study found that immigrants generally consumed less fat, more carbohydrate and less alcohol than the indigenous population (Pomerleau et al 1998). Rabinerson et al (2000) suggested that the incidence of hyperemesis gravidarum may increase amongst Muslim women at times of fasting, such as during Ramadan. Fasting and dieting may adversely affect the amniotic fluid volume (Wolman et al 2000), which also needs to be taken into consideration during religious festivals. In addition to the nutritional value of foods eaten during pregnancy, there is some evidence to suggest that childhood preferences for different foods commence with intrauterine exposure (Menella et al 2001), which may explain cultural variations in food preferences.

Preconceptional weight of the mother and excessive or inadequate weight gain during pregnancy may adversely affect pregnancy outcome. In one survey of American obstetricians (Abraham 2001), none calculated the body mass index (BMI) of women at booking, very few weighed women routinely and, when weighing was carried out, many doctors failed to relate these measurements to body weight records. Of the 67 obstetricians surveyed, less than half considered the possibility of anorexia or other eating disorders in the women in their care. In the UK, nutritional monitoring is largely the responsibility of the midwife, and a booking BMI may be determined, although the practice of routinely weighing women is no longer undertaken. There appears to be a link between lower weight gain in pregnancy and producing a baby with a neural tube defect (NTD) (Shaw et al 2001), although the authors of this study suggested that it is less likely that increased risks of NTD indicate a causal association between reduced weight gain during pregnancy and abnormal development, and that less gain in weight is more likely to be due to carrying an NTD-affected fetus.

Box 3.1 Functions of vitamin B6

Metabolism of protein and amino acids
Metabolism of serotonin, histamine, hydroxytryptamine
Metabolism of sugars and essential fatty acids

Formation of vitamin B3 (niacinamide) from tryptophan
Formation of antibodies
Metabolism of magnesium, absorption of zinc

Box 3.2 Dietary sources of vitamin B6

Avocado
Bananas
Fish
Egg yolk
Green leafy vegetables
Meat
Nuts

Potatoes
Poultry
Seeds
Sweet potatoes
Tomatoes
Wholegrain cereal

Box 3.3 Factors which contribute to vitamin B6 deficiency

Oestrogen-containing contraceptive pill (?)
Premenstrual syndrome
Depression, anxiety, insomnia
Diabetes mellitus
Allergy to monosodium glutamate and tartrazine

Carpal tunnel syndrome
Renal disease, renal calculi
High alcohol consumption
Excessive vomiting

NUTRIENTS IMPLICATED IN GESTATIONAL NAUSEA AND VOMITING

Vitamin B6

Vitamin B6 was first discovered in the 1930s and comes in three closely related forms as pyridoxine, pyridoxal and pyridoxamine, all of which, in the presence of vitamin B2 and magnesium, are converted to the active compound pyridoxal 5 phosphate. The majority of supplement tablets are in the form of pyridoxine hydrochloride.

Vitamin B6 is primarily required for protein metabolism and its constituent amino acids, with greater consumption of protein requiring increased amounts of the vitamin. Metabolism of certain body chemicals, such as histamine, hydroxytryptamine and serotonin is also dependent on B6. As serotonin is required for normal brain function, a deficiency can potentially have adverse effects on mood and behaviour. During pregnancy, pyridoxine contributes to the embryonic development of the central nervous system and may influence brain development and cognitive function. It is also needed for sugar and essential fatty acid metabolism and the formation of vitamin B3 (niacinamide) from the amino acid, tryptophan. Mineral metabolism, particularly magnesium, relies on B6 and the absorption of zinc may be impaired if B6 levels are inadequate. The conversion of B6 to its active form in the body may be enhanced by exercise, whilst demand for the vitamin will be increased in people who smoke, use food additives or take drugs, whether medicinal or recreational. Adult men and women normally require a daily amount of 2mg of vitamin B6; during pregnancy this increases to 2.5mg daily, although supplements may be useful to correct some of the biochemical abnormalities which may occur at this time (Davies & Stewart 1987).

Symptoms of vitamin B6 deficiency include

irritability, nervousness, weakness and insomnia. Physical signs include skin manifestations such as red, greasy, scaling or flaking skin, acne, especially on the forehead and seborrhoeic dermatitis around the nose. In more severe cases, the tongue may be sore, taste buds prominent, there is weight loss, reduced appetite, anaemia, lowered immunity and neurological disorder.

Use of the contraceptive pill has been thought to alter the body's ability to absorb pyridoxine (vitamin B6) from food. Davies and Stewart (1987:319) suggest that studies in the 1980s on the effects of oestrogen on tryptophan and B6 revealed conditions such as depression and other psychiatric problems, impaired glucose tolerance, peri-oral dermatosis and urinary tract carcinoma, but more recent searches of the literature failed to support this. Masse et al (1996) found that short-term use of the oral contraceptive did not appear statistically to cause pyridoxine deficiency, but a disturbance of vitamin B6 metabolism was detected. However, the authors acknowledged that their chosen evaluation of pyridoxal 5' phosphate (PLP) was insufficient and assessment of other aldehydic forms of vitamin B6 may be necessary.

No significant correlation has been shown in work by van der Vange et al (1989) who tested the effects of seven low-dose contraceptive preparations on vitamin B6 status in 55 women. PLP levels initially decreased in the first three months but a return to normal levels was found after six months. An additional measurement of erythrocyte glutamate oxaloacetate transaminase (EGOT) activity was included and its degree of in vitro stimulation. After six months, EGOT activity was increased but no changes were detected in the more reliable parameter of in vitro stimulation, and the team concluded that the low dose preparations investigated in the study did not have any adverse effect on the pyridoxine status. Similarly, Villegas-Salas et al (1997) conducted a randomised triple-blind controlled trial of 124 women to test the effects of a daily dose of 150mg of vitamin B6 to overcome nausea, headache, dizziness, irritability and depression associated with the commencement of a low dose oral contraceptive. Although the

---

Practice point
The maximum advised dose of vitamin B6 is 50mg per day; vitamin B6 should always be taken with vitamin B complex to aid absorption.

---

test group experienced a reduction in headaches and dizziness, decrease in symptoms was comparable between both groups and the researchers concluded that the effects were explained more as a result of a placebo effect than a pharmacological action.

Zinc

Zinc plays a vital role in a wide range of metabolic processes. It is needed for the metabolism of proteins, carbohydrates, and phosphorus and facilitates the release of stored vitamin A. It is essential for the normal growth of the skin, hair and skeleton, a healthy immune system and the repair of body tissues. In both extrauterine and intrauterine life it is required for cell development in the brain, liver, kidneys, lungs and prostate and thryroid glands.

Inadequate serum zinc levels can predispose to poor physical growth and retarded mental development, fatigue and impaired mental alertness. Wounds may be slow to heal, susceptibility to infection is increased, skin lesions arise and hair loss is apparent. Signs and symptoms of early zinc deficiency include white spots on the fingernails and a metallic taste in the mouth. Night blindness and an impaired sense of smell may occur. There may be delayed sexual maturity, reduced libido or infertility, particularly in men, in whom normal semen contains large quantities of zinc. As with other mineral elements, such as calcium and iron, hair analysis reveals both deficiencies and the effects of supplementation (Leung et al 1999).

Zinc requirements rise by approximately 30% during pregnancy, to provide for the development of the fetal central nervous system, and by 40% in lactating women. Absorption is enhanced by adequate intakes of calcium, copper, vitamins A, B6, B12 and C and certain

---

Box 3.4 Functions of zinc

Metabolism of vitamin A, essential fatty acids and conversion to prostaglandins	Muscle function
	Mental development and health
Cell formation	Vision, taste, olfaction
Healthy formation of spermatazoa	Wound healing
Prevention of miscarriage	Hair growth
Healthy functioning of immune system	

Box 3.5 Dietary sources of zinc

Almonds	Oats
Beans	Oysters
Brazil nuts	Parsley
Buckwheat	Pecans
Carrots	Pork chops
Chicken	Potatoes
Clams	Rye
Corn	Shrimps
Egg yolk	Steak
Garlic	Turnips
Ginger	Walnuts
Green peas	Wheatgerm
Hazelnuts	Wholewheat bread
Lima beans	Yeast
Milk (raw)	

Box 3.6 Factors which contribute to zinc deficiency

Inadequate intake of zinc in the diet
Strict vegetarians
Restricted protein diets
Inborn errors of metabolism requiring special diets e.g. phenylketonuria
Anorexia nervosa

Inadequate absorption of zinc from the diet
High fibre diets, including a lot of bran
Iron supplementation
Deficiency of hypochloric acid

Foods which adversely affect zinc absorption
Coffee, tea, alcohol

Cow's milk, cheese
Soya based milk and soya meat substitutes
Hamburgers
Wholewheat and brown bread, bran
Celery, lemon

Zinc loss from the body despite adequate intake
High levels of stress
Contraceptive pill, laxatives, diuretics, steroids, penicillamine
Diabetics
Women with chronic blood loss
Alcoholics
Women with liver disease or inflammatory bowel disease

---

amino acids. Zinc retention, in order to meet fetal demands, appears to be increased by adjustments in zinc absorption. Absorption and utilisation is impaired by tea, coffee, alcohol, processed grains, iron tablets, the contraceptive pill, and by excess levels of phytates, found in bran and some cereals, and calcium, as well as by gastrointestinal pathology (King 2000). Jew-

ish women may be deficient in zinc, due to the presence of phytates in unleavened bread. Zinc neutralises the toxic effects of cadmium, a contributory factor in hypertension, but, conversely, high levels of cadmium, found in large amounts in cigarettes, some processed and canned foods, some instant coffees and gelatine, will inhibit the action of zinc. Excessive sweating can cause a loss of up to 3mg of zinc per day and zinc is lost in the urine at times of stress and during increased diuresis such as following high alcohol consumption.

During pregnancy, low zinc intake or absorption may lead to poor outcome, including intrauterine growth retardation and preterm labour (Scholl et al 1993). Goldenberg et al (1995) conducted an investigation of 580 women in Birmingham, Alabama. Women with below-normal plasma zinc levels at a median 19 weeks' gestation were randomised to receive either 25mg of zinc daily or a placebo. Those who received supplementation delivered infants of higher birth weights and with greater head circumferences than those who were given the placebo. This was particularly marked in women with a body mass index of less than 26. Garg et al (1993) also demonstrated increased birth weight and gestational age with prenatal zinc supplementation, which was related to the duration of zinc therapy. Further work by Garg et al (1994) appeared to show that antenatal administration of zinc improved haemoglobin levels without depressing serum copper concentrations.

However, more recent work by some members of the same team (Tamura et al 2000) found that plasma zinc levels were not a predictor of pregnancy outcome in 3448 women of a low socioeconomic background. Similar investigations in Peru by Caulfield et al (1999) supported this conclusion. Danish researchers also found no particular benefits of additional zinc administration (Jonsson et al 1996). Tamura et al (2000) showed that zinc concentrations decline as gestation progresses, and indeed, earlier work by Fehily et al (1986) found an association between *higher* plasma zinc and copper concentrations and lower birth weight babies. In the light of concerns about dosage and the possibility of micronutrient interactions, Shah and Sachdev (2001) consider that zinc supplementation should not be advocated as a routine until more data are available regarding its safety. However this is disputed by Osendarp et al (2001) who found a reduction in the health risks of infants up to six months of age who had been of low birth weight and whose mothers had received

---

Practice point
Zinc absorption and bioavailability is finely balanced with iron, therefore excessive iron supplementation may result in zinc deficiency.

zinc supplements antenatally. Interestingly, this was not seen in infants who were of normal weight at birth, even when their mothers had taken zinc supplements. A follow-up study by the same team (Hamadani et al 2002) found no significant effect of zinc supplementation on growth or behaviour of infants, but a surprising deficit in mental development compared to those in the control groups. A review of trials in the Cochrane Database by Mahomed (2000) found insufficient evidence to support the routine use of zinc supplements during pregnancy but suggested that its effects on preterm labour should be further evaluated. Postnatally, the role of zinc in lactating women has also not been determined (Moser-Veillon & Reynolds 1990).

Magnesium

Intracellular magnesium is second in amount only to potassium and its distribution across cell membranes is related to the metabolism of calcium and phosphorus. Adults have, on average, 20-30g of magnesium, most of which is within teeth and bones, the remaining 30% being found within the cells. 400-800mg is considered a normal daily requirement but this may increase in certain circumstances, such as high intake of protein, calcium, phosphorus or vitamin D. Magnesium is essential for a number of metabolic processes, particularly the mechanisms responsible for the distribution of sodium, potassium and calcium across cell membranes. Metabolism of vitamins B1 and B6 are also dependent on magnesium. Deficiency may be exacerbated by a diet high in refined and processed foods, or if bran is added to the diet, as this binds with the limited amounts of magnesium and affects absorption. Early signs of deficiency include appetite loss, apathy and weakness, constipation, insomnia and premenstrual symptoms. This is followed by

---

Box 3.7 Functions of magnesium

Blood sugar maintenance
Cardiological functioning
Enhances calcium absorption from food
Enzyme action
Maintenance of neurological functioning

Regulation of calcium storage in skeleton
Sodium, potassium and calcium distribution across cell membranes
Vitamin B1, B6 and phosphorus metabolism and utilisation

Box 3.8 Dietary sources of magnesium

Green leafy vegetables (contained in the chlorophyll)
Nuts
Shrimps

Soya beans
Tap water in hard water areas
Whole grains – bread, cereals etc.

Box 3.9 Factors which contribute to magnesium deficiency

Alcohol intake
Cardiac disease
Diabetes mellitus, hypoglycaemia

Diuretics
Renal calculi

---

nausea and vomiting, hypoglycaemia, numbness and tingling in the extremities, memory impairment, difficulty in swallowing and the eyes are seen to blink and the tongue flicks uncontrollably. Finally, in extreme cases, there is confusion and disorientation followed by muscle cramps and twitching leading to convulsions, epilepsy and tetany and abnormal cardiac rhythms and ECG. Hypertension and renal damage may also develop, and the use of magnesium sulphate for pre-eclampsia, which has long been standard practice in the USA, has more recently been adopted in UK obstetric practice (Magpie Trial Collaborative Group 2002; Sheth & Chalmers 2002).

However the case for antenatal magnesium supplementation is unproven, either to prevent possible intrauterine growth retardation resulting from maternal deficiency or to avoid preterm labour (Hussain & Sibley 1993), although Spatling et al (1989) suggested that routine administration could overcome the 25% increase in renal excretion of magnesium, thus prolonging pregnancy and avoiding hospitalisation for preterm labour.

Practice point

If magnesium supplementation is required, a dose of 100-300mg is usually sufficient; excessive doses may cause diarrhoea.

Copper

The potential for people to be copper deficient has been known for almost 60 years, with inadequate levels leading to anaemia, skeletal defects, neurological degeneration, infertility and pregnancy loss, cardiovascular conditions including raised cholesterol levels and pigmentation and hair structural defects. Normal hormonal activity during pregnancy increases copper levels or the body's ability to absorb it from food, and can exacerbate any zinc deficiency, as can being on the contraceptive pill, which increases serum copper levels. However, although copper is essential for normal metabolism, it is relatively easy to absorb it to excess, which can lead to lowered levels of zinc, in which many people are already deficient (see above). The average adult absorbs about 0.6-

---

Box 3.10 Functions of copper

Blood cholesterol regulation
Brain metabolism and production of brain chemicals
Immunity against disease

Neurological functioning
Oxidation of vitamin C
Skin pigmentation, hair structure

Box 3.11 Dietary sources of copper

Dried beans, peas, lentils
Liver
Kidneys
Nuts
Oysters

N.B. The copper content of foods depends on the copper content of the soil in which vegetables are grown, including the grazing land for animals, as well as the copper content of the water in which foods are prepared.

Box 3.12 Factors which contribute to copper deficiency

Excessive zinc, vitamin C or calcium levels
Exposure to mercury, lead or sulphide
Ingestion of raw meat
Metal of domestic water pipes (usually copper but may

be lead in older houses); hot water contains higher copper levels due to increased solubility of copper at higher temperatures.

1.6mg from the daily food intake and has approximately 60-110mg of copper in the body, being fairly equally distributed in thirds between the brain, the liver and the rest of the body (Davies and Stewart 1987:74). Copper is excreted via the biliary tract although excess intake will result in increased storage.

Antioxidants

Antioxidants, including beta-carotene, vitamins A, C and E, selenium-containing amino acids such as cystine and a range of enzymes – gluathione reductase, peroxidase and superoxide dismutase – provide a means of protecting cells in the body against the effects of oxidation, in which free radicals are produced and which are thought to be responsible for a variety of auto-immune, inflammatory and degenerative ill-nesses. A link between reduced plasma glutathione levels and hyperemesis gravidarum, compared to pregnant, non-emetic and non-pregnant controls, has been suggested by Fait et al (2002), implying that oxidative stress is associated with the condition. The plasma glu-

Practice point

Copper and zinc work on a finely attuned balancing mechanism; an excess of one will lead to a deficiency of the other.

tathione levels appear to be significantly lower during the period of hyperemesis, returning to normal levels on cessation of vomiting. Glutathione requires selenium for effective use, while other antioxidants require other nutrients – superoxide dismutase needs copper, manganese and zinc. Deficiencies of selenium, copper, manganese and zinc can result in increased susceptibility to free radical damage of the fat component of cell membranes, while excess copper can also cause free-radical peroxidation (Chan et al 1998). Oxidative stress can be exacerbated by environmental toxins, including cigarette smoke, pollutants and chemical processes which produce oxidants such as nitrogen dioxide, nitrates and hydrocarbon-derived free radicals (Davies & Stewart 1987:151-2). It has also been shown to be affected in generally healthy human beings who undertake high levels of physical exercise, particularly in cold climates at moderate altitude (Schmidt et al 2002).

Women can be encouraged to eat foods containing beta-carotene (a vitamin-A type compound), selenium, zinc, manganese and other nutrients: this should avoid the tendency to overdose with over-the-counter supplements, which are not necessary in the majority of women who are eating a well-balanced diet. Sources of vitamin A/beta-carotene include animal and fish livers, kidneys, eggs, milk, butter and margarine. Most green, yellow or orange-coloured fruits and vegetables also contain beta-carotene, with greater amounts being found in those of darker pigmentation. However, while deficiency of vitamin A may be associated with poor fetal growth and defects such as transposition of the cardiac vessels (Rondo et al 2001; Botto et al 2001) and with maternal morbidity and mortality in developing countries (van den Broek et al 2002; Schmidt et al 2001), excessive amounts can be detrimental to the mother and routine self-administration is discouraged (Azais-Braesco & Pascal 2000; Voyles et al 2000). Conversely, vitamin A, given to Nepalese women, together with beta-carotene, in an attempt to reduce maternal mortality, was also found to reduce third trimester nausea, although beta-carotene did not (Christian et al 2000). The amino acid cystine is found in animal protein sources, but women who are vegetarian must ensure a balance of different amino acids by mixing their vegetable protein sources, for example five parts rice to one part beans. Dietary selenium is found in grains, fish and most wholefoods, and as a therapeutic agent, may be helpful in the treatment of mercury toxicity (Davies & Stewart 1987:86). By inference, therefore, a woman who has unwittingly consumed seafood thought to contain higher than normal levels of mercury could take a prophylactic course of selenium, in the form of selenomethionine in brewer's yeast.

THE EUROPEAN SITUATION

At the time of writing, regulation regarding vitamin and mineral supplements is being debated, since the Food Supplements Directive was passed through the European Parliament and became law in July 2002. This arose from claims that the EU member states were restricting or prohibiting the marketing of nutritional supplements on the grounds of public safety. Concern has been expressed by some complementary medical organisations and commercial supplement producers about the potential restrictions on the use and availability to the general public of nutritional supplements within Britain, although most of those commonly self-administered have already been approved for use within the EU. The EU's Scientific Committee on Food has compiled a list of permitted vitamin and mineral sources, but many practitioners believe it to be extremely limited. Additions to the list will only be approved subject to presentation by the manufacturing companies of a comprehensive dossier for individual ingredients and toxicological profiles, which has similarities with pharmaceutical preparation approval procedures. Further dispute over recommended daily allowances may continue over the three-year consultation period up to July 2005.

The most convenient way of ingesting vitamins and minerals would obviously be to consume foods containing the required elements, but women who are feeling nauseated and constantly vomiting may be unable to do so. The following discussion therefore debates the theoretical principles of appropriate supplements, but in the future, obstetricians and GPs may need to prescribe supplements as medicines rather than direct women to purchase their own supplies from health food stores.

NUTRITIONAL MANAGEMENT OF NAUSEA AND VOMITING IN PREGNANCY

The concept of nutrition as a therapeutic intervention is not generally considered by pregnant women, and although they spontaneously make adaptations in their diet in accordance with their symptoms, they may not readily take vitamins and minerals unless prescribed, and these

---

Case 3.1

A 24-year-old nulliparous woman attended the complementary therapy antenatal clinic for persistent nausea and vomiting at 22 weeks' gestation. She was also complaining of heartburn, constipation and backache, and pre-existing eczema had worsened. She had experienced a miscarriage earlier in the year but had been shocked to discover she was pregnant again, and had poor social circumstances. During the initial assessment, the midwife questioned the woman about her diet and discovered that she seemed to survive solely on a daily repetitive diet of chicken and pasta, with little fruit, except juice, and no vegetables. The mother steadfastly refused to acknowledge that her diet could be a contributing factor to most of her complaints, not only due to the lack of essential nutrients, but possibly also as a result of allergies. The midwife explained the need to work in partnership, but the woman was obviously unwilling to concede to making any dietary changes. As the philosophy of the CT clinic requires women to take some responsibility for their condition, the midwife merely provided suggestions for a few natural remedies which might alleviate her problems, but declined to see the mother again, referring her to her GP if symptoms persisted.

---

may be with the advised intention of preventing damage to fetal DNA (Park et al 1999) or aimed specifically at reducing the severity of complications such as pre-eclampsia (Wanchu et al 2001; Atallah et al 2000). However, amongst those who resort to complementary and alternative therapies, nutritional supplementation may be used for nausea and vomiting, often in conjunction with herbal remedies, by up to 60% (Hollyer et al 2002), although other surveys put this figure much lower (Ranzini et al 2001) and may be related to sociodemographic and health behaviour factors (Messerer et al 2001). Those already taking multivitamin supplements prior to conception may, in fact, experience less severe sickness (Niebyl & Goodwin 2002).

Much can be achieved to relieve nausea and vomiting through the judicious adaptation of the diet, although conventional dietary advice tends to focus on restoring and maintaining blood sugar levels, particularly on waking. Some women may conceive whilst being malnourished, and in others, constant vomiting will cause a depletion of essential vitamins and minerals, thus exacerbating any pre-existing nutritional deficiencies. Normal midwifery and obstetric care incorporates advice regarding optimum nutrition, although this depends on women working in partnership to follow this advice. Those who are already deficient in essential nutrients may include women who smoke or who abuse alcohol or drugs, and it may be more difficult to encourage them to desist in order to provide a more favourable intrauterine environment for the fetus. However, women suffering from persistent nausea and vomiting are *usually* motivated to comply with dietary advice in order to reduce the severity of their symptoms (see Case 3.1).

General dietary information related to nausea and vomiting is offered by midwives and obstetricians on the use of complex carbohydrates, rather than more rapidly utilised simple sugars, which may initiate a cycle of peaks and troughs of blood sugar. Many women are advised to eat a carbohydrate snack before rising and to eat little and often throughout the day (Dilorio et al 1994), but this is certainly not sufficient for all expectant mothers. Power et al's survey of American obstetricians (2001) found that over 95% advised women to take small, frequent meals and almost 90% suggested the consumption of soda crackers. Broussard and Richter (1998) advocated similar advice in conjunction with reassurance that the condition is transient, with a good prognosis, although this is not always so.

In general, being pregnant appears to legitimise increased food intake, without causing undue concern to women about weight gain, even in those who were weight conscious prior to conception (Clark & Ogden 1999). Total weight gain during pregnancy is normally between 11 and 15kg (Kolassa & Weismiller 1997) but may vary according to diet, activity and gestational factors such as physiological sickness or multiple pregnancy. Women with nausea and vomiting frequently experiment to find foods which suit them best and eliminate those which make the condition worse. However, this sometimes leads them to express concern and to experience immense feelings of guilt that they are failing their unborn babies because they are not eating 'nourishing' food. In most women, the condition will resolve spontaneously, often by the second trimester, and they should be 'given permission' to eat foods which will not be regurgitated, with the proviso, of course, that they are not known to be directly harmful to the fetus. It is highly probable that these women, once relieved of the constant nausea, will compensate in later pregnancy by eating greater quantities of better quality.

Cravings for particular foods may be the body's attempt to replace nutrients being lost from vomiting, and often include demands for sour foods, sharp fruit or sweet substances (Wijewardene et al 1994), although the theory that food *aversion* is a protective mechanism was not upheld by Brown et al (1997). An interesting revelation, more marked in Caucasian than Asian people, is the preference of salt and salty foods in the offspring of mothers who have experienced pregnancy sickness (Hudson & Distel 1999; Crystal & Bernstein 1995), suggesting that a gestational event may be a determinant of salt intake and preference in adulthood. Further work by Crystal and Bernstein (1998) led them to reaffirm the hypothesis that the dehydration from frequent vomiting in pregnancy results in an enhanced preference for salt in the babies of these women, although it is not thought that these are mediated by familial dietary practices (Crystal et al 1999). Although the majority of nauseated women will abhor the odour of cigarette smoke, the incidence of nausea may be less in those who smoke (Meyer et al 1994).

There is some suggestion that eating protein-rich foods can assist in reducing gastric slow wave tachygastria or bradygastria (Jednak et al 1999). Protein is metabolised to amino acids, transported to the liver and converted to a more usable form by amino acid transferases in a process requiring vitamin B6; consequently, a high protein intake will require an increase in vitamin B6 intake. Women with mild to moderate nausea and vomiting demonstrate an increased incidence of gastric dysrhythmias, found to be reduced more significantly after protein-rich meals than after meals predominating in carbohydrates or fats (Jednak et al 1999). Liquid meals appear to have a greater effect on the reduction in dysrhythmias than solid meals.

The value of vitamin B6 to reduce nausea and vomiting may lie in its role in glucose metabolism, with supplementation decreasing the hypoglycaemic effects on the body, generally held to be one of the main causes of 'morning sickness', although hypoglycaemia does not appear to be predictive of adverse perinatal outcome (Calfee et al 1999). However, supplements of vitamin B6 and folic acid do seem to have a favourable effect on fetal growth in women with a history of pre-eclampsia and/or fetal growth restriction (Leeda et al 1998). Daily doses of 2-3mg of vitamin B6 during pregnancy have also been shown by Chang (1999) and Chang and Kirksey (2002) to have a growth benefit on the neonate. Additionally, the glucocorticoid-antagonistic effect of pyridoxal phosphate may reduce the risk of hypertension, insulin resistance syndrome and coronary events associated with intrauterine growth retardation. This fact led McCarty (2000) to advocate the antenatal supplementation of high-dose pyridoxine in selected women, but Masin and Kahle (2002) advise caution in dosage, since excessive vitamin B6 intake may have adverse effects on maternal neurological functioning, while the effects on the fetus are unknown. A Cochrane review of trials of vitamin B6 supplementation during pregnancy (Mahomed & Gulmezoglu 2000) found one study suggesting that pyridoxine may also be associated with a reduced incidence of dental decay in expectant women, while Bryan et al (2002) highlighted a possible effect on memory performance in women, although this was not directly related to expectant mothers.

Schuster et al (1985) investigated the vitamin B6 status of 180 women with pregnancy sickness but found no significant difference in the plasma PLP levels, nor those of erythrocyte aspartate aminotransferase activity between women who experienced sickness and those who did not. Sahakian et al's (1991) randomised double-blind, placebo-controlled study of 59 women demonstrated minimal effect in women who took vitamin B6 for mild to moderate nausea and vomiting, but those with severe sickness responded significantly. A prospective study by Emelianova et al (1999) found a significant correlation between severity of vomiting and lack of vitamin B6 supplementation prior to the sixth week of pregnancy, although the authors suggest that further work is required to determine the biological basis of this.

Smith (1982) found a reduction of nausea and vomiting of all degrees following vitamin B6 supplementation, whilst Vutyavanich et al (1995) suggest that pyridoxine can be useful in relieving the severity of the nausea, but found no statistical significance in its effects on episodes of vomiting. Czeilel et al (1992) advocate periconceptional administration of multivitamins to prevent or reduce the severity of sickness. It is however interesting to note that an increased intake of niacin (vitamin B3) in early pregnancy may have a correlation with lower birthweights (Tierson et al 1986), although no more recent work on this has been found.

Trace elements have been found to be suboptimal in women with hypermesis gravidarum, particularly zinc and magnesium, and although it is unclear whether these deficiencies are a cause or an effect of severe vomiting, supplementation to hospitalised women may have a beneficial effect (Teksen et al 2001). This team compared plasma zinc, copper and magnesium levels between pregnant women with and without hyperemesis gravidarum and with nonpregnant women. Zinc concentrations were markedly lower in women with severe vomiting than in those without sickness, but not significantly different from non-pregnant women. Copper and magnesium levels in those with hyperemesis also appeared to be lower than in normal pregnant and in non-pregnant women.

Zinc supplements for women with low plasma zinc concentrations should be considered as this may be associated with low birthweight (Fehily et al 1986). Smithells et al (1980) identified an increased risk of neural tube defects in women who were zinc deficient, and there is more recent evidence to suggest that it may assist in improving infant neurobehavioural development and immune function (Shah & Sachdev 2001), although whether there is sufficient evidence for the routine use of zinc alone has been challenged by Hamadani et al (2002) and Osendarp et al (2001).

Goldenberg et al (1995) demonstrated that women with low zinc levels in *early* pregnancy may produce babies with reduced birthweights and head circumferences, particularly those with a Body Mass Index of less than 26. However, later work by members of the same team disputed this (Neggers et al 1997). Tamura et al (2000) indicates that zinc levels naturally decline as gestation progresses, and, from the late first trimester, do not appear to be a predictor of pregnancy outcome.

Dietary management of other symptoms associated with nausea and vomiting

Women with pregnancy sickness often report mouth problems such as excessive salivation, ulcers and cold sores and an unpleasant taste in the mouth, which result from continued nutritional deficiencies and impaired immunity. Heartburn, or reflux oesophagitis, although commonly cited as a third trimester disorder, frequently accompanies the nausea, and constipation and flatulence may develop due to poor food intake and dehydration. Straining to defaecate may trigger the prolapse of internal haemorrhoids. In combination, these complaints contribute to the woman's overall sense of distress and may significantly reduce her ability to cope with the nausea and vomiting. However, it may be difficult for women to respond to any suggestions for dietary change to resolve these problems, as the foods containing the relevant nutrients may not appeal to them.

The most fundamental advice to any woman with sickness, particularly when she is also suffering constipation, is to increase her fluid intake, preferably drinking at least two litres of water daily. The usual dietary advice for constipation includes increasing the fibre content, but it is not wise to advocate the use of bran unless the woman also doubles her fluid intake, as it absorbs fluid from the colon and hardens the stool (Stapleton & Tiran 2000:116). Similarly the overuse of laxatives is inadvisable, and some, such as senna, are rather too purgative during pregnancy. Women can be informed about high fibre foods, but this should be accompanied by advice to reduce or eliminate refined carbohydrates, sugars and added salt. Linseeds, one spoonful daily, or sprinkled on food, are a good source of fibre. Both tea and milk also contribute to constipation, as may a magnesium deficiency (Davies & Stewart 1987: 207; 225). Coffee and spicy, greasy or rich foods will exacerbate heartburn.

Flatulence may be reduced by eating food slowly, reducing the amount of wheat products in the diet and not drinking fluids at the same time. If the mother can eat them, garlic and onions have a beneficial effect on the veins and may assist in reducing haemorrhoids.

CONCLUSION

Dietary advice is a normal component of midwifery and obstetric care. Professionals generally feel comfortable informing women about nutritional requirements, and women seem to expect to discuss their diet, appetite, cravings and other issues related to food intake. It would therefore appear to be a logical step towards more successful treatment of women with gestational nausea and vomiting for staff to consider more comprehensively whether or not symptoms can be relieved by dietary changes or nutritional supplements, although administration of the latter should not be routine.

This chapter has explored some of the research on nutritional aetiology and management of pregnancy sickness, although the debate is somewhat inconclusive. Where there is little evidence regarding potential harmful effects of specific nutrients, judicious administration may be a useful adjunct to care, but women should be encouraged to view any supplementation as a form of medical treatment and not presume to self-administer vitamins and minerals routinely.

REFERENCES

Abraham S 2001 Obstetricians and maternal body weight and eating disorders during pregnancy. Journal of Psychosomatic Obstetrics and Gynecology 22 (3): 159-163

Alfaham M, Woodhead S, Pask G et al 1995 Vitamin D deficiency: a concern in pregnant Asian women. British Journal of Nutrition 73 (6): 881-887

Atallah A N, Hofmeyr G J, Duley L 2000 Calcium supplementation during pregnancy for preventing hypertensive disorders and related problems. Cochrane Database Systematic Review (2): CD 001059

Azais-Braesco V, Pascal G 2000 Vitamin A in pregnancy: requirements and safety limits. American Journal of Clinical Nutrition 71 (suppl 5): S1325-1333

Barker D J P 1999 Foetal and childhood growth and cardiovascular disease in adult life. Journal of Paediatrics, Obstetrics and Gynaecology 25 (6): 5-8

Bishai R, Mazzotta P, Atanackovic G et al 2000 Critical appraisal of drug therapy for nausea and vomiting of pregnancy. II: efficacy and safety of diclectin (doxylamine B6). Canadian Journal of Clinical Pharmacology 7 (3): 138-143

Botto L D, Loffredo Scanlon K S et al 2001 Vitamin A and cardiac outflow tract defects. Epidemiology 12 (5): 491-496

Botto L D, Mulinare J, Erickson J D 2002 Occurrence of omphalocele in relation to maternal multivitamin use: a population-based study. Pediatrics 109 (5): 904-908

Bronner Y 2000 Cross-cultural issues during pregnancy and lactation: implications for assessment and counselling. In: Story M, Stang J (eds) Nutrition and the pregnant adolescent. University of Minnesota Centre for Leadership Education and Training in Maternal and Child Nutrition, Minneapolis MN

Broussard C N, Richter J E 1998 Nausea and vomiting of pregnancy. Gastroenterology Clinics of North America 27 (1): 123-151

Brown J E, Kahn E S, Hartman T J 1997 Profet, profits and proof: do nausea and vomiting of early pregnancy protect women from 'harmful' vegetables? American Journal of Obstetrics and Gynaecology 176 (Pt 1): 179-181

Bryan J, Calvaresi E, Hughes D 2002 Short-term folate, vitamin B12 or vitamin B6 supplementation slightly affects memory performance but not mood in women of various ages. Journal of Nutrition 132 (6): 1345-1356

Calfee E F, Rust O A, Bofill J A et al 1999 Maternal hypoglycemia: is it associated with adverse perinatal outcome? Journal of Perinatology 19 (5): 379-382

Cattalano P M 1999 Pregnancy and lactation in relation to

range of acceptable carbohydrate and fat intake. European Journal of Clinical Nutrition 53 (suppl 1): S124-S135

Caulfield L E, Zavaleta N, Figueroa A et al 1999 Maternal zinc supplementation does not affect size at birth or pregnancy duration in Peru. Journal of Nutrition 129 (8): 1563-1568

Chan S, Gerson B, Subramaniam S 1998 The role of copper, molybedenum, selenium and zinc in nutrition and health. Clin Lab Med 18 (4): 673-685

Chang S J 1999 Adequacy of maternal pyridoxine supplementation during pregnancy in relation to the vitamin B6 status and growth of neonates at birth. Journal of Nutrition and Scientific Vitaminology (Tokyo) 45 (4): 449-458

Chang S J, Kirksey A 2002 Vitamin B6 status of breastfed infants in relation to pyridoxine HCl supplementation of mothers. Journal of Nutritional Science and Vitaminology (Tokyo) 48 (1): 10-17

Christian P, West K P Jr, Khatry S K et al 2000 Vitamin A or beta-carotene supplementation reduces symptoms of illness in pregnant and lactating Nepali women. Journal of Nutrition 130 (11): 2675-2682

Cikot R J L M, Steegers-Theunisson R P M Thomas C M G et al 2001 Longitudinal vitamin and homocysteine levels in normal pregnancy. British Journal of Nutrition 85 (1): 49-58

Clark M, Ogden J 1999 The impact pf pregnancy on eating behaviour and aspects of weight concern. International Journal of Obesity and Related Metabolic Disorders 23 (1): 18-24

Cohen M, Bendich A 1986 Safety of pyridoxine: a review of human and animal studies. Toxicology Letters 34: 129

Crystal S R, Bernstein I L 1995 Morning sickness: impact on offspring salt preference. Appetite 25 (3): 231-240

Crystal S R, Bernstein I L 1998 Infant salt preference and mother's morning sickness. Appetite 30 (3): 297-307

Crystal S R, Bowen D J, Bernstein I L 1999 Morning sickness and salt intake, food cravings and food aversions. Physiology and Behaviour 67 (2): 181-187

Czeilel A, Dudas I, Fritz G et al 1992 The effect of periconceptional multivitamin-mineral supplementation on vertigo, nausea and vomiting in the first trimester of pregnancy. Archives of Gynecology and Obstetrics 251 (4): 181-185

Davies S, Stewart A 1987 Nutritional medicine. Pan, London

Dilorio C, van Lier D, Manteuffel B 1994 Recommendations by clinicians for nausea and vomiting of pregnancy. Clinical Nurse Research 3 (3): 209-227

Dolk H M, Nau H, Hummler H et al 1999 Dietary vitamin A and teratogenic risk: European Teratology Society discussion paper. European Journal of Obstetrics and Gynecology and Reproductive Biology 83 (1): 31-36

Doyle W, Crawford M A, Srivastava A et al 1999 Interpregnancy nutrition intervention with mothers of low birthweight babies living in an inner city area: a feasibility study. Journal of Human Nutrition and Dietetics 12 (6): 517-528

Emelianova S, Mazzotta P, Einarson A et al 1999 Prevalence and severity of nausea and vomiting of pregnancy and effect of vitamin supplementation. Clinical Investigation in Medicine 22 (3): 106-110

Eskenazi B, Stapleton A L, Kharrazi M et al 1999 Associations between maternal decaffeinated and caffeinated coffee consumption and fetal growth and gestational duration. Epidemiology 10 (3): 242-249

Fait V, Sela S, Ophir E et al 2002 Hyeremesis gravidarum is associated with oxidative stress. American Journal of Perinatology 19 (2): 93-98

Fehily D, Fitzsimmons B, Jenkins D et al 1986 Association of fetal growth with maternal plasma zinc concentration in human pregnancy. Human Nutrition and Clinical Nutrition 40 (3): 221-227

Fernandez-Ballart J, Murphy M M 2001 Preventive nutritional supplementation throughout the reproductive life cycle. Public Health and Nutrition 4 (6A): 1363-1366

Food Standards Agency 2002 Agency issues precautionary advice on eating shark, swordfish and marlin [press release]. Food Standards Agency, London

Garg H K, Singhal K C, Arshad Z 1994 Effect of oral zinc supplementation on copper and haemoglobin levels in pregnant women. Indian Journal of Physiology and Pharmacology 38 (4): 272-276

Garg H K, Singhal K C, Arshad Z 1993 A study of the effect of oral sonc supplementation during pregnancy on pregnancy outcome. Indian Journal of Physiology and Pharmacology 37 (4): 276-284

Goldenberg R l, Tamura T, Neggers Y et al 1995 The effect of zinc supplementation on pregnancy outcome. Journal of the American Medical Association 274 (6): 463-468

Grandjean P, Bjerve K S, Weihe P et al 2001 Birthweight in a fishing community: significance of essential fatty acids and marine food contaminants. International Journal of Epidemiology 30 (6): 1272-1278

Hamadani J D, Fuchs G J, Osendarp S J et al 2002 Zinc supplementation during pregnancy and effects on mental development and behaviour of infants: a follow-up study. Lancet 360 (9329): 290-294

Harding J 1999 Nutritional causes of impaired fetal growth and their treatment. Journal of the Royal Society of Medicine 92 (12): 612-615

Harding J E 1997 Nutrition and fetal growth. Journal of the Society of Obstetricians and Gynaecologists of Canada 19 (13): 1393-1396

Hollyer T, Boon H, Georgousis A et al 2002 The use of CAM by women suffering from nausea and vomiting during pregnancy. Complementary and Alternative Medicine 2 (1): 5

Hudson R, Distel H 1999 The flavour of life: perinatal development of odor and taste preferences. Schweiz Med Wochenschr 129 (5): 176-181

Hussain S M, Sibley C P 1993 Magnesium and pregnancy. Mineral and Electrolyte Metabolism 19 (4-5): 296-307

Jednak M A, Shadigian E M, Kim M S et al 1999 Protein meals reduce nausea and gastric slow wave dysrhythmic activity in first trimester pregnancy. American Journal of Physiology 277 (4 Pt 1): G855-861

Jewell D, Young G 2000 Interventions for nausea and vomiting in early pregnancy. Cochrane Database Systematic Reviews 2000 (2): CD 000145

Jones G, Riley M D, Dwyer T 2000 Maternal diet during pregnancy is associated with bone mineral density in children: a longitudinal study. European Journal of Clinical Nutrition 54 (10): 749-756

Jonsson B, Hauge B, Larsen M F et al 1996 Zinc supplementation during pregnancy: a double-blind randomised controlled trial. Acta Obstetrica Gynecologica Scandinavia 75 (8): 725-729

Kesmodel U, Wisborg K, Olsen S F et al 2002 Moderate alcohol intake during pregnancy and the risk of stillbirth and neonatal death in the first year of life. American Journal of Epidemiology 155 (4): 305-312

King J C 2000 Determinants of maternal zinc status during pregnancy. American Journal of Clinical Nutrition 71 (suppl 5): S1334-1343

Kolassa K M, Weismiller D G 1997 Nutrition during pregnancy. American Family Physician 56 (1): 205-212

Kramer M S 1999 Nutritional advice in pregnancy (Date of most recent substantive amendment: 29 April 1996) Cochrane Library Oxford Software Update issue 1

Kulier R, de ONis M, Gulmezoglu A M et al 1998 Nutritional interventions for the prevention of maternal morbidity. International Journal of Gynecology and Obstetrics 63 (3): 231-246

Leeda M, Riyazi N, de Vries J I et al 1998 Effects of folic acid and vitamin B6 supplementation on women with hyperhomocysteinaemia and a history of preeclampsia or fetal growth restriction. American Journal of Obstetrics and Gynecology 179 (1): 135-139

Leung P L, Huang H M, Sun D Z et al 1999 Hair concentrations of calcium, iron, and zinc in pregnant women and effects of supplementation. Biol Trace Elem Res 69 (3): 269-282

Magpie Trial Collaborative Group 2002 Do women with pre-eclampsia, and their babies, benefit from magnesium sulphate? The Magpie Trial: a randomised placebo-controlled tria.l Lancet 359 (9321): 1877-1890

Mahomed K 2000 Zinc supplementation in pregnancy. Cochrane Database Systematic Review (2): CD 000230

Mahomed K, Gulmezoglu 2000 Pyridoxine (vitamin B6) supplementation in pregnancy Cochrane Database Systematic Review (2): CD 000179

Masin S A, Kahle J S 2002 Vitamin B6 therapy during childbearing years – cause for caution? Nutrition in Neuroscience 5 (4): 241-242

Masse P G, van der Berg H, Duguay C et al 1996 Early effect of a low dose (30 micrograms) ethinyl estradiol-containing Triphasil on vitamin B6 status. A follow up study on six menstrual cycles. International Journal of Vitamin and Nutritional Research 66 (1): 46-54

Mathews F, Yudkin P, Smith R F et al 2000 Nutritional intakes during pregnancy: the influence of smoking status and age. Journal of Epidemiology and Community Health 54 (1): 17-23

Mathews F, Yudkin P, Neil A 1999 Influence of maternal nutrition on outcome of pregnancy: prospective cohort study. British Medical Journal 319 (7206): 339-343

Mathews F, Neil H A W 1998 Nutrient intakes during pregnancy in a cohort of nulliparous women. Journal of Human Nutrition and Dietetics 11 (2): 151-161

Mazzotta P, Magee L A 2000 A risk-benefit assessment of pharmacological and non-pharmacological treatments for nausea and vomiting of pregnancy. Drugs 59 (4): 781-800

McCarty M F 2000 Prenatal high-dose pyridoxine may prevent hypertension and syndrome X in-utero by protecting the fetus from glucocorticoid activity. Medical Hypotheses 54 (5): 808-813

Menella J A, Jagnow C P, Beauchamp G K 2001 Prenatal and postnatal flavour learning by human infants. Pediatrics 107 (6): E88

Messerer M, Johanson S E, Wolk A 2001 Sociodemographic and health behaviour factors among dietary supplement and natural remedy users. European Journal of Clinical Nutrition 55 (12): 1104-1110

Meyer L C, Peacock J L, Bland J M et al 1994 Symptoms and health problems in pregnancy: their association with social factors, smoking, alcohol, caffeine and attitude to pregnancy. Paediatric and Perinatal Epidemiology 8 (2): 145-155

Moser-Veillon P B, Reynolds R D A longitudinal study of pyridoxine and zinc supplementation on lactating women .American Journal of Clinical Nutrition 52 (1): 135-141

Niebyl J R, Goodwin T M 2002 Overview of nausea and vomiting of pregnancy with an emphasis on vitamins and ginger. American Journal of Obstetrics and Gynecology 185 (5 Suppl Understanding): S253-255

Neggers Y H, Goldenberg R L, Tamura T et al 1997 The relationship between maternal dietary intake and infant birthweight. Acta Obstet Gynecol Scand Suppl 165: 71-75

Olsen S F 2001 Commentary: mercury, PCB and now eicosapentaenoic acid: still another reason why pregnant women should be concerned about eating seafood? International Journal of Epidemiology 30 (6): 1279-1280

Olsen S F, Secher N J 2002 Low consumption of seafood in early pregnancy as a risk factor for preterm delivery. British Medical Journal 324 (7335): 447-450

Osendarp S J, van Raaij J M, Darmstadt G L et al 2001 Zinc supplementation during pregnancy and effects on growth and morbidity in low birthweight infants: a randomised placebo-controlled trial. Lancet 357 (9262): 1080-1085

Otto S J, van Houwelingen A C, Badart-Smook A et al 2001 Changes in the maternal essential fatty acid profile during pregnancy and the relation of the profile to diet. American Journal of Clinical Nutrition 73 (2): 302-307

Park E, Wagenbichler P, Elmadfa I 1999 Effects of multivitamin/mineral supplementation , at nutritional doses, on plasma antioxidant status and DNA damage estimated by sister chromatid exchanges in lymphocytes in pregnant women. International Journal of Vitamin and Nutritional Research 69 (6): 396-402

Pearson S, Dimond H, Ford F et al 1996 A survey of pre-pregnancy nutritional knowledge in family planning clinics. British Journal of Family Planning 22 (2): 92-94

Pomerleau J, Ostbye T, Bright-See E 1998 Place of birth and dietary intake in Ontario: energy, fat, cholesterol, carbohydrate, fiber and alcohol. Preventive Medicine 27 (1): 32-40

Pope J F, Skinner J D, Carruth B R 1997 Adolescents' self-reported motivation for dietary changes during pregnancy. Journal of Nutrition Education 29 (3): 137-144

Power M L, Holzman G B, Schulkin J 2001 A survey on the management of nausea and vomiting in pregnancy by obstetricians/gynecologists. Primary Care Update in Obstetrics and Gynecology 8 (2): 69-72

Rabinerson D, Dicker D, Kaplan B et al 2000 Hyperemesis gravidarum during Ramadan. Journal of Psychosomatic Obstetrics and Gynaecology 21 (4): 189-191

Ranzini A, Allen A, Lai Y 2001 Use of complementary medicines and alternative therapies among obstetric patients. Obstetrics and Gynecology 97 (4 Suppl 1): S46

Reid M, Adamson H 1997 Opportunities for and barriers to good nutritional health in women of childbearing age, pregnant women, children under 1 and children aged 1 to 5. Department of Health publication. HMSO, London

Reifsnider E, Gill S L 2000 Nutrition for the childbearing years. Journal of Obstetric, Gynecologic and Neonatal

Nursing 29 (1): 43-55

Rondo P H C, Abbott R, Tomkins A M 2001 Vitamin A and neonatal anthropometry. Journal of Tropical Pediatrics 47 (5): 307-310

Rudman D, Williams P J 1983 Megadose vitamins: use and misuse. New England Journal of Medicine 309: 488

Sahakian V, Rousse D, Sipes S et al 1991 Vitamin B6 is effective therapy for nausea and vomiting of pregnancy: a randomized double-blind placebo-controlled trial. Obstetrics and Gynecology 78 (1): 33-36

Satter N, Berry C, Greer I A 1998 Essential fatty acids in relation to pregnancy complications and fetal developments. British Journal of Obstetrics and Gynaecology 105 (12): 1248-1255

Schaumburg K et al 1983 Sensory neuropathy from pyridoxine abuse: a new megavitamin syndrome. New England Journal of Medicine 309: 445

Schmidt M C, Askew E W, Roberts D E et al 2002 Oxidative stress in humans training in a cold, moderate altitude environment and their response to a phytochemical antioxidant supplement. Wilderness and Environmental Medicine 13 (2): 94-105

Schmidt M K, Muslimatun S, West C E et al 2001 Vitamin A and iron supplementation of Indonesian pregnant women benefits vitamin A status of their infants. British Journal of Nutrition 86 (5): 607-615

Scholl T O, Hedigeer M L, Schall J I et al 1993 Low zinc intake during pregnancy: its association with very preterm and preterm delivery. Abstract of paper presented at 5th Annual Meeting of Society for Pediatric Epidemiology Research Minneapolis 1992. Paediatric and Perinatal Epidemiology 7 (1): A2

Schuster K, Bailey L B, Dimperio D et al 1985 Morning sickness and vitamin B6 status of pregnant women. Human Nutrition Clinical Nutrition 39: 75

Shah D, Sachdev H P 2001 Effect of gestational zinc deficiency on pregnancy outcomes: summary of observation studies and zinc supplementation trials. British Journal of Nutrition 85 (Suppl 2): S101-108

Shaw G M, Todoroff K, Carmichael S L 2001 Lowered weight gain during pregnancy and risk of neural tube defects among offspring. International Journal of Epidemiology 30 (1): 60-65

Shaw G M, Todoroff K, Schaffer D M et al 1999 Periconceptional nutrient intake and risk for neural tube defect-affected pregnancies. Epidemiology 10 (6): 711-716

Sheth S S, Chalmers I 2002 Magnesium for preventing and treating pre-eclampsia: time for international action. Lancet 359 (9321): 1872-1873

Siega-Riz A M, Bodnar L M, Savitz D A 2002 What are pregnant women eating? Nutrient and food group differences by race. American Journal of Obstetrics and Gynecology 186 (3): 480-486

Siega-Riz A M, Herrman T S, Savitz D A et al 2001 Frequency of eating during pregnancy and its effect on preterm delivery. American Journal of Epidemiology 153 (7): 647-652

Smithells R W, Sheppard S, Schorah C J et al 1980 Possible prevention of neural tube defects by periconceptional vitamin supplementation. Lancet 1 (8164): 339-340

Spatling L, Disch G, Classen H G 1989 Magnesium in pregnant women and the newborn. Magnesium Research 2 (4): 271-280

Stapleton H, Tiran D 2000 Herbal medicine. In: Tiran D, Mack S (eds) Complementary therapies for pregnancy and childbirth, 2nd edn. Elsevier Science, Edinburgh

Stephenson T, Symonds M E 2002 Maternal nutrition as a determinant of birth weight. Archives of Diseases in Childhood: Fetal and Neonatal Edition 86 (1): F4-6

Stoll C, Dott B, Alembik Y et al 1999 Maternal trace elements, vitamin B12, vitamin A, folic acid and fetal malformations. Reproductive Toxicology 13 (1): 53-57

Tamura T, Goldenberg R L, Johnston K E 2000 Maternal plasma zinc concentrations and pregnancy outcome. American Journal of Clinical Nutrition 71 (1): 109-113

Tierson F D, Olsen C L, Hook E B 1986 Nausea and vomiting of pregnancy and association with pregnancy outcome. American Journal of Obstetrics and Gynecology 1555 (5): 1017-1022

Teksen F, Dokmeci F, Kavas G et al 2001 Copper, zinc and magnesium status in hyperemesis gravidarum. Journal of Obstetrics and Gynaecology 21: 46-48

Urgell M R, Benavides J F, Laborda R G A et al Maternal nutritional factors: significance for the fetus and the neonate. Early Human Development 53 (suppl 1): S61-76

Van den Broek N, Kulier R, Gulmezoglu A M et al 2002 Vitamin A supplementation during pregnancy. Cochrane Database Issue 4 (22.8.02)

van der Vange N, van der Berg H, Kloosterboer H J et al 1989 Effects of seven low-dose combined contraceptives on vitamin B6 status. Contraception 40 (3): 377-384

Villegas-Salas E, Ponce de Leon R, Juarez-Perez M A et al 1997 Effect of vitamin B6 on the side-effects of a low dose combined oral contraceptive. Contraception 55 (4): 245-248

Voyles L M, Turner R E, Lukowski M J et al 2000 High levels of retinol intake during the first trimester of pregnancy result from use of over-the-counter vitamin/mineral supplements. Journal of the American Dietetic Association 100 (9): 1068-1070

Vutyavanich T, Wongtra Ngan S, Ruangsri R 1995 Pyridoxine for nausea and vomiting of pregnancy: a randomized double-blind, placebo-controlled trial. American Journal of Obstetrics and Gynecology 173 (3 part 1): 881-884

Wanchu M, Malhotra S, Khullar M 2001 Calcium supplementation in pre-eclampsia. Journal of the Association of Physicians in India 49: 795-798

Wijewardene K, Fonseka P, Goonaratne C 1994 Dietary cravings and aversions during pregnancy. Indian J Public Health 38 (3): 95-98

Winkvist A, Habicht J P, Rasmussen K M 1998 Linking maternal and infant benefits of a nutritional supplement during pregnancy and lactation. American Journal of Clinical Nutrition 68 (3): 656-661

Wolman I, Groutz A, Gull I et al 2000 Is amniotic fluid volume influenced by a 24 hour fast? Journal of Reproductive Medicine 45 (8): 685-687

4

Acupuncture and the Traditional Chinese Medicine approach

Stimulation of the Pericardium 6 acupuncture point on the inner wrist is now a well-known technique for relieving nausea and vomiting. This chapter discusses the theory behind the technique and evaluates some of the evidence into its efficacy and safety. Its use in isolation from the holistic perspective of Traditional Chinese Medicine is also debated.

INTRODUCTION

The word 'acupuncture' is derived from the Latin *acus* or needle, and *punctura*, punctured. The therapy originated amongst the ancient Chinese who recognised that arrow punctures sustained in battle apparently cured long-term illnesses, and began to map out various points on the body which, when punctured, would treat illnesses. Over nearly three thousand years, the techniques have been developed and refined, and in China, acupuncture is an accepted component of general healthcare.

Traditional Chinese Medicine (TCM) utilises the principle of energy channels, or meridians, which flow beneath the skin and through the body, each of the twelve major meridians passing through an organ, from which it takes its name. There are also eight additional primary channels, which follow a set route through the body. When the whole person – the body, mind and spirit – are in total equilibrium, energy (called Qi, pronounced 'chee') flows unimpeded along the meridians and assists in maintaining

Figure 4.1 Map of meridians and tsubos

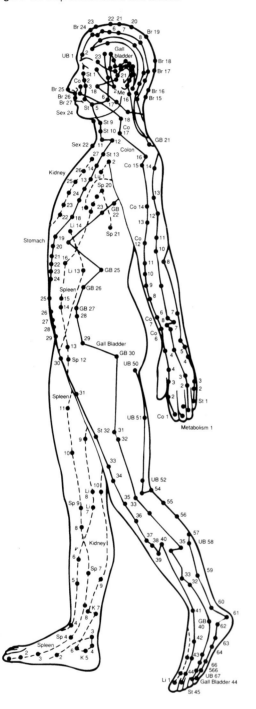

From Budd, in Tiran and Mack, 2000, with permission of WB Saunders

circulation and temperature and in resisting or fighting disease. However, in times of physical, mental, emotional or spiritual disharmony, or dis-ease, the energy flow is interrupted, resulting in stagnation or hyperactivity of Qi at certain points along the meridians. These energy focus points are called *tsubos* and it is at one or more of these points that treatment is given, by inserting needles (acupuncture), by thumb and finger pressure (acupressure, or the similar, more recent, Japanese technique, shiatsu), or by other methods such as moxibustion (using a heat source over the tsubos) or cupping to stimulate, sedate or regulate the flow of energy. More recently, electro-acupuncture has also been used. There are over two thousand tsubos, although in practice, only about 200 are used regularly (see Figure 4.1). A complete set of acupuncture points is also found on the ear and on the tongue (Wong et al 2001) and these offer alternative means of rebalancing Qi. Needles may be used, or tiny studs or seeds may be inserted into the relevant acupuncture point in the ear and left *in situ*.

TCM is a complete system of medicine which also utilises diet, exercise, special massage (*tuina*) and Chinese herbs to treat the person holistically. The theoretical basis of TCM is that each separate part of an individual is fundamentally inter-related with the whole. The Chinese use the principle of two opposing forces, Yin and Yang, which must remain in balance for optimum health and wellbeing. Yin energy is related to cold, darkness, sluggishness, passivity and negative aspects, whereas Yang energy focuses on warmth, light, activity, expression and positive aspects. An organ showing signs of Yin energy will be sluggish or static and will accumulate waste; an organ which is too Yang will generate heat and shows signs of being overactive and out of control. Other principles are also used to assist in diagnosis and treatment of disease, by grouping of symptoms into categories: empty – full; hot – cold; excessive – deficient. Treatment aims to correct these principles so that the whole person is rebalanced. Emphasis is also placed on the interaction between body, mind, spirit and the external environment, including the impact of weather changes on health and wellbeing.

In contemporary western medicine, acupuncture has been used increasingly in the last three decades, and is one of very few aspects of complementary medicine considered by medical practitioners to be reputable. This is somewhat surprising, given that there remains continual debate as to exactly how acupuncture works, yet the British Medical Association (1993), the Foundation for Integrated Medicine (1997) and the House of Lords (2000) have all favoured acupuncture over other, more easily comprehensible, therapies such as aromatherapy. This may be because acupuncture is sometimes practised alongside conventional medicine as an adjunct to other strategies, for example as a means of treating people with illnesses which result in chronic pain. There are over 2000 medically qualified acupuncturists in the UK (BMAS 2001) and over 1200 physiotherapists registered with the Acupuncture Association of Chartered Physiotherapists (AACP 2001). Controversy currently persists however, regarding the classification of western-style acupuncture into group 1 of the House of Lords report (2000) (see Chapter 2), while TCM is relegated to group 3. This is in part due to the perceived lack of evidence of efficacy and safety as well as concerns about the herbal medicine aspect of TCM, which is not regulated and standardised in the same way as pharmaceutical preparations. However, while it is commonly believed that there is a clear distinction between traditional and western styles of acupuncture, there are commonalities in the two approaches (Birch 1998).

It is not fully understood how acupuncture works although various studies have been undertaken, especially in the latter half of the 20th century. The use of a medical language which is different from that of healthcare practitioners in the west has caused particular difficulties in communicating the results of research, for western trained doctors are unfamiliar with the concept of 'energy', 'meridians' and 'channels'. Many centuries of successful TCM experience in China is challenged by scientists and conventional doctors clamouring for evidence

of both efficacy and safety, in terms that they can understand. The diagnostic techniques used in TCM, such as tongue examination and measurement of energy in numerous pulses around the body to determine the current health status of the patient constitute an alien concept in western medicine.

It has been shown that acupuncture has various physiological effects on the recipient. Its analgesic effects are well known, although more often attributed by western doctors to the neurological pathways and the gate control mechanism, or to trigger points, similar to the concept of referred pain (Baldry 1993), than to TCM theories of reduced vasoconstriction and gastric acidity (Bensoussan 1991:20). It is now thought that acupuncture stimulates peripheral nerves in muscles to send impulses to the central nervous system, with the spinal cord, midbrain and hypothalamus/pituitary gland being activated to release endorphins and encephalins, which intercept pain impulses (Pomeranz 2000).

The use of acupuncture for anaesthesia began only in 1958, with early work concentrating on relatively short surgical procedures, such as tonsillectomy (Needham & Lu 1980). There are also numerous early reports of the success of acupuncture in relieving labour pain (Hyodo & Gega 1977; Ledergerber 1976; Wallis et al 1974) and in inducing labour (Zhu et al 1986; Tsui et al 1977; Yip et al 1976), and a more contemporary study by Rabl et al (2001) seemed to confirm the use of tsubos traditionally used to stimulate uterine action. Altered haemodynamics have occurred following acupuncture, including improved cardiovascular and respiratory function (Chen et al 1984; Omura 1975), biochemical changes have been noted (Han & Terenius 1982) and other work has elicited the effects of needling on the immune system (Brown et al 1974). Sedative effects and improvement in psychological wellbeing have also been shown (Ceccherelli et al 1981).

Although the concept of energy channels seems implausible to many practitioners of western orthodox medicine, experiments to confirm the existence of these meridians have been undertaken. Several studies focused on attempting to find an anatomical correspondence between the acupuncture points and nerves, blood and lymph vessels. Zhang et al (1982) dissected 324 acupuncture points and found that 304 corresponded to superficial nerves, 155 to deep cutaneous nerves and 137 points were supplied with both; in a similar study, Gong et al (1985) showed that 24 points were directly above arterial branches and 262 were in close proximity (half a centimetre) to either arterial or venous branches. Other work has demonstrated the anatomical existence of tsubos using radio-isotopes (Bossy 1984; Tiberiu et al 1981) although Simon et al's 1983 investigation disputed these earlier studies. Bensoussan (1991:68-9) discusses a bioelectric theory of action, in which the tsubos and meridians exhibit an electromagnetic nature, needling stimulates changes in their electromagnetic properties and electromagnetic fields influence physiological functions.

Recent research techniques are much more sophisticated and, for example, appear to demonstrate that acupuncture has quantifiable effects on brain structures by stimulating gene expression of neuropeptides (Kaptchuk 2002). Litscher et al (2002a) employed near infrared spectroscopy to monitor cerebral haemodynamic changes which were found to occur during manual acupuncture stimulation of the Large Intestine 4 tsubo. Lee et al (2001) investigated the relationship between the meridians, tsubos and viscera using neuroanatomical tracers and confirmed a specific link between central neural pathways to the stomach and the Zusanli or Stomach 36 tsubo; Cho et al (1998) used functional magnetic resonance imaging to identify a correlation between tsubos traditionally used to treat eye disorders and brain cortices for vision. Litscher et al (2002b) conducted a randomised, placebo-controlled crossover study to show statistically significant differences between fingertip skin perfusion following acupuncture at the Neiguan point (Pericardium 6) and at a placebo (dummy) point, using laser Doppler perfusion imaging.

The number of clinical studies in acupuncture may be higher than in many other complementary therapies, although much of the work is undertaken in China, making an objective evaluation of the standards of methodology difficult. Acupuncture for pain relief after dental surgery has been shown to be more effective than placebo (Lao et al 1999; 1995; Kitade & Ohyabu 2000), but the limited and predictable course of oral pain in these circumstances may have a positive impact on the results, whereas other studies on postoperative pain have employed diverse techniques, variable methodology and small sample sizes (Chen et al 1998; Christensen et al 1993; Martelete & Fiori 1985). There is also conflicting evidence from randomised controlled studies on the use of acupuncture in the treatment of chronic pain, including backache (Cherkin et al 2001; Franke et al 2000), headache (White et al 2000; Karst et al 2000) and chronic pelvic pain in pregnancy (Wedenberg et al 2000; Thomas & Napolitano 2000). However, Wedenberg et al (2000) found acupuncture to be more effective in reducing chronic low back pain in pregnancy than physiotherapy. Studies on patients with asthma are also of variable size, quality and effectiveness (Medici 1999; Joos et al 2000; Kleijnen et al 1991; Linde et al 2001). The majority of RCTs have not been reproduced and currently offer limited insight into the mechanisms, efficacy or, indeed, safety of acupuncture.

TRADITIONAL CHINESE MEDICINE THEORIES ABOUT SICKNESS IN PREGNANCY

The Chinese believe that gestational sickness occurs as a result of imbalances in the energies of the mother as her body is attempting to adapt to the major changes occurring as the embryo/fetus grows. The Ren and Chong channels are essential to conception and nourishment of the fetus. The Directing and Penetrating Vessels, Blood Essence and Kidney energy are all required to provide nourishment for the growing fetus and, in some women, the effort required to maintain this function can lead to a deficiency of blood and an excess of Yang energy. If, in addition to the changes of pregnancy,

Box 4.1 Identification of QI levels

	STOMACH & SPLEEN DISHARMONY	LIVER & STOMACH DISHARMONY	LIVER & GALL BLADDER DISHARMONY
TIME OF DAY	Morning	Afternoon	Continuous
EFFECT OF EATING	Poor appetite; better after eating	No change after eating	Worse after eating
EFFECT OF ACTIVITY	Weak/lethargic/fatigued; better if resting	Restless; better with slight exercise	
NATURE OF NAUSEA AND VOMITING	Nausea slight; vomits later after eating		Severe nausea; vomiting soon after eating
CONTENT OF VOMIT	Thin watery fluids	Retention of food, vomiting of bile	Undigested foods
EFFECT ON NAUSEA	Worse after vomiting	No change after vomiting	Better after vomiting
MOUTH	Absence of thirst; pale tongue with white coating	Thirst without desire; bitter taste in mouth	Intensely thirsty for cold fluids
PAIN	Dull pain	Distending epigastric pain; diarrhoea	Severe pain in hypochondrium; fullness in chest
EMOTION	Miserable, tearful, worried	Anger; long-term emotional issues	Depression and irritability
POINTS TO BE USED	Pericardium 6; Stomach 36; Bladder 20/21 Conception Vessel 12; Spleen 4 (2nd Rx) N.B. moxa can be used instead	Pericardium 6; Liver 3, Bladder 17 & 19; Stomach 36 & 34 (2nd Rx); Stomach 21 & Conception Vessel 13	Pericardium 6; Liver 3; Stomach 36 (2nd Rx); Stomach 4; Liver 14 (hypochondrial pain); Gall Bladder 34

there are also emotional, spiritual or lifestyle difficulties or a constitutional weakness, nausea and vomiting may be reactive consequences. Qi in pregnancy may be affected by disharmony in three principle organs: the spleen, kidneys or liver.

Stomach disharmony, as a result of this organ's link to the Penetrating Vessel, is a common trigger for nausea. This is because blood accumulates in the Ren and Chong channels to nourish the fetus, the latter being connected to the Yang Ming which facilitates the descent of Stomach Qi. Both of these channels are linked to the Stomach 30 point, but if there is a pre-existing weakness in the stomach and spleen energies, blood and Qi may counterflow upwards, which results in the symptom of nausea.

The Chinese also put great emphasis on the state of the mother's emotions at this time, due to their links with specific organs. Worry will cause Qi congestion and food retention, as a result of the emotions on the spleen and stomach meridians. These energy lines are also affected by tiredness, especially if caused by overexertion and work, and will lead to a deficiency of stomach Yin energy, as well as dull pain, muscle weakness, abdominal distension and loss of appetite. The mother is likely to look tired, lethargic and miserable and her tongue will be pale and white-coated. She may report that the sickness is worst in the morning but improves after eating. Stomach and spleen disharmony is the most commonly observed amongst pregnant women with nausea and vomiting. Anger will cause stagnation of the liver Qi, which will also affect the spleen and lead to diarrhoea. As a result of this, stomach Qi is prevented from descending and triggers obstruction (of energy), epigastric pain, belching and nausea.

Optimum liver Qi is vital as this meridian disseminates upwards and outwards in all directions and will affect many other organs. It is thought that the root cause of liver and stomach disharmony may be long-term emotional problems. As well as the nausea, the mother may experience a bitter taste in the mouth, regurgitation of bile, thirst, restlessness and congestion or pain in the chest, abdomen and hypochondrium. This latter, together with the bitter oral taste, are classic signs of liver and stomach disharmony.

Where there is disharmony of the liver and gall bladder meridians, nausea and bile regurgitation are accompanied by irritability and depression. Again, there may be a feeling of fullness in the chest and/or pain in the hypochondium. Fear adversely inhibits the ability of the Kidney channels to control the Ren and Chong channels, and because these are essential for fetal nourishment, deficiency may lead to spontaneous abortion.

Unlike western obstetrics, in which the symptom of gestational sickness is dismissed as a single, physiological entity, Traditional Chinese Medicine practitioners view it as a complex, significant symptom of the whole person. It is therefore important to elicit sufficient information from which to make an accurate diagnosis of the cause, which will then determine the most appropriate management. Various questions are asked in order to assess whether the symptom is a result of Qi deficiency, stagnation or excess, and which meridians are affected (see Table 4.1).

TRADITIONAL CHINESE MEDICINE TREATMENT

Acupressure or acupuncture on the Pericardium 6 tsubo (also called the Neiguan point) has been used in a variety of clinical settings and many research studies have been conducted on the effect of stimulation of the P6 point for nausea and vomiting, either from physiological causes such as pregnancy or motion sickness, or from idiopathic aetiology such as surgery, chemotherapy or radiotherapy. In TCM terms it assists in relaxing the chest and diaphragm and removing stagnant Qi to reduce the symptoms. Isolating its use in a reductionist western medical manner may be one of the reasons for lack of success in some trials, when TCM theory has not been applied to the nature of the symptoms and the selection of appropriate points to stimulate or sedate the unbalanced Qi.

Other tsubos which may require acupuncture or acupressure include Stomach 36 where stomach Qi is deficient, particularly in combination with Pericardium 6 and Conception Vessel 12. Where spleen and stomach Qi is deficient Conception Vessel 12 treatment can be effective; when food is being regurgitated, Conception Vessel 10, which helps to control the cardiac sphincter at the top of the stomach, can be stimulated in conjunction with P6. Conception Vessel 14 is useful when there are emotional problems. Stomach meridian tsubos which may have a therapeutic effect include Stomach 19 or 20 if there is a feeling of epigastrial congestion relieved by vomiting; Stomach 34 when excess stomach Qi results in hyperemesis and other stomach points in relation to heat, cold or damp (extrapolated from West 2001) (see Table 4.1).

When a woman's condition is severe and persistent, West (2001:79) cites an effective combination from Macocia (1998), using Spleen 4 on the right and Pericardium 6 on the left, as a last resort but urges caution as it is considered a strong treatment. In cases of hyperemesis gravidarum, when the woman is dehydrated, vomiting excessively, particularly bile and may be receiving intravenous fluids, West (2001:84) advocates acupuncture to the P6 point, combined with Liver 3, Conception Vessel 12 and Kidney 21, leaving the needles in place for up to an hour.

Although heartburn and indigestion are normally considered to be complaints of the second and third trimester, they frequently occur in conjunction with nausea and vomiting, especially when the latter continues past the first trimester. The Traditional Chinese Medicine approach to heartburn relates the symptoms to weak stomach Qi, with stomach heat and retention of food. Chinese dietary advice includes eating cooling foods to reduce the heat, such as apples, bananas, watermelon, cucumber, celery, cabbage, courgettes, broccoli, cauliflower and spinach, as well as consuming teas made from peppermint, nettle or lemon balm. A range of acupuncture points might require needling in order to reduce heat, strengthen stomach Qi and eliminate stagnation, although West (2001:91) states that abdominal points are contraindicated during pregnancy.

RESEARCH EVIDENCE ON PERICARDIUM 6 (P6) ACUPUNCTURE AND ACUPRESSURE

The specific points discussed above would provide a comprehensive treatment of women with identified differences in their symptoms but the full acupuncture treatment can only be carried out by a qualified and experienced practitioner. On the other hand, Pericardium 6 acupressure or acupuncture, in isolation from other points, is a well-known strategy for sickness of all aetiologies. The P6 or Neiguan point is located on the inner wrist, three cun (Chinese inches) up from the junction of the hand with the arm. Accurate location involves a mental division of the length of the upper, inner arm into 12 which identifies the cun specific to the individual. An estimation of three twelfths up from the wrist crease between the tendons should locate the P6 point. More easily, three fingers of one hand of the woman should be placed on the opposite

Practice point
Accurate location of the Pericardium 6 point is vital to its effectiveness; if medical staff need to insert a cannula for intravenous rehydration, care should be taken to reposition the acupressure wristbands correctly.

Figure 4.2 Location of Pericardium 6 point

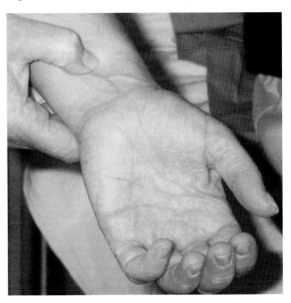

inner wrist and the P6 point is found between two and three finger breadths up from the wrist crease (see Figure 4.2). A slight indentation may be felt and the point may feel tender on palpation, although Janovsky et al (2000) did not confirm the TCM theory that tsubos are more tender in women than in men.

Most of the research on Neiguan point stimulation for nausea and vomiting has involved acupressure rather than acupuncture, presumably as this is a more practical method of treatment and does not require the presence of a practitioner trained in the insertion of needles. Commercially-produced wristbands are readily available and frequently used by pregnant women, although their effectiveness appears variable, perhaps partially dependent on correct siting on the P6 tsubo of the button on the inside of the band. Women often complain that the bands are uncomfortable, leading them to wear the bands intermittently, or to displace them from the P6 point, or to discontinue use altogether. Where women are admitted to hospital for fluid replacement in cases of hyperemesis gravidarum, siting of the intravenous cannula can sometimes mean that the wristbands are inadvertently adjusted and not replaced on the correct point, thus reducing their effectiveness. West (2001) suggests that, if needles are inserted at the P6 point, this may be unilateral, although more commonly women choose to wear them on both wrists.

An early randomised controlled trial by Dundee et al (1988) showed that manual acupressure was only partially effective for pregnancy sickness when compared with sham acupressure or control. They found that pressure needed to be applied for five minutes every two hours, although it was felt that there may be a psychological element to this. Later work by Dundee and Yang (1990) and Dundee and McMillan (1990) suggests that regular pressing for five minutes every two hours on the stud of the elasticated wristband will provide more effective acupressure stimulation. This was felt to be especially beneficial for cancer patients receiving chemotherapy, although the effects may only last for a mean eight hours. However, while some improvement was demonstrated in the incidence and severity of nausea and vomiting in women receiving chemotherapy for breast cancer, the results of Dibble et al's (2000) study were inconclusive. Another small American study of terminally ill patients in a hospice failed to show effectiveness of P6 wristbands but this may have been due in part to the difficulty in obtaining complete data from patients and their relatives (Brown et al 1992).

Two early Chinese studies appeared to be successful in using Pericardium 6 stimulation to treat gestational sickness, although no control group was used in either study, implying that the placebo effect may have had a bearing on the results (Zhao 1988; 1987). A study by Hyde (1989) compared the use of acupressure wristbands with a control group and demonstrated relief of morning sickness symptoms in 75% of the test subjects, together with a reduction in anxiety and depression, measured by standard psychometric tools. Steele et al's (2001) and Norheim et al's (2001) investigations found comparable effects of nausea reduction between the acupressure and placebo groups but a significantly longer duration of relief in those receiving Pericardium 6 stimulation. Knight et al (2001) concluded that Pericardium 6 stimula-tion was *at least as effective* as a sham procedure, but did not demonstrate significant differences between groups.

Evans et al (1993) used sensory afferent stimulation, or electroacupuncture versus no intervention and found improvement in nausea and vomiting in 87% of the experimental group and 43% of the control. It is interesting to note that, in dogs, electroacupuncture has been found to accelerate gastric emptying, possibly due to improvement in gastric slow-wave activity, with some involvement of the vagal pathway (Ouyang et al 2002).

De Aloysio and Penacchioni (1992) conducted a crossover trial using unilateral, bilateral and placebo acupressure, each for three days, and found a 65% to 69% reduction in pregnancy sickness when using acupressure compared to 29% to 31% with placebo. However Bayreuther et al (1994) also used a crossover design with acupressure wristbands and placebo but found only a reduction in nausea ($p = 0.0019$) and no effect on vomiting. There were similar findings in a replicated trial by Belluomini et al (1994) and O'Brien et al (1996) found no improvement in either nausea or vomiting between groups using true or sham acupressure or the control. More recent work by Werntoft and Dykes (2001) involved a pilot trial of 60 healthy women with 'normal' gestational sickness and found the duration of relief to be significantly greater in the acupressure group than in the placebo group.

Carlsson and colleagues in Sweden (2000) conducted a placebo-controlled, randomised, single-blind, crossover trial on 33 women with hyperemesis gravidarum in which they compared the effects of either deep Pericardium 6 acupuncture or superficial (placebo) needling. Women were asked to score the impact on nausea and vomiting using a visual analogue scale and results showed a greater, more rapid improvement in those who had received deep acupuncture than in those who received placebo treatment. It was suggested that, in conjunction with conventional management, hyperemesis could be relieved faster using acupuncture, presumably also reducing the time of hospital inpatient stay.

Postoperative nausea and vomiting has also been found to respond to Pericardium 6 stimulation. Barsoum et al (1990) considered that the incidence of postoperative vomiting amongst 162 general surgery patients was reduced, together with the need for non-elective intramuscular antiemetics, although the findings were not statistically significant. Women undergoing gynaecological surgery of more than six hours' duration were given acupressure by Gieron et al (1993). This produced a consequent reduction of nausea from 53% in the control group to 23% in the acupressure group, lasting up to six hours.

A double-blind randomised controlled trial by Alkaissi et al (1999) compared women having outpatient gynaecological surgery in three groups: bilateral Pericardium 6 acupressure; bilateral placebo (sham) acupressure; and a control group, in an attempt to investigate the 'true' or placebo effects of Pericardium 6 stimulation. They found that placebo acupressure reduced nausea after 24 hours but that vomiting and the need for antiemetic medication was reduced only by acupressure at the correct (Pericardium 6) tsubo. Postoperative vomiting was also shown to be reduced from 42% to 19% in women who received acupressure following laparoscopy and dye investigations (Harmon et al 1999). A more recent study of postoperative patients found direct acupressure to the P6 point more effective than wristbands, but these were significantly better at reducing nausea and vomiting than the control, with a wide variation in overall efficacy from a 73% reduction in nausea to 43% and in vomiting from 90% to 43% (Ming et al 2002). A Korean study compared the Korean hand point K-D2 with the Pericardium 6 acupoint and placebo, using capsicum plaster, a Yang remedy, and found both treatment points to reduce post-hysterectomy nausea and vomiting more effectively than placebo, with a consequent decrease in the use of antiemetic medication (Kim et al 2002).

Conversely however, Allen at al (1994) found no difference in the incidence of nausea and vomiting between a control and a trial group of women undergoing laparotomy for major gynaecological surgery. Interestingly there were less requests for antiemetic medication in the group receiving Pericardium 6 acupressure although there was no difference in the total morphine usage between the two groups. Similarly, no reduction in nausea and vomiting occurred when using acupressure wristbands, either in children undergoing tonsillectomy (Shenkman et al 1999) or after endoscopic urological procedures (Agarwal et al 2000).

Intra-operative nausea and vomiting during Caesarean section in women receiving spinal anaesthesia has been investigated. Stein et al's (1997) randomised controlled double-blinded trial demonstrated that Pericardium 6 acupressure was at least as effective as metoclopramide and more effective than a placebo. Harmon et al (2000) found a reduction in Caesarean intraoperative nausea and vomiting from 53% to 23% and in postoperative symptoms from 66% to 36%, while in a Chinese study by Ho et al (1996), women requiring post-Caesarean analgesia in the form of epidural morphine were found to have less iatrogenic nausea and vomiting when given Pericardium 6 acupressure than when receiving sham acupressure. The incidence reduced from 43% to 3% in the control group and from 27% to 0% in the trial group.

Traditional acupuncture, incorporating a range of points based on a full assessment of the expectant mothers, has been shown to be marginally better than Pericardium 6 acupuncture alone, with sham acupuncture and control groups faring less well, although a time-related placebo effect was also demonstrated in some women (Smith et al 2002). In another, paediatric, study, Schlager et al (2000) effectively used Korean hand acupressure of the Kidney 9 point to reduce postoperative vomiting in children having ophthalmic surgery. Children requiring treatment for vomiting after ophthalmic surgery have been found to respond well to acuplasters positioned at the Bladder 10, Bladder 11 and Gall Bladder 34 points, suggesting a possible inter-related mechanism between the three points resulting in a diminution of the parasympathetic stimulation caused by surgical traction of the eye muscles (Chu et al 1998).

Case 4.1

Jackie worked as a midwife on the labour ward. She was 9 weeks' pregnant with her second child and suffering severe nausea and vomiting, but was managing to continue to work by using Pericardium 6 acupressure wristbands which she found normally kept the symptoms to within manageable limits. One day she arrived at work but had forgotten to bring her wristbands with her and was beginning to experience severe nausea and a desire to vomit. She asked the Complementary Therapy midwife for help, who gathered together gauze, cotton wool balls, tape and two plastic 'butterflies' used for intravenous fluids, from which she cut and discarded the small length of tubing. She then wrapped the gauze swabs over Jackie's inner wrists, placed the 'butterflies', covered in gauze, precisely over the Pericardium 6 points, applied cotton wool balls over the top and taped the entire package firmly in place. Although this rather 'Heath Robinson' effort was uncomfortable and bulky, Jackie felt considerably better and was able to complete her shift without being sick.

This does bring into question the precise method of acupressure used by each research team, both in the siting of needles or pressure band and in the technique. Some use direct needling rather than pressure, whilst others use wristbands with or without buttons on the inner surface (Barsoum et al 1990), beads (Shenkman et al 1999) or metal bullets (Gieron et al 1993) taped to the tsubo. A more recent development is the use of tiny magnetised coils which are taped to the Pericardium 6 point; it is believed that the magnetic energy enhances the effect on the acupuncture point. Evans et al (1993) used continuous electroacupuncture, in which needles are attached to an energy source which can then be adjusted to provide additional stimulation at the relevant point. In an attempt to determine whether or not interaction between the patient and the clinician affected the relief obtained, Shen et al (2000) conducted a study comparing electroacupuncture with minimal needling, sham acupuncture and placebo for women receiving chemotherapy for breast cancer and found electroacupuncture to be most effective, but for a limited duration, while postoperative nausea, but not vomiting, was reduced in laparoscopic cholecystectomy patients who received Pericardium 6 transcutaneous electrical nerve stimulation (Zarate et al 2001). Lee and Done (1999) reviewed a series of studies in which the Pericardium 6 point was stimulated, finding stimulation overall more effective than placebo in preventing early postoperative nausea and vomiting in adults, but not in children. The reviewed sources of stimulation included acupuncture, electroacupuncture, transcutaneous nerve stimulation, direct acupoint stimulation and acupressure.

Stimulation may be intermittent (Belluomini et al 1994) or continuous (Stein et al 1997; Ho et al 1996). Some acupressure was applied before induction of anaesthetic and/or opioid injections, which Dundee and McMillan (1990) postulate is the most effective; they suggest that the antiemetic effect can be negated by local anaesthesia. In one surgically-related study the beads were replaced with acupuncture needles after the patients were anaesthetised (Shenkman et al 1999). Transcutaneous electrical nerve stimulation (TENS) equipment has also been used at the Pericardium 6 point, but only one meta-analysis appears to have been undertaken, comparing acupuncture and TENS effectiveness, in this case for the treatment of dysmenorrhoea (Proctor et al 2002). In practice, any method of applying pressure to the Pericardium 6 point may be effective (see Case 4.1).

Some research teams use unilateral acupressure, whilst others use bilateral bands. Most studies compare true acupressure with placebo and control. Windle et al (2001) compared Pericardium 6 acupressure and placebo both unilaterally and bilaterally and produced inconclusive results, although they suggest that the

---

Practice point

Women need to be given consistently correct advice about how to position the acupressure wristbands; a consensus should be reached within each maternity unit, where encouragement is given, to ensure that women use them accurately.

results must be viewed with caution due to the inadequate sample sizes and recommend further studies.

Many of the studies used a crossover design, including Hyde et al (1989), Bayreuther et al (1994) and Evans et al (1993); all were randomised and controlled. One small study (n=9) on motion sickness (Bertolucci & DiDario 1995) used acupressure wristbands on either the Pericardium 6 point or a wrist placebo; these were later switched over on each subject. The results demonstrated an improvement in seasickness, only when the wristband was correctly positioned at the Pericardium 6 tsubo. Another investigation on the effects of acupressure bands worn on the wrist or forearm achieved a reduction in both the severity of motion sickness symptoms and in abnormal gastric activity, although the variations in siting of the bands may have been a placebo effect.

SAFETY OF ACUPUNCTURE AND ACUPRESSURE DURING PREGNANCY

In common with other systems of complementary medicine, contemporary belief in the value of Pericardium 6 acupressure/acupuncture appears to take precedence over any challenge to its relative safety and an assumption is made that its benefits are greater than its risks. This may, of course, be the case, particularly when compared to the risk-benefit assessment of pharmacological preparations for nausea and vomiting (see Chapter 1). Certainly, when considering the effectiveness of Pericardium 6 stimulation, healthcare professionals have the option of resuming conventional care in the event of a negative response to acupuncture or acupressure. Vickers (1996) suggests that more practical questions need to be asked, once the effectiveness of the technique has been adequately demonstrated, including challenging its safety. What is not known is whether or not Pericardium 6 stimulation could potentially cause any harm to mother or fetus, and although Slotnick (2001) demonstrated successful use of Pericardium 6 electroacupuncture,

---

Practice point
Certain acupuncture points are contraindicated during pregnancy as they may stimulate uterine contractions.

with no incidence of neonatal congenital abnormality, a search of the literature has failed to reveal studies specifically evaluating the safety, either to mother or fetus.

There are few reports on the dangers of acupuncture, although there are specific points which should be avoided during pregnancy as these might stimulate uterine contractions. These include the Gall Bladder 21 point across the top of the trapezius muscle, Large Intestine 4 in the webbing of the thumbs and forefingers, Stomach 36 on the inner lower leg and a range of points in the sacral area. Some authorities also advocate avoiding points which may, at certain gestations, adversely affect the growth, development and health of the fetus, for example, the points on the abdomen from 24 to 32 weeks of pregnancy (West 2001). Experienced practitioners of acupuncture or acupressure will be aware of these contraindicated points as they are taught as part of accepted theory of pre-registration training. Indeed, it is more likely that enthusiastic amateurs, including poorly educated massage therapists, could inadvertently over-stimulate contraindicated points, for example by vigorous petrissage of the shoulders or lower back.

Many healthcare professionals express concern about the potential for the transmission of blood-borne infections such as hepatitis and HIV, either to other patients or to the acupuncture practitioner. However, the vast majority of acupuncturists use disposable needles, and those who do not will autoclave re-usable needles. The needles are extremely fine and no reports could be found in the literature of needlestick injuries to practitioners, leading one to assume that the incidence of risk is, at most, no greater than that to midwives and doctors administering injections. Sermoneta-Gertel et al (2001) investigated the incidence of Hepatitis C

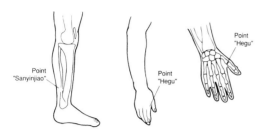

Figure 4.3 Acupuncture points contraindicated in pregnancy

From Budd, in Tiran and Mack, 2000, with permission of WB Saunders

virus infection amongst employees in a large Israeli hospital and found no evidence of a link between presence of the virus and either current occupation and exposure to blood, or acupuncture or tattooing. In institutional settings, safe storage is particularly important to avoid the risk of accidental trauma from poorly sealed packages, as well as to keep the needles locked away from patients and visitors and staff who are not approved to use them.

An interesting study comparing the practice of ancient and modern theories on the depth of needle insertion was carried out by Lin (1997). The safety depth of acupoints was found to be different between those on the back and those on the chest although these appeared to correspond to original teachings for the treatment of adults, but wider variations for the treatment of neonates was revealed. The depth at which De-Qi (therapeutic needling sensation) was achieved differed between male and female patients, and appears to be related to the amount of adipose tissue, rather than to electrical resistance. Accidental retention of needles has been reported in several reviews (MacPherson et al 2001; Yamashita et al 2001; Bensoussan et al 2000; Yamashita et al 1999) and pain and bleeding around the point of insertion has been revealed in others (Ernst & White 2001).

There are isolated reports of complications assumed to have arisen following acupuncture treatment, including increased pain, nausea and vomiting and fainting (Bensoussan et al 2000). A case of contact vesicular dermatitis in a woman who had received acupuncture for

headache and shoulder stiffness is reported by Morimoto et al (2000), and granuloma occurring after acupuncture in a woman with silicone implants is discussed by Alani and Busam (2001). More serious complications are rare but include spinal cord lesions (Peuker & Gronemeyer 2001), acute intracranial haemorrhage (Choo & Yue 2000) and cardiac tamponade (Cheng 2000). Several authorities mention pneumothorax as a possible consequence of stab injuries and inaccurate needle insertion, including the case of a woman who had acupuncture in the region of the thoracic vertebrae (Ramnarain & Braams 2002). De Groot (2001) cites an inquiry of Norwegian medical acupuncturists which revealed 250 cases of pneumothorax before 1995. However, more recently, Ernst and White (2001) found only two cases of pneumothorax in almost 250,000 treatments. Indeed, Peuker and Gronemeyer (2001) suggest that improved, and better applied, knowledge of anatomy and physiology amongst acupuncturists could prevent the occurrence of traumatic injuries during or following treatment. There is also a need for practitioners who use electrical acupuncture to be adequately trained, and for improved calibration of the electrostimulator output, as Lytle et al (2000) found several devices with measured safety parameters outside the levels claimed by the manufacturers.

Acupuncture is commonly used as an adjunct to conventional pain management for patients with chronic medical conditions. Increases in systolic blood pressure were shown in three out of fifteen acupuncture patients at risk of developing autonomic dysreflexia following spinal cord injury above the level of the eighth thoracic vertebra, including one with concomitant essential hypertension, leading the authors to recommend the need for careful monitoring of patients with hypertension or spinal cord injury during acupuncture (Averill et al 2000). If this concern is applied to obstetrics, it may be wise to be cautious in offering acupuncture as pain relief in labour to women with severe pre-eclampsia. A patient with Marfan's syndrome and a prosthetic valve *in situ* developed valve endocarditis following acupuncture, indicating the need for prophylactic antibiotics in patients with prosthetic valves who require or request acupuncture treatment (Nambiar & Ratnatunga 2001). Filshie (2001) suggests that acupuncture may mask the state of tumour progression in oncology patients and that it should be avoided in those with coagulation disorders, neutropenia and lymphoedema, and advocates practitioners having a comprehensive understanding of the disease process and of current orthodox treatment.

Bensoussan et al (2000) conducted a comprehensive Australian survey of all practitioners of Traditional Chinese Medicine, or of acupuncture alone, including both government-registered and unregistered practitioners, and found an incidence of adverse reactions of 1:633 consultations, although it was postulated that the reporting rate of unregistered or non-medical practitioners may be lower than registered medical acupuncturists, thus masking a true reflection of the incidence of complications. MacPherson et al (2001) found a rate of 1.3 adverse reactions per 1,000 treatments in a survey of over 34,000 consultations with British acupuncturists, although this figure included adverse effects from moxibustion (e.g. burns). However, there were no serious complications requiring hospital admission or prolonged hospital stay or leading to permanent disability or death.

Yamashita et al (2001) reviewed case reports of adverse events from acupuncture in Japan between 1987 and 1999. 124 cases from 89 papers were considered, showing 48 incidents of needle breakage and 10 cases of injury from self-treatment. There were also 25 cases of pneumothorax, 18 cases of spinal cord injury, 11 cases of acute hepatitis and 10 cases of localised argyria. Two fatalities occurred as a result of infection. Recommendations focused on improved training for therapists, including medical practitioners, and on discouraging people from unsupervised self-treatment. Ernst and White (2001) also reviewed a series of surveys into the safety of acupuncture and concluded that, while the incidence of minor adverse events may be relatively high, serious complications appear to be rare, although still further

work is required by teachers of acupuncture to ensure that complications remain minimal. This is supported by the work of Yamashita et al (1999) who found no cases of severe complications in over 65,000 treatments carried out in a Japanese acupuncture training institution, and who suggest that most published cases of adverse reactions are actually a result of negligence. Informed consent of patients is vital and could be facilitated by the provision of a leaflet developed from a consensus of the three main UK professional acupuncture organisations (White et al 2001). This could also include information on the risks of driving immediately after treatment, which may leave the patient drowsy and euphoric. Dr Vivienne Nathanson at the British Medical Association raised this issue at a meeting of the Parliamentary Advisory Council for Transport Safety, suggesting that driving after acupuncture could be as dangerous as drink-driving (McNeil 2002).

Biley (2002) expresses concern about the incidence of adverse effects within complementary therapies in general and advocates the establishment of an adverse events register, similar to that already in existence for pharmaceutical preparations, and in keeping with systems being considered for conventional medical practices as a means of reducing risk to patients. There is currently no national method of reporting of side-effects or complications from medical techniques or use of technology, these being largely dealt with at a local level, but wider collation could prove a positive benefit to patients and practitioners in conventional healthcare. Similarly, in complementary therapies, there may be 50,000 independent practitioners of at least 25 therapies (even counting only those included in the House of Lords report (2000)) as well as 10,000 conventional healthcare professionals incorporating complementary therapies into their practice and as many as five million people receiving complementary treatment (Biley 2002), thus the incidence of adverse events may be not inconsiderable.

Until, and unless, such an adverse events register can be established it is vital that practitioners work within accepted boundaries, based

---

Box 4.1 Safety factors in relation to acupuncture and acupressure for pregnancy sickness

- Knowledge of contraindicated acupoints during pregnancy
- Safe storage and disposal of acupuncture needles
- Reporting of needlestick injuries from acupuncture needles
- Check number of needles removed against number inserted
- Mother's informed consent re. possibility of 'normal' reactions to treatment
- Mother advised to report headaches, worsening nausea, pain, inflammation or infection at needle

insertion site
- Cautious use by experienced practitioner if mother is pre-eclamptic
- Avoid acupuncture in mothers who have coagulation disorders
- ? Use gloves if mother is HIV/hepatitis carrier – or ? avoid acupuncture
- Regular checking of electroacupuncture equipment if used
- Local collation of reported adverse reactions or events

---

on contemporary evidence and knowledge. As complementary medicine increasingly becomes integrated into conventional specialisms, an even more cautious approach is required in order to apply generic principles to specific client groups. This is particularly pertinent to systems such as Traditional Chinese Medicine, the theories of which are not readily comprehended by conventional practitioners.

CONCLUSION

Acupuncture and acupressure are well-accepted forms of complementary medicine, with a relatively low incidence of adverse effects. Their use in pregnancy for relief of nausea and vomiting has been extensively researched with many positive results, and acupressure wristbands in particular offer women a simple, easily accessible, harm-free and self-administered means of alleviating their symptoms. The application of Pericardium 6 stimulation, either by needling or by pressure, is worthy of further investigation as a cost-effective and practical treatment for hyperemesis gravidarum, either as an alternative or a complementary form of management.

REFERENCES

Acupuncture Association of Chartered Physiotherapists 2001 AACP website statistics www.aacp.uk.com (accessed 19.6.2001)

Agarwal A, Pathak A, Gaur A 2000 Acupressure wristbands do not prevent postoperative nausea and vomiting after urological endoscopic surgery. Canadian Journal of Anaesthetics 47 (4): 319-324

Alkaissi A, Stalnert M, Kalman S 1999 Effect and placebo effect of acupressure (P6) on nausea and vomiting after outpatient gynaecological surgery. Acta Anaesthesiology Scandinavia 43 (3): 270-274

Alani R M, Busam K 2001 Acupuncture granulomas. Journal of the American Academy of Dermatology 45 (6 Suppl): S225-226

Allen D L, Kitching A J, Nagle C 1994 P6 acupressure and nausea and vomiting after gynaecological surgery. Anaesthetics and Intensive Care 22 (6): 691-693

Averill A, Cotter A C, Nayak S et al 2000 Blood pressure response to acupuncture in a population at risk for autonomic dysreflexia. Archives of Physical and Medical Rehabilitation 81 (11): 1494-1497

Baldry P E 1993 Acupuncture, trigger points and musculoskeletal pain. Churchill Livingstone, London

Barsoum G, Perry E P, Fraser I A Postoperative nausea is relieved by acupressure. Journal of the Royal Society of Medicine 83 (2): 86-89

Bayreuther J, Lewith G, Pickering R 1994 A double-blind crossover study to evaluate the effectiveness of acupressure at Pericardium 6 (P6) in the treatment of early morning sickness (EMS). Complementary Therapies in Medicine 2: 70

Belluomini J, Litt R C, Lee K A et al 1995 Acupressure for nausea and vomiting of pregnancy: a randomized blinded study. Obstetrics and Gynecology 85 (1): 159-160

Bensoussan A 1991 The vital meridian. Churchill Livingstone, Melbourne

Bensoussan A, Myers S P, Carlton A L 2000 Risks associated with the practice of traditional Chinese medicine: an Australian study. Archives of Family Medicine 9 (10): 1071-1078

Bertolucci L E, DiDario B 1995 Efficacy of a portable acustimulation device in controlling seasickness. Aviation Space and Environmental Medicine 66 (12): 1155-1158

Birch S 1998 Diversity and acupuncture. In: Vickers A J (ed)

1998 Examining complementary medicine. Stanley Thornes, Cheltenham

Bossy J 1984 Morphological data concening the acupuncture points and channel network. Acupuncture and Electrotherapeutics Research 9: 79-106

Bowie R A 1999 Acupressure and prevention of nausea and vomiting. British Journal of Anaesthesia 83 (3): 542

Brill J R 1995 Acupressure for nausea and vomiting of pregnancy: a randomised blinded study. Obstetrics and Gynecology 85 (1): 159-160

British Medical Acupuncture Society 2001 BMAS website statistics www.medical-acupuncture.co.uk (accessed 19.6.2001)

British Medical Association 1993 Complementary medicine: new approaches to good practice. Oxford University Press, Oxford

Brown M L, Ulett G A, Stern J A 1974 The effects of acupuncture on white cell counts. American Journal of Chinese Medicine 2 (4): 383-398

Brown S, North D, Marvel M K et al 1992 Acupressure wristbands to relieve nausea and vomiting in hospice patients: do they work? American Journal of Hospice and Palliative Care 9 (4): 26-29

Carlsson C P, Axemo P, Bodin A et al 2001 Manual acupuncture reduces hyperemesis gravidarum: a placebo-controlled randomized single-blind crossover study. Journal of Pain Symptom Management 20 (4): 273-279

Ceccherelli F, Manai G, Ambrosio F et al 1981 Influence of acupuncture on the postoperative complications following ketamine anaesthesia. The importance of manual stimulation of point R and Shenman. Acupuncture and Electrotherapeutics Research 6: 255-264

Chen L, Tang J, White P F et al 1998 The effect of location of transcutaneous electrical nerve stimulation on postoperative opioid analgesia requirement: acupoint versus non-acupoint stimulation. Anesthesia and Analgesia 87: 1129-1134

Cheng T O 2000 Cardiac tamponade following acupuncture. Chest 118 (6): 1836-1837

Cherkin D, Eisenberg D, Sherman K et al 2001 Randomised trial comparing traditional Chinese medical acupuncture, therapeutic massage, and self-care education for chronic low back pain. Archives of Internal Medicine 161: 1081-1088

Cho Z H, Chung S C, Jones J P et al 1998 New findings of the correlation between acupoints and corresponding brain cortices using functional MRI. Procedures of the National Academy of Science of USA 95 (5): 2670-2673

Choo D C, Yue G 2000 Acute intracranial haemorrhage caused by acupuncture. Headache 40 (5): 397-398

Chow A E 1998 Treatment of postoperative nausea and vomiting by acupressure. British Journal of Anaesthesia 81 (1): 102

Christensen P A, Rotne M, Vedelsdal R et al 1993 Electroacupuncture in anaesthesia for hysterectomy. British Journal of Anaesthesia 71: 835-838

Chu Y C, Lin S M, Hsieh Y C et al 1998 Effect of BL-10 (tianzhu), BL-11 (Dazhu) and GB-34 (yanglinquan) acuplaster for prevention of vomiting after strabismus surgery in children. Acta Anaesthesiology Sinica 36 (1): 11-16

De Aloysio D, Penacchioni P 1992 Morning sickness control in early pregnancy by Neiguan point acupressure. Obstetrics and Gynecology 80(5): 852-854

De Groot M 2001 Acupuncture: complications, contraindications and informed consent. Forsch Komplementarmed Klass Naturheilkd 8 (5): 256-262

Dibble S L, Chapman J, Mack K A 2000 Acupressure for nausea: results of a pilot study. Oncology Nurses Forum 27 (1): 41-47

Dundee J W, Sourial F B, Bell P F 1988 P6 acupressure reduces morning sickness. Journal of the Royal Society of Medicine 81: 456

Dundee J W, McMillan C M 1990 Clinical uses of P6 acupuncture antiemesis. Acupuncture Electrotherapy Research 15 (3-4): 211-215

Dundee J W, Yang J 1990 Prolongation of the antiemetic action of P6 acupuncture by acupressure in patients having cancer chemotherapy. Journal of the Royal Society of Medicine 83 (6): 360-362

Ernst E, White A R 2001 Prospective studies of the safety of acupuncture: a systematic review. American Journal of Medicine110 (6): 481-485

Evans T et al 1993 Suppresion of pregnancy-induced nausea and vomiting with sensory afferent stimulation. Journal of Reproductive Medicine 38: 603

Fan C F, Tanhui E, Joshi S et al 1997 Acupressure treatment for prevention of postoperative nausea and vomiting. Anesthesia and Analgesia 84 (4): 821-825

Filshie J 2001 Safety aspects of acupuncture in palliative care. Acupuncture in Medicine 19 (2): 117-122

Foundation for Integrated Medicine 1997 Integrated healthcare: a way forward for the next five years? FIM, London

Franke A, Gebauer S, Franke K et al 2000 Acupuncture massage vs Swedish massage and individual exercise vs group exercise in low back pain sufferers – a randomised controlled clinical trial in a 2 x 2 factorial design. Forsch Komplementarmed Klass Naturhelikd 7: 286-293

Gieron C, Wieland B, von der Laage D et al 1993 Acupressure in the prevention of postoperative nausea and vomiting. Anaesthetist 42 (4): 221-226

Gong Q H, Xiang Y M, Cao J R et al 1985 Studies on the relationship between the channels and the lymphatic system. TCM Digest 1 (2): 1-10

Han J S, Terenius L 1982 Neurochemical basis of acupuncture analgesia. Annual Review of Pharmacology and Toxicology 22: 193-220

Harmon D, Gardiner J, Harrison R et al 1999 Acupressure and the prevention of nausea and vomiting after laparoscopy. British Journal of Anaesthesia 82 (3): 387-390

Harmon D, Ryan M, Kelly R et al 2000 Acupressure and prevention of nausea and vomiting during and after spinal anaesthesia for caesarean section. British Journal of Anaesthesia 84 (4): 463-467

Ho C M, Hseu S S, Tsai S K et al 1996 Effect of P-6 acupressure on prevention of nausea and vomiting after epidural morphine for post-cesarean section pain relief. Acta Anaesthesiology Scandinavia 40 (3): 372-375

House of Lords Select Committee on Science and Technology 2000 Sixth report on complementary and alternative medicine. HMSO, London

Hyde E 1989 Acupressure therapy for morning sickness: a controlled clinical trial. Journal of Nursing and Midwifery 34: 171

Hyodo M, Gega O 1977 The use of acupuncture analgesia for normal delivery. American Journal of Chinese

Medicine 5 (1): 63-69

Janovsky B, White A R, Filshie J et al 2000 Are acupuncture points tender? A blinded study of Spleen 6. Journal of Alternative and Complementary Medicine 6 (2): 149-155

Joos S, Schott C, Zou H et al 2000 Immunomodulatory effects of acupuncture in the treatment of allergic asthma: a randomised controlled study. Journal of Alternative and Complementary Medicine 6: 519-525

Kaptchuk T J 2002 Acupuncture: theory, efficacy and practice. Annals of Internal Medicine 136 (5): 374-383

Karst M, Rollnik J, Fink M et al 2000 Pressure pain threshold and needle acupuncture in chronic tension-type headache – a double-blind placebo-controlled study. Pain 88: 199-203

Kim K S, Koo M S, Jeon J W et al 2002 Capsicum plaster at the Korean hand acupuncture point reduces postoperative nausea and vomiting after abdominal hysterectomy. Anesthesia and Analgesia 95 (4): 1103-1107

Kitade T, Ohyabu H 2000 Analgesic effects of acupuncture on pain after mandibular wisdom tooth extraction. Acupuncture and Electrotherapeutics Research 25: 109-115

Knight B, Mudge C, Openshaw S et al 2001 Effect of acupuncture on nausea of pregnancy: a randomised controlled trial. Obstetrics and Gynecology 97 (2): 184-188

Lao L, Bergman S, Hamilton G et al 1999 Evaluation of acupuncture for pain control after oral surgery: a placebo-controlled trial. Archives of Otolaryngology Head Neck Surgery 125: 567-572

Ledergerber C P 1976 Electroacupuncture in obstetrics. Acupuncture and Electrotherapeutics Research 2: 105-118

Lee A, Done M L 1999 The use of non-pharmacological techniques to prevent postoperative nausea and vomiting: a meta-analysis. Anesth Analg 88 (6): 1362-1369

Lee C H, Jung H S, Lee T Y et al 2001 Studies of the central neural pathways to the stomach and Zusanli (ST36). American Journal of Chinese Medicine 29 (2): 211-220

Lin J G 1997 Studies of needling depth in acupuncture treatment. Chinese Medical Journal [English] 110 (2): 154-156

Litscher G, Wang L, Huber E 2002a Changes in cerebral near infrared spectroscopy parameters during manual acupuncture needle stimulation. Biomedical Technology (Berlin) 47 (4): 76-79

Litscher G, Wang L, Huber E 2002b Changed skin blood perfusion in the fingertip following acupuncture needle introduction as evaluated by laser Doppler perfusion imaging. Lasers in Medical Science 17 (1): 19-25

Lytle C D, Thomas B M, Gordon E A et al 2000 Journal of Alternative and Complementary Medicine 6 (1): 37-44

Macocia G 1998 Obstetrics and gynaecology in Chinese medicine. Churchill Livingstone, Edinburgh. Cited in West Z 2001 Acupuncture in pregnancy and childbirth. Churchill Livingstone, Edinburgh

MacPherson H, Thomas K, Walters S et al 2001 A prospective study of adverse events and treatment reactions following 34,000 consultations with professional acupuncturists. Acupuncture in Medicine 19 (2): 93-102

Martelete M, Fiori A M 1985 Comparative study of the analgesic effect of transcutaneous nerve stimulation (TNS) electroacupuncture (EA) amd meperidine in the treatment of postoperative pain. Acupuncture and Electrotherapeutics Research 10: 183-193

McNeil R 2002 Acupuncture could be as dangerous for drivers as alcohol. Evening Standard [London] 24 October 2002: 22

Medici T 1999 Acupuncture and bronchial asthma. Forsch Komplementarmed 6: 26-28

Ming J L, Kuo B I, Lin J G 2002 The efficacy of acupressure to prevent nausea and vomiting in postoperative patients. Journal of Advanced Nursing 39 (4): 343-351

Morimoto M, Kawata K, Tsuchiya N et al 2000 A case of acupuncture needle dermatitis. Masui 49 (8): 887-889

Nambiar P, Ratnatunga C 2001 Prosthetic valve endocarditis in a patient with Marfan's syndrome following acupuncture. Journal of Heart Valve Disease 10 (5): 689-690

Needham J, Lu G D 1980 Celestial lancets: a history and rationale of acupuncture and moxibustion. Cambridge University Press, Cambridge

Norheim A J, Pedersen E J, Fonnebo V et al 2001 Acupressure treatment of morning sickness in pregnancy. A randomized double-blind placebo-controlled study. Scandinavian Journal of Primary Health Care 19 (1): 43-47

O'Brien B, Relyea M J, Taerum T 1996 Efficacy of P6 acupressure in the treatment of nausea and vomiting during pregnancy. American Journal of Obstetrics and Gynecology 19: 138

Omura Y 1975 Pathophysiology of acupuncture treatment: effects of acupuncture on cardiovascular and nervous systems. Acupuncture and Electrotherapeutics Research 1: 511

Ouyang H, Yin J, Wang Z et al 2002 Electroacupuncture accelerates gastric emptying in association with changes in vagal activity. American Journal of Physiology, Gastroenterology and Liver Physiology 282 (2): 390-396

Peuker E, Gronemeyer D 2001 Rare but serious complications of acupuncture: traumatic lesions. Acupuncture in Medicine 19 (2): 103-108

Pomeranz B 2000 Acupuncture analgesia. In: Stux G, Hammerschlag R (eds) Clinical acupuncture: scientific basis. Springer, Berlin

Proctor M L, Smith C A, Farquhar C M et al 2002 Transcutaneous electrical nerve stimulation and acupuncture for primary dysmenorrhoea. Cochrane Database Systematic Review (1): CD 002123

Rabl M, Ahner R, Bitschnau M et al 2001 Acupuncture for cervical ripening and induction of labour at term – a randomised controlled trial. Wiener Kliniks Wochenschrift 113 (23-24): 942-946

Ramnarain D, Braams R 2002 Bilateral pneumothorax in a young woman after acupuncture. Nederlands Tijdschrift Geneeskunde 146 (4): 172-175

Schlager A, Boehler M, Puhringer F 2000 Korean hand acupressure reduces postoperative vomiting in children after strabismus surgery. British Journal of Anaesthesia 85 (2): 267-270

Sermoneta-Gertel S, Donchin M, Adler R et al 2001 Hepatitis C virus infection in employees of a large university hospital in Israel. Infection Control and Hospital Epidemiology 22 (19): 754-761

Shen J, Wenger N, Glaspy J et al 2000 Electroacupuncture for control of myeloblastic chemotherapy-induced emesis: a randomised controlled trial. Journal of the American Medical Association 284 (21): 2755-2761

Shenkman Z, Holzman R S, Kim C et al 1999 Acupressure-acupuncture antiemetic prophylaxis in children undergoing tonsillectomy. Anesthesiology 90 (5): 1311-1316

Simon J, Guiraud G, Esquerre J P et al 1988 Acupuncture meridians demystified. Contribution of radiotracer methodology. Press Medicale 17 (26): 1341-1344

Slotnick R N 2001 Safe, successful nausea suppression in early pregnancy with P-6 acustimulation. Journal of Reproductive Medicine 46 (9): 811-814

Smith C, Crowther C, Beilby J 2002 Acupuncture to treat nausea and vomiting in early pregnancy: a randomised controlled trial. Birth 2991: 1-9

Steele N M, French J, Gatherer-Boyles J et al 2001 Effect of acupressure by Sea Bands on nausea and vomiting of pregnancy. Journal of Obstetric, Gynecological and Neonatal Nursing 30 (1): 61-70

Stein D J, Birnbach D J, Danzer B I et al 1997 Acupressure versus intravenous metoclopramide to prevent nausea and vomiting during spinal anesthesia for cesarean section. Anesthesia and Analgesia 84 (2): 342-345

Stern R M, Jokerst M D, Muth E R et al 2001 Acupressure relieves the symptoms of motion sickness and reduces abnormal gastric activity. Alternative Therapies in Health and Medicine 7 (4): 91-94

Thomas C T, Napolitano P G 2000 Use of acupuncture for managing chronic pelvic pain in pregnancy. A case report. Journal of Reproductive Medicine 45 (11): 944-946

Tiberiu R, Gheorghe G, Popescu I 1981 Do meridians of acupuncture exist? A radio-active tracer study of the bladder meridian. American Journal of Acupuncture 9 (3): 251-256

Tsui J J, Lai Y, Sharma S D 1977 The influence of acupuncture stimulation during pregnancy: the induction and inhibition of labour. Obstetrics and Gynaecology 50 (4): 479-488

Vickers A 1996 Can acupuncture have specific effects on health? A systematic review of acupuncture antiemesis trials. Journal of the Royal Society of Medicine 89 (6): 303-311

Wallis L, Schnider S, Palahniuk R J et al 1974 An evaluation of acupuncture analgesia in obstetrics Anesthesiology 41 (6): 596-601

Wedenberg K, Moen B, Norling A 2000 A prospective randomised study comparing acupuncture with physiotherapy for low back pain and pelvic pain in pregnancy. Acta Obstetrics Gynecology Scandinavia 79:331-5

Werntoft E, Dykes A K 2001 Effect of acupressure on nausea and vomiting during pregnancy. A randomised placebo-controlled pilot study. Journal of Reproductive Medicine 46 (9): 835-839

West Z 2001 Acupuncture in pregnancy and childbirth. Churchill Livingstone, Edinburgh

White A, Cummings M, Hopwood V et al 2001 Informed consent for acupuncture – an information leaflet developed by consensus. Acupuncture in Medicine 19 (2): 123-129

Windle P E, Borromeo A, Robles H et al 2001 The effects of acupressure on the incidence of postoperative nausea and vomiting in postsurgical patients. Journal of Perianaesthetic Nursing 16 (3): 158-162

Wong V, Sun J G, Wong W 2001 Traditional Chinese medicine (tongue acupuncture) in children with drooling problems. Pediatric Neurology 25 (1): 47-54

Yamashita H, Tsukayama H, White A R 2001 Systematic review of adverse events following acupuncture: the Japanese literature. Complementary Therapies in Medicine 9 (2): 98-104

Yamashita H, Tsukayama H, Tanno Y et al 1999 Adverse events in acupuncture and moxibustion treatment: a six year survey at a national clinic in Japan. Journal of Alternative and Complementary Medicine 5 (3): 229-236

Yip S K, Pang J C K, Sung M L 1976 Induction of labour by acupuncture electrostimulation. American Journal of Chinese Medicine 4 (3): 257-265

Youngs P J 2000 Acupressure and prevention of nausea and vomiting. British Journal of Anaesthesia 85 (5): 807-808

Zarate E, Mingus M, White P F et al 2001 The use of transcutaneous acupoint electrical stimulation for preventing nausea and vomiting after laparoscopic surgery. Anesthesia and Analgesia 92 (3): 629-635

Zhang K 1982 A morphological study on the receptors of acupuncture points. Journal of Traditional Chinese Medicine 2 (4): 251-260

Zhao C X 1988 Acupuncture treatment of morning sickness. Journal of Traditional Chinese Medicine 8: 228

Zhao R J 1987 39 cases of morning sickness treated with acupuncture. Journal of Traditional Chinese Medicine 7: 25

Zhu R L, Gao X H, Zhou Y L et al 1986 The induction of labour by electroacupuncture stimulation – analysis of 771 cases. In: Zhang X T (ed) 1986 Research on acupuncture, moxibustion and acupuncture anaesthesia. Science Press, Beijing

FURTHER READING

Budd S 2000 Acupuncture. In: Tiran D, Mack S (eds) Complementary therapies for pregnancy and childbirth, 2nd edn. Bailliere Tindall, London

West Z 2001 Acupuncture in pregnancy and childbirth. Churchill Livingstone, Edinburgh

5

The phytotherapeutic approach

This chapter deals with the western form of herbal medicine, including aromatherapy, both of which act primarily pharmacologically. A general discussion regarding the safety of herbal remedies and essential oils in pregnancy is followed by an exploration of the use of specific remedies for gestational sickness.

INTRODUCTION

Herbal medicine utilises whole or parts of plants in different forms and is the precursor of contemporary pharmaceuticals, many of which are derived from different plants (for example the contraceptive pill from the wild yam). Herbal remedies contain pharmacologically active ingredients which are thought to act at a molecular level, each type of which has different chemical effects. These effects may result from one or a combination of active constituents, which, once known, are used to standardise preparations. Herbs may be administered as teas and tisanes or infusions made from the fresh or dried plant, or in manufactured tablets, capsules and creams (see Glossary).

Although there is some similarity between herbal remedies and manufactured drugs, the active ingredients of herbal remedies work in combination and synergy with one another, whereas conventional medicines involve the isolation and synthetic production of one active constituent. Unfortunately it is this isolation of a single therapeutic component which is likely to produce unpleasant side-effects, whereas the combination of constituents in herbal remedies acts as a balance to prevent adverse effects, when used appropriately. An example of this is the use by herbalists of the willow bark, from which is derived salicylate, the precursor of aspirin: its interaction and synergy with other constituents within the plant extract counteract the gastritis effects of salicylate which its isolation and synthetic manufacture by pharmaceutical companies often produce.

Aromatherapy is a specific element of herbal medicine although it usually enjoys a reputation as a discrete therapy, in which the essential oil components of plants are extracted by steam distillation, cold expression, carbon dioxide or solvent extraction (see Glossary). These essential oils are highly concentrated, with the chemical constituents having a range of therapeutic properties. (See Tiran 2000 for a more comprehensive exploration of the clinical use of aromatherapy in pregnancy.)

Although the chemical constituents of the essential oils work pharmacologically, many practitioners of aromatherapy view it as an holistic form of complementary medicine, with the oils also having psychological and spiritual effects. Certainly, research has focused on what *exactly* makes the oils work – whether it is the chemicals, the power of the aroma, the method of administration (especially touch as in massage), or whether it is simply the effect of the time and attention which clients/patients receive.

In Britain, herbal medicine has been classified as one of the top five therapies (BMA 1993; FIM 1997), and is in group 1 of the House of Lords report (2000). Other forms of botanical medicine are not so fortunate: aromatherapy, which the House of Lords report saw as having less of a body of evidence to support its claims, is in group 2 (supportive therapies), whilst traditional systems of healing incorporating plants, such as Traditional Chinese Medicine and Indian Ayurvedic medicine, are relegated to group 3a. A statutory regulation working party has been set up by the government to explore a range of options for statutory self-reg-

ulation of the herbal medicine professions, and is expected to produce its report in early 2003 (FIM 2002).

The situation in Britain is currently somewhat uncertain, as there are moves within the European Union to standardise the regulations regarding herbal and dietary supplements. In May 2000 the European Commission published a proposal, aimed at ensuring a high level of health protection and free circulation of the products concerned. It followed the submission of a substantial number of complaints to the Commission, claiming restriction or prohibition on marketing of supplements within member states, on grounds of protecting public health (Atkinson 2002). Many herbal medicines, which have been freely available without the need to go through the process of approval that is required by the Medicines Control Agency for drugs, could potentially lose their licences as the directives take effect, unless the individual companies are prepared to fund research to demonstrate efficacy and safety to the satisfaction of the Commission.

American terminology incorporates both herbal medicines and vitamin and mineral supplements, sometimes referred to as the former, but more commonly grouping herbal remedies as 'nutritional supplements'. This can be confusing to practitioners in the UK, both in terms of legal classifications, and in relation to extrapolating evidence about one or other form of natural medicine from reports which encompass both. In the USA herbal products are marketed without the proof of efficacy and safety that is demanded of drugs by the Food and Drug Administration (FDA); the Dietary Supplement and Health Education Act of 1994 places responsibility for safety on the manufacturers of herbal remedies without submission of formal documentation. However, although companies may identify the physiological effects of a particular herbal substance, they may not make claims for treatment or cure of specific conditions. Thus there is little publicly accessible information on the efficacy, safety, precautions, contraindications or interactions, for either patients or doctors (Valli & Giardina 2002; Cupp 1999).

USE OF HERBAL REMEDIES AND ESSENTIAL OILS IN PREGNANCY

Pinn (2001) suggests that the use of herbal remedies, particularly phytoestrogens for menopausal symptoms, is 'fashionable' amongst women, although there is very little real evidence of safety. Wagner et al (1999) identify reasons why people use herbal medicines, especially St John's wort, as ease of access and an unquestioning belief in their 'safety' as opposed to the 'dangers' of drugs. However, the incidence of use of herbal remedies and essential oils by pregnant women is not truly known, although 55% of a small survey of 229 women in South Africa (Mabina et al 1997) had self-administered herbal remedies, but there appeared to be an associated higher risk of meconium staining during labour, and resulting Caesarean section, compared to controls. A questionnaire distributed by Tsui et al (2001) in San Francisco found that 20% of 150 women surveyed used herbal remedies, with echinacea being the most popular (9%) and ginger being used by 6.7%. The most common reason was to relieve nausea and vomiting and other gastrointestinal symptoms, although Gibson et al's Rhode Island survey (2001) found that the use of herbal medicines in pregnancy was associated with prior knowledge and use. In Hepner et al's survey (2002), 7.1% of women reported the antenatal use of herbal remedies, and interestingly, those in the 41-50 years age group had the highest rate of usage (17.1%). Many of the women in this study had commenced taking herbal medicines *during* pregnancy on the recommendation of health professionals. 12% of pregnant women in Pinn and Pallett's Australian study (2002) used herbal medicines, superseded only by the number of women taking vitamin supplements.

Many medical practitioners are interested in alternative remedies and are keen to be seen to be responding to patient demands. In one study in Toronto, 54% of 242 physicians were prepared to discuss natural medicines with patients although only one doctor actually recommended a herbal product to a pregnant woman

(Einarson et al 2000). The use of herbs by American nurse-midwives appears to be about 10% (McFarlin 1999), although Allaire et al (2000) found that, of the 10% of nurse-midwives advocating complementary therapies in general, herbal medicine accounted for over 73%.

In Britain, midwives are more likely to use complementary therapies such as aromatherapy, massage or reflexology, which can readily be incorporated into their normal practice, whereas the administration of herbs is less widespread, requiring, as it does, a specialised knowledge of diagnosis and herbal medicine prescription. Where complementary therapies are being integrated into midwifery practice, this is most commonly aromatherapy (Ager 2002; Burns et al 1999; Tiran 2001) as it is relatively inexpensive and easy to implement. Although no figures could be found for the self-use of aromatherapy by pregnant women, it is known that many women report informally that they use essential oils at home, usually added to the bath water or in a room vaporiser. This is, however, of concern, since the possible side-effects and/or complications of inappropriate use in pregnancy go largely unacknowledged, both by the women and, more worryingly, by healthcare professionals.

Yarnell (1997) stresses the need for pregnant women wishing to use herbal remedies to seek expert advice from practitioners experienced in both botanical medicine and maternity care, especially for conditions which are not physiological symptoms of pregnancy. Women frequently self-administer herbal remedies and aromatherapy oils on the advice of friends or as a result of information gleaned from a variety of consumer sources. However, Ernst and Schmidt (2002) surveyed websites and email addresses offering information over the Internet on the use of herbs for pregnancy sickness and revealed that 45% of respondents recommend-

Practice point
'Natural' does not necessarily mean 'safe'.

ed ginger, of which 21% did not mention possible adverse effects, and 17% suggested raspberry leaf with no mention of precautions. Fortunately, none of the respondents recommended gestational use of juniper and 29% actually cautioned against its use. The researchers expressed concern about advice offered to pregnant women via the Internet, suggesting that it is misleading and sometimes dangerous.

Concern has often been expressed in the professional literature about the safety of herbal remedies, especially during pregnancy (Tsui et al 2001; Simpson et al 2001; Vaes & Chyka 2000; Wilkinson 2000). The effect of herbal medicines on embryonic development is unknown, as is the risk of fetal loss. Pradeepkumar et al (1996) go so far as to attribute a suspected case of fetal alcohol syndrome to first trimester use of a 'herbal health tonic' containing up to 14% alco-

> **Practice point**
>
> Women anticipating an elective Caesarean section should be advised to discontinue taking any herbal remedies at least two weeks prior to surgery.

hol, although the mother was unaware of this. Expectant women should be encouraged to inform their conventional healthcare practitioners if they are using *any* form of natural remedy, particularly herbal medicines and essential oils, and Kuhn (2002) recommends enquiring about the use of herbal teas (Johanns et al 2002) and culinary herbs.

The issue of potential interactions with prescribed drugs is also a matter of concern (Scott & Elmer 2002; Maliakal & Wanwimolruk 2001;

Box 5.1 Potential herb-drug interactions

HERB	DRUG	INTERACTION
Echinacea	Cyclosporine	Decrease in immuno-suppression (Miller 1998)
Evening primrose oil	Phenothiazines	Induces fits in epileptics
Feverfew	Platelet inhibitors	Potentiates effects
Garlic	Warfarin	Augments anticoagulant effect (Miller 1998; Fugh Berman 2000)
Ginger	Cardiac, anticoagulant or anti-diabetic therapy	May potentiate *or* reverse effects
Ginkgo biloba	Platelet inhibitors; warfarin	Potentiates effects (Miller 1998; Fugh Berman 2000)
Ginseng	Cardiac, anticoagulants sedatives/tranquillisers, hypo/hypertensives, MAOIs, hypo/hyperglycaemics	Potentiates or reverses effects
Juniper	Lithium	Reduces lithium clearance, potentiates effects
Kava kava N.B. Now withdrawn from sale in UK	Benzodiazepines, barbiturates, antipsychotics, alcohol	Excessive sedation, coma (Miller 1998)
Liquorice	Oral contraceptive	Hypertension, oedema, hypokalaemia
Passiflora	Propranolol	Hallucinations
St John's wort	Serotonin re-uptake inhibitors	Serotonin excess syndrome

(Extrapolated from Shaw 1997; Kelly 2002)

Box 5.2 Possible adverse effects of herbal medicines

HERBAL REMEDY	POSSIBLE ADVERSE EFFECT
Comfrey	Liver failure, pulmonary hypertension (Winship 1991)
Ginkgo biloba	Subarachnoid haemorrhage, subdural haematoma (Vale 1998), gastrointestinal upset, hypotension
Ginseng	Vaginal bleeding, mastalgia (Greenspan 1983; Punnonen & Lukola 1980), insomnia, hypoglycaemia, affects blood pressure
Juniper	Irritant, abortifacient
Kava kava	Sedation, lingual dyskinesia, torticollis, oculogyric crisis, exacerbation of Parkinson's disease (Cupp 1999)
Liquorice	Hypertension, hypokalaemia, ventricular fibrillation (D'Arcy 1991)
Ma huang (ephedra) NB prohibited in food supplements in UK but may be present in imported herbal remedies	Insomnia, nervousness, headaches, tremors, fits, cardiac arrhythmia, cerebrovascular accident, death (Cupp 1999)
Nutmeg	Hallucinations, psychosis (Brown 2000)
Valerian	Hepatitis (D'Arcy 1991), hypnotic effects, may be addictive with alcohol

(Extrapolated from Shaw 1997; Kelly 2002)

Ang-Lee et al 2000; Cupp 1999; Miller 1998). In particular, obstetricians, midwives and anaesthetists should enquire about women's use of herbal medicines near term if there is a likelihood of requiring anaesthesia in labour. Women for whom an elective Caesarean section is planned should be advised to discontinue any herbal medicines at least two weeks prior to surgery (Hodges & Kam 2002). The theoretical risk of haematoma after epidural or spinal anaesthesia should also be considered in women taking ginger, ginkgo biloba or excessive amounts of garlic (Hodges & Kam 2002).

N.B. This does not apply to homeopathic remedies (see Chapter 6).

Some authorities, in the absence of adequate safety data, caution against the use of almost all herbal remedies preconceptionally and antenatally (Ernst & Pittler 2002). Langmead and Rampton (2001) and Fleming (2001) identified approximately 900 plants contraindicated in pregnancy. Klepser and Klepser (1999) suggest that there is a need for improved education of both healthcare professionals and consumers about herbal medicines, as well as quality control legislation and further controlled studies to establish safety and efficacy of the various remedies. Wilkinson's review (2000) also revealed a lack of evidence for safety and a plethora of conflicting information, and thus advocates cautious use of herbal remedies during pregnancy, notably ginger, raspberry leaf, camomile and peppermint. One case report (Cahill et al 1994) associated multiple follicular development in a woman undergoing in vitro fertilisation with hyperstimulation resulting from concomitant use of vitex agnus castus in the fourth cycle; the use of this herb to promote normal ovarian function is not recommended.

Some herbal medicines are contraindicated during the preconception phase, pregnancy and breastfeeding (Klier et al 2002), since they may

---

Practice point

Pregnant women and those planning to conceive should be encouraged to inform their GP, gynaecologist, family planning doctor, midwife, practice nurse or health visitor if they are using *any* herbal remedies or essential oils.

be abortifacient, emmenagoguic, teratogenic or excessively laxative. Many essential oils are also contraindicated, as they are highly concentrated; on occasions it is safer to use the fresh herbs, for example in cooking, than the essential oil. However, a worrying lack of awareness amongst the general public unfortunately leads many women to continuing to use essential oils during the preconception period and first trimester, without recognising that they are administering chemicals which are absorbed into the body, metabolised, utilised and excreted in much the same ways as pharmaceutical preparations, and, indeed, may interact with certain drugs, either medically prescribed or self-administered. Individual constituents of the essential oils may have embryotoxic effects (Araujo et al 1996) or have differing excretion times affected by physiological changes, such as occur in the renal tract, during pregnancy (Li et al 1998)

SPECIFIC HERBAL MEDICINES AND THEIR SAFETY IN PREGNANCY

Although this section does not deal specifically with herbal medicines for nausea and vomiting, information is included here about the safety in pregnancy of a variety of herbal remedies as examples of the issues of concern for practitioners who may be asked for information.

St John's wort

St John's wort, one of the most popular of herbal remedies (Einarson et al 2000) is advocated as an antidepressant, although the evidence of efficacy is contradictory (Kalb et al 2001; Shelton et al 2001; Schrader 2000). It should not, however, be taken by breastfeeding mothers with self-diagnosed postnatal depression, and should be discontinued by those who have used it for symptoms of premenstrual tension (Stevinson & Ernst 2000), once attempting to conceive. Damage to oocytes may occur with St John's wort in high concentrations (as also with echinacea and ginkgo biloba) (Ondrizek et al 1999a) and sperm motility may be inhibited (Ondrizek

et al 1999b). A study on the effects of St John's wort on the neurobehavioural development of mice produced smaller offspring, although growth impairment was not long-term; there was, however, no adverse effect on their ability to perform specified developmental tasks and locomotor activities (Rayburn et al 2001; 2000). Conversely, Cado et al (2001) found minimal effects on fetal development in rats exposed to St John's wort.

Minor side-effects to St John's wort include allergy, fatigue, anxiety, gastrointestinal symptoms and the possibility of photosensitivity. The absorption of iron may be inhibited by the presence of tannins, predisposing women to anaemia (Miller 1998). It would be wise, therefore, when taking an antenatal booking history, to take account of a woman's use of St John's wort immediately prior to conception, and to consider the aetiology of any pre-existing anaemia.

The potential for interactions with a number of drugs has been considered. St John's wort induces the CYPA3 enzymes, through which approximately 50% of drugs are metabolised. Thus the half-life of certain drugs may be reduced (Wargovich et al 2001). Both the contraceptive pill (Ratz et al 2001) and diabetic medication may be less effective, and antihypertensives may be potentiated (Ernst et al 2001:189,191,192). It is possible that St John's wort works by inhibiting re-uptake of serotonin, dopamine and noradrenaline and by modulating interleukin-6 activity (Singer et al 1999; Nathan 1999), but, as the mechanism of action remains unclear, it should be avoided by those on monoamine oxidase inhibitors (Deltito & Beyer 1998).

New evidence was presented to the UK Committee on the Safety of Medicines (2000) regarding the risk of interaction of St John's

---

Practice point

St John's wort interferes with the action of the contraceptive pill and may cause breakthrough bleeding; it is contraindicated prior to and during pregnancy and breastfeeding.

Practice point

Prolonged use of echinacea may lead to toxicity of the liver.

---

wort with a range of drugs, including warfarin, digoxin (Johne et al 1999), theophylline, HIV medication and drugs used to prevent rejection in transplant patients, as well as those already mentioned. This prompted the UK Department of Health to advise GPs, gynaecologists and relevant physicians to counsel caution to patients likely to be affected.

Echinacea

Major complications can arise from inadvertently inaccurate or inappropriate use, or abuse, of herbal medicines. For example, *echinacea*, an immunostimulant often used prophylactically against the common cold (Schulten et al 2001), could lead to hepatotoxicity if used for longer than eight weeks; conversely it should be avoided if the person is also taking immunosuppressants such as corticosteroids (Miller 1998). Although advocated by the media for the treatment of recurrent genital herpes, no statistically significant benefit over placebo was found in a year-long study of echinacea by Vonau et al (2001). Its safety prior to and during pregnancy has not been confirmed although Gallo and Koren (2001) and Gallo et al (2000) suggest that the incidence of major embryonic malformations is no greater than in non-users. However, as the sample size was small, the validity of this trial has been challenged by Scialli and Fugh-Berman (2001).

Ginseng

Ginseng, commonly used to boost energy and vitality, immune function and sexual performance, may alter bleeding time and is contraindicated with concomitant warfarin use, with oestrogens, anti-hypertensives, corticosteroids, MAOIs or digitalis; additionally it may affect serum glucose levels and should be avoided by

patients with diabetes mellitus (Miller 1998). There is some question of its effect on MCF-7 cells, with associated risk of breast cancer, notably in women using it for menopausal symptoms (Amato et al 2002).

A report of 88 women who had used ginseng antenatally appeared to relate to an increased risk of adverse outcome (Chin 1991) although animal studies do not support this (Hess 1982). Minor side-effects include diarrhoea, vaginal bleeding, swollen, tender breasts, dizziness, tachycardia, insomnia and headaches, and in more severe cases, mania. One problem for consumers is that proprietary products often combine Siberian with Asian or Korean ginseng so the constituents of one product may be different from those of another. The evidence for safety is inconclusive and this suggests caution, at the very least, during the organogenic phase of pregnancy, while Ernst (2002) states that there is insufficient evidence of safety or efficacy, from a range of well-conducted trials, to advocate the use of ginseng for any condition.

Blue cohosh and black cohosh

Blue cohosh (Caulophyllum thalictroides) and black cohosh (Cimicifuga racemosa) are used by some women to facilitate uterine efficiency in labour, but may cause minor side-effects such as nausea, meconium-stained liquor or transient fetal heart irregularities. More major complications, as a result of the saponin constituents which are vasoconstrictive and cardiotoxic (Irikura & Kennelly 1999), have also been reported, including neonatal myocardial infarction and congestive cardiac failure (Jones & Lawson 1998). An attempt to induce uterine contractions with black and blue cohosh has reportedly caused neonatal hypoxic ischaemia (Gunn & Wright 1996). McIntyre (2001) states that it is this possibility of fetal

---

Practice point

Ginseng should be avoided by women taking oestrogens and during the preconception and antenatal periods.

> **Practice point**
>
> Several reports of fetal malformations or neonatal cardiac problems suggest that black cohosh should be used with caution during pregnancy and labour; blue cohosh should be avoided because of the potential to cause fetal hypoxia.

hypoxia which has led medical herbalists to discontinue the use of *blue* cohosh in particular. Another constituent of blue cohosh is anagyrine, although it is thought that teratogenicity will occur only if metabolised by rumen microflora, i.e. in cows (Betts et al 1998; Keeler 1988). However, a possible link between infant vascular and skeletal abnormalities and maternal consumption of anagyrine-containing goat's milk has been suggested by Ortega and Lazerson (1987).

Ginkgo biloba

Ginkgo biloba, popularly used to stimulate cognitive functioning, may initiate epileptiform convulsions when taken in large amounts by children (Ernst et al 2001:115). Kajiyama et al (2002) report the case of a two-year-old who ingested a large amount of ginkgo seeds and presented to the emergency department with diarrhoea, vomiting, afebrile convulsions and an excessively high serum concentration of 4-metoxypyridoxine, who was fortunately treated successfully with pyridoxal phosphate.

Ginkgo may also upset the balance of the coagulation mechanism (Fessenden et al 2001). McIntyre (2001) cites a 2000 study in which it was claimed that the use of ginkgo biloba during pregnancy may cause fetal harm due to the accumulation of colchicine in the placenta, although the American Botanical Council later found the research methodology of this particular study to be flawed. However, Petty et al (2001) also found significantly higher levels of colchicine in the placentae of women who had used non-prescription herbal supplements during pregnancy and suggest that ginkgo should be avoided at this time.

SAFETY OF ESSENTIAL OILS IN PREGNANCY

Similarly, aromatherapy essential oils should also be used with care, especially during the first trimester, as little is known regarding their safety or the potential teratogenic, mutagenic or abortifacient properties (Tiran 2000), although Tisserand and Balacs (1995) state that there is no real reason why extra caution should be employed solely in the first three months.

The oils are absorbed into the body through the skin, mucus membranes and gastrointestinal tract, depending on the method of administration, and via the respiratory tract, irrespective of the primary method of administration. Essential oils are fat-soluble and are absorbed via lipid-rich cell membranes, including those in the central nervous system (CNS) and brain. Much research has focused on the CNS effects of oils, including the sedative action of oils such as *Lavandula angustifolia* (lavender) and *Citrus bergamia* (bergamot), which have also been found to be anticonvulsant (Yamada et al 1994; Occhiuto et al 1995), whereas *Salvia officinale* (sage) and *Hyssopus officinalis* (hyssop) have a convulsive action (Millet et al 1981) and are contraindicated in pregnancy.

Essential oils may play a part in regulating immune function by lodging in leucocyte membranes and may affect nerve function as do anaesthetic drugs (Balacs 1991). The circulatory stimulation of massage enhances absorption through the skin, particularly when the epidermis is damaged or diseased. Cardiovascular effects include the hypotensive action of oils such as *Lavandula angustifolia* (lavender) (Buchbauer et al 1991; 1993), the hypertensive effect of *Salvia sclarea* (clary sage) (Tisserand & Balacs 1995: 65) and a cholesterol-lowering action of *Nigella sativa* (black onion seed) (El Tahir et al 1993). Essential oils reach the liver via the bloodstream, and can have an impact on the urinary tract (Falk-Filipsson 1993), biliary tract (Trabace et al 1992), pancreas (Al-Hader et al 1994) and retina (Recsan et al 1997).

There are many reports of skin sensitivity to specific oils, including the increasingly popular

Melaleuca alternifolia (tea tree) (Southwell et al 1997; De Groot & Weyland 1993) and *Chamomilla recutita* (camomile) (Giordinano-Labadie et al 2000; McGeorge & Steele 1991). Camomile has also been reported to cause anaphylaxis (Reider et al 2000), in one case, fatally when used in an enema during labour (Jensen-Jarolim et al 1998), and has been found to possess weak oestrogenic agonist activity, as has grapeseed, an oil frequently used as a carrier for the essential oils (Rosenberg Zand et al 2001). Others, such as *Citrus limonum* increase susceptible individuals to photosensitivity when exposed to strong sunlight (Naganuma et al 1985).

Although essential oils are sometimes administered as oral medications in countries such as France, this is under the strict control of appropriately trained doctors; in the UK, oral administration is actively discouraged and obtaining adequate insurance cover is difficult for practitioners. There is therefore a lack of data about the safety or efficacy of oral administration, but collation of case reports in which accidental or intentional overdose has caused illness or even death contribute to the body of knowledge. For example, accidental overdose of *Eucalyptus globulus* (eucalyptus) has been reported on several occasions (Gurr & Scroggie 1965; Spoerke et al 1989), yet an Australian review of 41 cases of eucalyptus oil poisoning found no fatalities, even when small children had ingested large quantities (Webb & Pitt 1993).

Certain oils have the potential to interact with drugs due to competition for plasma albumin binding sites. For instance, the myristicin component of *Myristica fragrans* (nutmeg), an oil sometimes used for relief of pain in labour, may potentiate the action of pethidine, since it is thought to inhibit monoamine oxidases, with which pethidine is contraindicated (Reynolds 1993). Theoretically, liver enzyme activity may be increased by some essential oils, as with certain drugs, implying that essential oils may exacerbate drug metabolism, although this is unlikely, given the low percentages of essential oils used in clinical aromatherapy. The safrole content of *Cinnamomum zeylanicum* (cinnamon) oil is thought to cause an increase in cytochrome P450, enhancing the effects of drugs such as paracetamol (Boyland & Chasseur 1970). Transdermal penetration of drugs may be affected by administration of essential oils via the skin, as in massage, which may be of relevance to gynaecologists prescribing skin patches for women requiring postmenopausal hormone replacement therapy. On a more positive note, all essential oils have some anti-infective properties, but some are particularly effective as anti-viral or antibacterial agents (Domokos et al 1997; Viollon et al 1996; Carson et al 1996).

Many essential oils are classified, in aromatherapy literature, as emmenagoguic, although this does not automatically infer that they are also abortifacient. However, those which were traditionally used to self-induce abortion, such as pennyroyal oil, with its high pulegone content, are categorically contraindicated for clinical use in all circumstances. This is actually less to do with the supposed abortifacient action, but rather that excessive use of the oil results in hepatic, renal and cardiac toxicity, frequently being ultimately fatal (Balacs 1992).

The ethical and practical difficulties of conducting randomised controlled clinical trials on women who may, themselves, not yet be aware of their pregnancies, means that opportunities to determine statistically whether or not specific essential oils are safe, are limited to single case reporting of problems arising from inadvertent self-administered overdose.

The teratogenic effects of essential oils are also difficult to determine definitively with human research; where studies on pregnant mice or rats have shown possible fetal effects, the essential oils have usually been administered in such large doses that comparable amounts in humans would be systemically toxic rather than specifically teratogenic. Additionally, animal trials frequently study the impact of single chemical constituents rather than whole essential oils, in which those same specific constituents may work in synergy with other chemicals, or be in low enough percentages as to be relatively harmless. For example, the high levels of sabinyl acetate in *Juniperus communis* (juniper) have been thought to be the cause of abortion

---

Practice point

Essential oils should be treated with the same caution as pharmaceutical preparations, since they are absorbed, metabolised, utilised and excreted by the same mechanisms as drugs.

---

fetal abnormality in mice (Agrawal et al 1980) yet no adverse effects on mice offspring were found in Pages et al's work (1990) on *Eucalyptus globulus* (eucalyptus) which also contains sabinyl acetate, but in much lower proportions.

An additional issue related to the use of aromatherapy in pregnancy is that of *olfaction*, as the volatile essential oils possess aromas in varying strengths, which may, in some women, be off-putting, especially when they are feeling nauseous, although this may differ, given the wide day-to-day variation in olfactory sensitivity (Krone et al 2001), cultural and age differences (Hudson & Distel 1999; Ayabe-Kanamura et al 1998; Wysocki & Pelchat 1993). Aromas appear to be processed by the brain in different ways, according to which nostril the odour molecules enter the respiratory tract (Kobal et al 1992), with olfactory 'labelling' being attributed to the left frontal brain (Kline et al 1999; Lorig et al 1993). Odours can have a negative or positive effect on the mood and sense of wellbeing (Masago et al 2000; Knasko 1992), and certain essential oil aromas have been shown to affect neurological function (Millot et al 2002; Santos et al 1996; Manley 1993; Karamat et al 1992; Kikuchi et al 1991).

The choice of essential oils for antenatal use is entirely subjective, and, in relation to nausea and vomiting, may be rejected by women whose symptoms are exacerbated by any odours. Despite an extensive literature search, little data could be found on the effect of pregnancy on the sense of olfaction, although numerous women anecdotally report changes in their sense of smell and become noticeably sensitive to strong odours, such as food cooking and tobacco. Certainly, in pubescent males, endocrine changes do not appear to have an impact on odour preference (Laing & Clark 1983), although different factors may have an effect in females. Erick (1995) suggests that there may be a hyperolfactory mechanism associated with hyperemesis gravidarum, the purpose of which may be to encourage women to seek appropriately hygienic, peaceful and safe environments as a protection for the fetus. Heinrichs (2002) also found a reduced incidence of severe nausea and vomiting amongst pregnant women with congenital anosmia, suggesting an olfactory trigger for gestational sickness. He also postulated on the feasibility of a common aetiological mechanism between hyperemesis gravidarum and migraine headaches, possibly based on allelic variation in the dopaminergic receptor gene. Olfactory receptors, types of odours and MHC antigens are closely related and, as the protective role of pregnancy nausea and vomiting and the MHC antigen appear to overlap in women with recurrent abortion, it implies that an olfactory mechanism may be involved in positive pregnancy outcomes.

It is worthwhile, here, considering the impact on the fetus, as it has been found that the behavioural effects of early (i.e. fetal/neonatal) exposure to specific odours may last into adulthood (Coopersmith & Leon 1986), especially as strong odours such as garlic have been found to cross the placental barrier and to be detectable in amniotic fluid and fetal blood (Nolte et al 1992). Hudson and Distel (1999) also found, in rabbits, that preferences appear to develop as a result of intrauterine exposure to pleasant and unpleasant odours and tastes, and Marlier et al (1998) demonstrated similar reactions in human infants.

Very few trials have, therefore, been carried out on pregnant women, and those where essential oils have been used have *assumed* the relative safety of the oils, based on applied research findings and on the absence of evidence of harmful effects. Generally, aromatherapy is offered by midwives as a means of relaxation rather than for a specific pharmacological action, although Dale and Cornwell (1994) investigated the possible postpartum perineal wound healing properties of *Lavandula angustifolia* (lavender). Their results were inconclusive

Box 5.3 Herbal medicines contraindicated during pregnancy

The following herbal medicines/essential oils are generally contraindicated during pregnancy or should be used with caution and prescribed only by an experienced practitioner; they are referred to by both the common and the Latin names.

arbour vitae	*Thuja occidentalis*
barberry	*Berberis vulgaris*
basil oil	*Ocimum basilicum*
beth root	*Trillium erectum*
black cohosh	*Cimicifuga racemosa*
blue cohosh	*Caulophyllum thalictroides*
cinchona	*Cinchona spp.*
clary sage oil	*Salvia sclarea*
	(can be used in labour)
cotton root bark	*Gossypium hebaceum*
fennel oil	*Foeniculum vulgare*
ginseng (Siberian)	*Eleuterococcus senticosus*

golden seal	*Hydrastis candensis*
greater celandine	*Chelidonium majus*
hyssop oil	*Hyssopus officinalis*
juniper – herb and oil	*Juniperus communis*
marjoram	*Origanum vulgare*
meadow saffron	*Crocus sativus*
motherwort	*Leonorus cardiaca*
mugwort	*Artemesia vulgaris*
nutmeg oil	*Myristica fragrans*
	(can be used in labour)
pennyroyal	*Menthe pulegium*
poke root	*Phytolacca decandra*
rue	*Ruta graveolens*
sage – herb and oil	*Salvia officinalis*
squaw vine	*Mitchella repens*
St John's wort	*Hypericum perforatum*
tansy	*Tanacetum vulgare*
wormwood	*Artemesia absinthum*

with regards to speed of wound healing, but women reported less pain and an improved sense of relaxation, although Wiebe's (2000) exploration of the use of aromatherapy prior to termination of pregnancy found no significantly greater reduction in anxiety from specific essential oils than from any other pleasant odour.

Possibly the largest clinical aromatherapy study undertaken is that of Burns et al (1999) who offered aromatherapy to over 8,000 women in labour over a period of nine years. Ten essential oils were administered in various combinations via the skin and in inhalation and the findings suggested a significant reduction in maternal anxiety and fear, thus indirectly having a positive effect on their perception of pain; *Chamomilla reticulata* (camomile) and *Salvia sclarea* (clary sage) oils in particular appeared to be effective analgesics and there was a corresponding reduction in the use of systemic opioids. Maternal side-effects were less than 1%, all of which were minor (e.g. skin irritation, nausea), with none affecting the fetus. As the midwives offering aromatherapy to labouring women were those already designated to provide individualised intrapartum care, there was no increase in staffing required and aromatherapy proved an inexpensive additional care option.

THE USE OF HERBAL REMEDIES AND ESSENTIAL OILS FOR NAUSEA AND VOMITING IN PREGNANCY

Ginger (*Zingiber officinale*)

Some complementary strategies are now so well publicised that conventional healthcare practitioners may adopt the practice of advising a specific natural remedy without fully understanding its mode of action. Ginger is a herbal remedy long used in both European phytotherapy and in Traditional Chinese Medicine for its carminative properties. The therapeutic product is derived from the rhizome, believed to possess analgesic, anti-inflammatory, antithrombotic and cholesterol-lowering properties. Its antiemetic effects are thought to be due to anticholinergic and antihistamine actions (Quian & Liu 1992), rather than an effect on gastric emptying (Phillips, Hutchenson & Ruggier 1993; Stewart et al 1991). Ginger has also been found to have similar, but less pronounced effects than the serotonin receptor (5-HT3) antagonists to ondansetron and granisetron (Huang & Iwamoto 1991). The pharmacological action is likely to be a local gastrointestinal one rather than a central effect (Holtmann et al 1989; Grontved & Hentzer 1986).

A survey by Power et al (2001) in Washington DC found that female obstetricians were more likely to advise women to try ginger before prescribing antiemetic medication than their male counterparts. Women are aware of the potential value of ginger, but frequently resort to ginger biscuits, from which the surge in blood sugar causes only a temporary relief followed by a rapid reduction and a consequent worsening of symptoms. Crystallised ginger may have similar effects, and the alcohol content, albeit low, of ginger beer, precludes this as an option. A tea, made from grated ginger root steeped in boiling water, is the recommended means of administration, although the effort required to purchase the root and make the tea, together with the differences in taste and smell perception of pregnant women, may lead them to seek other means of dealing with their symptoms. Several tablet/capsule preparations of ginger are now commercially available and probably constitute the easiest and most effective means of administering ginger in a regulated dose, and Keating and Chez (2002) found ginger syrup to be effective and practical. Ginger essential oil may also be of use, although the mother's altered sense of olfaction may mean that she finds the aroma too strong.

There are many occasions when ginger may indeed be effective in combating sickness and several randomised double-blind studies support this hypothesis, although recent systematic reviews by Jewell and Young (2000) and Ernst and Pittler (2000) suggest that the evidence is insufficient. Some of the early work focused on relief of sickness caused by motion, although the methodology of Mowrey and Clayson's study showing the efficacy of ginger (1982) has been questioned. Grontved et al (1986) depicted no differences in incidence of nausea or rates of vomiting between test and control groups with artificially-induced vertigo and nystagmus, although later work by the same team (Grontved et al 1988), on the effects of ginger on seasickness rates amongst naval cadets, found that it was significantly better at reducing symptoms than a placebo. Wood et al (1988) compared placebo levels of ginger with

therapeutic levels of scopolamine and d-amphetamine and, unsurprisingly, found the drugs to be a more reliable form of prophylaxis against motion sickness.

Vutyavanich et al (2001) randomised 70 women, less than 17 weeks pregnant, to receive either ginger 1g per day or an identical placebo for four days, and measured the number of vomiting episodes per 24 hours and the severity of nausea, using visual analogue scales. There were significant improvements in both nausea and vomiting in the ginger group compared to the placebo group, leading them to conclude that ginger is an effective remedy for relieving nausea and vomiting of pregnancy. An earlier trial by Fischer Rasmussen et al (1991) demonstrated its effectiveness in alleviating hyperemesis gravidarum when compared to a placebo, although this study involved hospitalised women, for whom the environment itself may have had a placebo effect.

Postoperative nausea and vomiting was investigated by Bone et al (1990) who compared the use of ginger with metoclopramide and a placebo in a controlled study of 60 women following major gynaecological surgery. The incidence of nausea significantly decreased in both the ginger and metoclopramide groups, with antiemetic administration being greatest in the placebo group. Phillips, Ruggier & Hutchinson (1993) conducted a similar study for 120 women having day case gynaecological laparoscopy. The incidence of postoperative nausea and vomiting was found to be 21% in the study group, 27% in the metoclopramide group and 41% in the placebo group, with no difference in the incidence of potential side-effects such as itching, sedation, visual disturbance or abnormal movement.

On the other hand, an investigation by Arfeen and colleagues (1995) compared placebo with the administration of either 0.5g or 1.0g of ginger, all with oral premedication of diazepam, in three randomised groups of women having gynaecological laparoscopy. They found no significant differences in the relief of postoperative nausea and vomiting between the groups. Indeed, a slight but non-

---

> **Practice point**
>
> The maximum daily dose of ginger should probably not exceed one gram.

significant increase in nausea was noted with increasing doses of ginger. Visalyaputra et al (1998) also dispute the effectiveness of ginger for postoperative nausea.

Conversely, the use of ginger by some women, either orally or through inhalation, may exacerbate the nausea and vomiting, possibly contributing to a belief amongst obstetricians and general practitioners that it is, at best, ineffective and, at worst, harmful. A minor side-effect of heartburn has also been reported (Stewart et al 1991), which may be problematic for some women whose sickness is already compounded by indigestion and heartburn. However, theories of Traditional Chinese Medicine (TCM), in which body-mind-spirit harmony is achieved through a delicate balance of Yin and Yang energies (see Chapter 4), attribute the exacerbation of sickness by ginger to an inappropriate use of a 'hot' remedy (Yang) in women whose energies are already too Yang biased. Women for whom ginger compounds an already excess Qi are those whose nausea occurs at times other than in the mornings, is worse after eating and for whom vomiting of undigested food soon after eating improves their condition (West 2001). These women usually respond well to peppermint or spearmint which are considered 'cooling', or Yin, thereby reducing Yang energies. Similarly women who have no effect or a worsening of symptoms when using peppermint may gain relief from ginger which reduces Yin energies.

The safety of ginger in pregnancy has not been adequately investigated to date, although concerns have been expressed by some researchers. Traditional texts on herbal medicine quote ginger as a promoter of menstruation but this may not necessarily imply an emmenagoguic effect. Early work by Nagabhushan and Amonkar (1987) and Unnrikrishan and Kuttan (1988) suggests that certain constituents of *Zingiber officinale* are mutagenic while others have an anti-mutagenic effect. Fischer Rasmussen et al (1991) considered a theoretical link between ginger and sex steroid differentiation in the fetal brain due to its inhibitory action on thromboxane synthetase. Wilkinson's (2000) study identified an increased early embryo loss in rats given ginger, although an interesting increase in growth was demonstrated in surviving fetuses. However, Fulder and Tenne (1996) found no clinical evidence of adverse effects in human pregnancy, and in Weidner and Sigwart's (2001) study, no maternal or fetal developmental toxicity was shown in rats given daily doses of ginger up to 1,000mg/kg of body weight. Fetal effects may be dose dependent although Traditional Chinese Medicine dosages are usually much higher than those used in European phytotherapy (Bergner 1991) but caution suggests maintaining doses at a maximum of one gram per day. This is particularly pertinent given the potential adverse effects on the neurological system which have been shown in adults (Rudman & Williams 1983).

Ernst et al (2001:113, 185, 187) suggest that

> **Case 5.1**
>
> A woman came to the CT clinic at 18 weeks' gestation, complaining that she was still being sick and felt constantly nauseous, with symptoms worse in the afternoon and early evening. Her midwife had advised her to take ginger and she had been drinking ginger beer and eating ginger biscuits and crystallised ginger, but felt even worse. The CT midwife diplomatically suggested that neither the sugar-laden biscuits nor the mildly alcoholic beer were appropriate for her condition. She also questioned the mother and found that she was craving cold drinks and foods, suggesting an unconscious attempt to reduce the excessive 'heat' in her body. It was suggested that she tried peppermint tea and sucked sugar-free peppermints, and the following week the mother reported virtual cessation of vomiting and much more intermittent nausea, with which she felt able to cope. However, whether this response was due to the peppermint, the cessation of the ginger or the placebo effect of having had a professional validate the symptoms is difficult to identify.

> **Practice point**
>
> Women requiring anticoagulants or antihypertensives should refrain from taking ginger; those using ginger long-term may require regular coagulation studies to be undertaken.

patients taking ginger should have regular assessment for coagulation disorders. Potentiation of anticoagulants is a possibility, although a review of the evidence of possible interactions with warfarin was found to be insufficient to determine practice guidelines (Vaes & Chyka 2000). Fetrow (2000) claims that any reported interactions are based on antiplatelet effects (Verma et al 1993; Lumb 1994) and Janssen et al (1996) found no antithrombotic activity after one week's usage. Furthermore, as ginger does not appear to affect gastric emptying (Stewart et al 1991; Phillips, Hutchinson & Ruggier 1993), the possibility of interactions with drugs which are influenced by gastrointestinal transit time theoretically does not exist.

Peppermint (*Mentha piperata*)

It has already been suggested that, for those women whose nausea and vomiting is exacerbated by ginger, peppermint may offer a suitable alternative, based on the Chinese medicine theory of 'hot' and 'cold' remedies (see Chapter 4). Nauseated women often spontaneously reach for peppermint sweets to suck, ostensibly to disguise the unpleasant taste which they may have in the mouth, but they may also report a general improvement in symptoms.

Peppermint has long been known to be a carminative and anti-spasmodic, acting specifically on smooth muscle in the gastrointestinal and biliary tracts (Rees et al 1979; Duthie 1981; Giachetti et al 1988; Hills & Aaronson 1991; Hardcastle et al 1996). Peppermint is usually administered in the essential oil form, although this may be in a capsule; Mascher et al (2001) recommend enteric-coated capsules as being more readily tolerated by patients, although there may be some delay in bioavailability of the active constituents. It is certainly useful for people with the gastrointestinal symptoms associated with irritable bowel syndrome, including children (Kline et al 2001), although Jailwala et al's review (2000) advocates further studies be undertaken. It may have potential in the management of other gastrointestinal conditions, including duodenal ulcer (Micklefield et al 2000) and prior to procedures such as colonoscopy (Spirling & Daniels 2001; Asao et al 2001), as it has been shown to be effective in reducing oesophageal spasm (Pimentel et al 2001).

Dyspepsia responds well to peppermint and other similar oils such as caraway, and the effect is comparable with certain anti-dyspeptic drugs (May et al 2000; Madisch et al 2001; 1999). Peppermint also appears to have an analgesic effect, having been used to relieve post-herpetic neuralgia (Davies et al 2002), helps to reduce mental fatigue (Umezu et al 2001) and may alleviate nasal symptoms of allergic rhinitis (Inoue et al 2001). A Russian team investigated the antioxidant effects of peppermint and other plants in relation to acute toxic hepatitis in rats (Katikova et al 2001).

Despite an extensive search of the literature, little evidence could be found to suggest peppermint as a treatment for nausea, presumably as ginger is the herbal remedy of first choice. One study of postoperative gynaecological patients (Tate 1997) demonstrated superiority of peppermint over both placebo and control, with the experimental group requiring less pharmaceutical antiemetics, but more opioid analgesia.

The safety of peppermint in pregnancy has been debated frequently in the professional arena. The whole plant, as used in herbal medicine, contains between 50 and 85% essential oil (Kenner & Requena 1996), with the major constituents being 50% menthol, 19% menthone and between 0.1-2% *d*-pulegone, a recognised hepatotoxin (Tisserand & Balacs 1995:160; Nair 2001). Another constituent, menthofuran, has been likened to cytochrome P450 mono-oxygenase, found in the human liver (Bertea et al 2001; Lupien et al 1999). A proprietary product containing menthol has been reported as causing confusion and delirium (O'Mullane et al 1982), although this was not peppermint oil. Although there are some reports of neurotoxicity in rats administered peppermint oil (Olsen & Thorup 1984; Eickholt & Box 1965), doses were far in excess of those which would be administered to humans, either as a herbal remedy or in an essential oil blend for aromatherapy. The neurotoxic effects were attributed more to the pulegone and/or menthone content than the menthol (Thorup et al 1983) but the amount used in aromatherapy or herbal medicine is unlikely to cause adverse effects. Spearmint oil contains less pulegone and may be an acceptable alternative. Dermal and phototoxicity is minimal in peppermint oil (Schempp et al 2002; Nair 2001).

More significantly, menthol cord dressings administered to babies with a deficiency of glucose-6 phosphate dehydrogenase (G6PD) have triggered severe neonatal jaundice leading to kernicterus (Olowe & Ransome-Kuti 1980). Since detoxification of menthol is via a metabolic pathway involving G6PD, any deficiency will cause an accumulation of the substance, which may eventually lead to more serious neurological complications. Although the amount of peppermint oil used by pregnant woman to relieve nausea and vomiting will be minimal, it may be wise to avoid its use in women with a family history of G6PD.

Vasodilatation can occur when inhaling peppermint (Rakieten & Rakieten 1957) and bradycardia has occurred in a case of addiction to menthol cigarettes (de Smet et al 1992). It is recommended that anyone with cardiac fibrillation should avoid using peppermint oil (Tisserand & Balacs 1995:161), and Valli and Giardina (2002) suggest that cardiologists should become familiar with any available data on the impact of herbs on the cardiovascular system. However, it is the view of this author that *all* herbal medicines are contraindicated in pregnant women with any cardiac or other major medical condition, especially those which are pre-existing.

Other herbal remedies

Stapleton (2000) suggests several alternative herbal teas or medicines, including camomile,

Practice point
Peppermint oil is contraindicated in women with any cardiac condition, epilepsy and a family history of G6PD.

hops, fennel and slippery elm, possibly in combination. Camomile is a generic name for several different types, including German camomile (*Matricaria chamomilla*) and Roman camomile (*Anthemis nobilis*). Women could be advised to sip a tea made from the fresh or dried plant, but caution is advocated if the essential oil is used, particularly as nausea and vomiting most commonly occurs in the first trimester. Roman camomile is not approved by the German Commission E for safety reasons (Ernst et al 2002:178), although Tisserand and Balacs (1995:111) dispute the concerns. There is some suggestion that camomile may potentiate the action of anticoagulants (Ernst et al 2002:189); high concentrations of the essential oil on the skin may cause irritation (Van Ketel 1981), and a case of anaphylactic shock from the tea has been reported (ISA 1993:67).

Hops have a long history in traditional medicine as a sedative, and hop pillows are popular with people who have difficulty in sleeping, although only one study has been found to test this, in which the addition of valerian, another sedative plant (Gerhard et al 1996) may have complicated the picture. No suggestion of its use for sickness could be found in recent research-based literature. Ernst et al (2002:125) identify possible adverse effects such as allergy, leading to dermatitis or respiratory difficulties, and anaphylaxis, and a theoretical risk of menstrual cycle disruption; they advise against its use in pregnancy and lactation, and it is therefore best used only under the direction of a qualified medical herbalist. *Fennel*, similar to peppermint in action, may also cause allergic reactions (Ernst et al 2002: 168), but as there is also some suggestion that the oestrogenic action of the essential oil makes it emmenagoguic, this precludes its use during pregnancy. The evidence for the use of these other herbal remedies appears to be inconclusive, and although women will continue to purchase the teas such as camomile, it is professionally expedient to proceed cautiously with any advice about their benefits until more data are available regarding the possible hazards.

CONCLUSION

Herbal medicines and essential oils may provide additional strategies for helping women to cope with gestational sickness. However it is vital that they are made aware of the pharmacological nature of the remedies they wish to self-administer, and do not automatically assume that, because they are natural products, they are therefore safe. Ginger is a commonly used herbal remedy for sickness in pregnancy but is not appropriate for every woman and can occasionally exacerbate the problem; these women may respond better to peppermint. Healthcare professionals must appreciate the need to select the most appropriate remedy and ensure that any advice which they give to women is accurate and comprehensive, taking into account the potential hazards as well as the positive factors.

REFERENCES

Ager C 2002 A complementary therapy clinic: making it work. RCM Midwives Journal 5 (6): 198-200

Agrawal O P et al 1980 Antifertility effects of fruits of juniperus communis. Plant Medica 39: 98-101. Cited in Tisserand R, Balacs T 1995 Essential oil safety: a guide for health professionals. Churchill Livingstone, Edinburgh

Al-Hader A A, Hasan Z A, Aqel M B 1994 Hyperglycaemic and insulin release inhibitory effects of Rosmarinus officinalis. Journal of Ethnopharmacology 43: 217-221

Allaire A D, Moos M K, Wells S R 2000 Complementary and alternative medicine in pregnancy: a survey of North Carolina certified nurse-midwives. Obstetrics and Gynecology 95 (1): 19-23

Amato P, Christophe S, Mellon P L 2002 Estrogenic activity of herbs commonly used as remedies for menopausal symptoms. Menopause 992: 145-150

Ang-Lee M K, Moss J, Yuan C S 2001 Herbal medicines and perioperative care. Journal of the American Medical Association 286 (2): 208-216

Araujo I B, Souza C A, De-Carvalho R R et al 1996 Study of the embryofoetotoxicity of alpha-terpinene in the rat. Food and Chemical Toxicology 34 (5): 477-482

Arfeen Z, Owen H, Plummer J L et al 1995 A double-blind randomised controlled trial of ginger for the prevention of postoperative nausea and vomiting. Anaesthesia Intensive Care 23 (4): 449-452

Asao T, Mochiki E, Suzuki H et al 2001 An easy method for the intraluminal administration of peppermint oil before colonoscopy and its effectiveness in reducing colonic spasm. Gastrointestinal Endoscopy 53(2):172-7

Atkinson M 2002 Crisis in Europe – the European Directive on Food Supplements. Journal of the Complementary Medical Association August 2002

Ayabe-Kanamura S, Schicker I, Iasaka M at el 1998 Differences in perception of everyday odors: a Japanese-German cross-cultural study. Chemical Senses 23 (1): 31-38

Balacs T 1991 Essential issues. International Journal of Aromatherapy 3 (4): 23-5

Balacs T 1992 Safety in pregnancy. International Journal of Aromatherapy 4 (1): 12-15

Bergner P 1991 Is ginger safe in pregnancy? Medical Herbalism 3: 3

Bertea C M, Schalk M, Karp F et al 2001 Demonstration that menthofuran synthase of mint (Mentha) is a cytochrome P450 mono-oxygenase: cloning, functional expression and characterisation of the responsible gene. Archives of Biochemistry and Biophysiology 390 (2): 279-286

Betts J M et al 1998 Gas chromatographic determination of toxic quinolizidine alkaloids in blue cohosh Caulophyllum thalictroides (L). Phytochemical Analysis 9: 232-236

Bone M E, Wilkinson D J, Young J R et al 1990 Ginger root – a new antiemetic. The effect of ginger root on postoperative nausea and vomiting after major gynaecological surgery. Anaesthesia 45 (8): 669-671

Boyland E, Chasseur F 1970 The effects of some carbonyl compounds on rat liver glutathione levels. Biochemical Pharmacology 19: 1526-1528

British Medical Association 1993 Complementary medicine: new approaches to good practice. Oxford University Press, Oxford

Brown K 2000 Scary spice. New Scientist 168: 2270/2271: 53

Buchbauer G, Jirovetz L, Jager W et al 1991 Aromatherapy: evidence for sedative effects of the essential oil of lavender upon inhalation. Zeitschrift fur Naturforschung

C 46 (11-12): 1067-1072

Buchbauer G, Jirovetz L, Jager W et al 1993 Fragrance compounds and essential oils with sedative effects upon inhalation. Journal of Pharmaceutical Sciences 82 (6): 660-664

Burns E, Blamey C, Ersser S et al 1999 The use of aromatherapy in intrapartum midwifery practice: an observational study. OCHRAD, Oxford

Cada A M, Hansen D K, LaBorde J B et al 2001 Minimal effects from developmental exposure to St John's wort (Hypericum perforatum) in Sprague-Dawley rats. Nutrition in Neuroscience 4 (2): 135-141

Cahill D J, Fox R, Wardle P G et al 1994 Multiple follicular development associated with herbal medicine. Human Reproduction 9 (8): 1469-1480

Carson C F, Hammer K M, Riley T V 1996 In vitro activity of the essential oil of Melaleuca alternifolia against Streptococcus spp. Journal of Antimicrobial Chemotherapy 37 (6): 421-424

Chin R K 1991 Ginseng and common pregnancy disorders. Asia Oceania Journal of Obstetrics and Gynaecology 17: 379-380

Committee on Safety of Medicines 2000 Important interactions between St John's wort (Hypericum perforatum) preparations and prescribed medicines. Open letter to doctors and pharmacists. Department of Health, London

Coopersmith R, Leon M 1986 Enhanced neural response by adult rats to odors experienced early in life. Brain Research 371 (2): 400-403

Cupp M J 1999 Herbal remedies: adverse effects and drug interactions. American Family Physician 59 (5): 1239-1245

Dale A, Cornwell S 1994 The role of lavender oil in relieving perineal discomfort following childbirth: a blind randomised clinical trial. Journal of Advanced Nursing 19 (1): 89-96

D'Arcy P F 1991 Adverse reactions and interactions with herbal medicines. Part 1: adverse reactions. Adverse Drug Reactions and Toxicological Reviews 10 (4): 189-208

Davies S J, Harding L M, Baranowski A P 2002 A novel treatment of postherpetic neuralgia using peppermint oil. Clinical Journal of Pain 18 (3): 200-202

De Groot A C, Weyland J W 1996 Airborne allergic contact dermatitis from tea tree oil. Contact Dermatitis 35 (5): 304-305

Deltito J, Beyer D 1998 The scientific, quasi-scientific and popular literature on the use of St John's wort in the treatment of depression. Journal of Affective Disorders 51 (3): 345-351

De Smet P A G M, Keller K, Hansel R, Chandler R F (eds) 1992 Adverse effects of herbal drugs, volume 2. Springer-Verlag, Heidelberg

Domokos J D, Hethelyi E, Palinkas J et al 1997 Essential oil of rosemary (Rosmarinus officinalis) of Hungarian origin. Journal of Essential Oil Research 9: 41-45

Duthie H L 198 The effect of peppermint oil on colonic activity in man. British Journal of Surgery 68: 820

Eickholt T H, Box R H 1965 Toxicities of peppermint and Pycnanthemum albescens oils, Fam. Labiatae. Journal of Pharmaceutical Sciences 54: 1071-1072

Einarson A, Lawrimore T, Brand P et al 2000 Attitudes and practices of physicians and naturopaths toward herbal products, including use during pregnancy and lactation. Canadian Journal of Clinical Pharmacology 7 (1): 45-49

El Tahir K E H, Ashour M M S, Al-Harbi M M 1993 The cardiovascular actions of the volatile oil of the black seed (Nigella sativa) in rats: elucidation of the mechanism of action. General Pharmacology 24 (5): 1123-1131

Erick M 1995 Hyperolfaction and hyperemesis gravidarum: what is the relationship? Nutritional Review 53 (10): 289-295

Ernst E 2002 The risk-benefit profile of commonly used herbal therapies: Ginkgo, St John's wort, ginseng, echinacea, saw palmetto and kava. Annals of Internal Medicine 136 (1): 42-53

Ernst E, Pittler M H, Stevinson C et al 2001 The desktop guide to complementary and alternative medicine. Mosby, London

Ernst E, Pittler M H 2000 Efficacy of ginger for nausea and vomiting: a systematic review of randomised clinical trials. British Journal of Anaesthesia 84 (3): 367-371

Ernst E, Schmidt K 2002 Health risks over the Internet: advice offered by 'medical herbalists' to a pregnant woman Wiener Medizinische Wochenschrift 152 (7-8): 190-192

Falk-Filipsson A 1993 d-limonene exposure to humans by inhalation: uptake, distribution, elimination and effects on the pulmonary system. Journal of Toxicology and Environmental Health 38: 77-88

Fessenden J M, Wittenborn W, Clarke L 2001 Ginkgo biloba: a case report of herbal medicine and bleeding postoperatively from a laparoscopic cholecystectomy. American Surgery 67 (1): 33-35

Fetrow C W 2000 Hot topics in healthcare: ginger (zingiber officinale) for motion sickness http://www.ahcpub.com Accessed 9.1.02

Fischer Rasmussen W et al 1991 Ginger treatment of hyperemesis gravidarum. European Journal of Obstetrics, Gynecology and Reproductive Biology 38: 19

Fleming T 2001 Physician desk reference for herbal medicine, 2nd edn. Medical Economics Co, New Jersey

Foundation for Integrated Medicine 1997 Integrated healthcare: a way forward for the next five years? FIM, London

Foundation for Integrated Medicine 2002 Integrated Health: News 10: 3 April

Fugh Berman A 2000 Herb-drug interactions. Lancet 355 (9198): 134-138

Fulder S, Tenne M 1996 Ginger as an anti-nausea remedy in pregnancy: the issue of safety. Herbalgram 38: 47-50

Gallo M, Koren G 2001 Can herbal products be used safely during pregnancy? Focus on echinacea. Canadian Family Physician 47: 1727-1728

Gallo M et al 2000 Pregnancy outcome following gestational exposure to echinacea. Archives of Internal Medicine 160: 3141-3143

Giachetti D, Taddei E, Taddei I 1988 Pharmacological activity of essential oils on Oddi's sphincter. Plant Medica 54 (5): 389-392

Gibson P S, Powrie R, Star J 2001 Herbal and alternative medicine use during pregnancy: a cross-sectional survey. Obstetrics and Gynecology 97 (4 suppl 1): S44-45

Giordano-Labardie F, Schwarze H P, Bazex J 2000 Allergic contact dermatitis from camomile used in phytotherapy. Contact Dermatitis 42 (4): 247

Greenspan E 1983 Ginseng and vaginal bleeding. Journal of the American Medical Association 249 (15): 2018

Grontved A et al 1988 Ginger root against seasickness: a controlled trial in the open sea. Acta Otolaryngology105:

45-49

Grontved A, Hentzer E 1986 Vertigo-reducing effect of ginger root. Journal of Otorhinolaryngology Related Specialties 48: 282-286

Grush L R et al 1998 St John's wort during pregnancy. Journal of the American Medical Association 280: 1566

Gunn T R, Wright I M 1996 The use of black and blue cohosh in labour. New Zealand Medical Journal 109: 410-411

Gurr F W, Scroggie J G 1965 Eucalyptus oil poisoning treated by dialysis and mannitol infusion with an appendix on the analysis of biological fluids for alcohol and eucalyptol. Australasian Annals of Medicine 14 (3): 238-249

Hardcastle A B, Hardcastle P T, Taylor C J 1996 Influence of peppermint oil on absorptive and secretory processes in rat small intestine. Gut 39: 214-219

Heinrichs L 2002 Linking olfaction with nausea and vomiting of pregnancy, recurrent abortion, hyperemesis gravidarum and migraine headache. American Journal of Obstetrics and Gynecology 186 (5 suppl): S215-219

Hepner D L, Harnett M, Segal S et al 2002 Herbal medicine use in parturients. Anesthesia and Analgesia 94 (3): 690-693

Hess F G Jr et al 1982 Reproduction study in rats of ginseng extract. Food Chemistry and Toxicology 20: 189-192

Hills J M, Aaronson P I 1991 The mechanism of action of peppermint oil on gastrointestinal muscle. An analysis using patch clamp electrophysiology and isolated tissue pharmacology in rabbit and guinea pig. Gastroenterology 10 (1): 55-65

Holtmann S et al 1989 The anti-motion sickness mechanism of ginger: a comparative study with placebo and dimenhydrinate. Acta Otolaryngology 108: 168-174

House of Lords Select Committee on Science and Technology 2000 Sixth report on complementary and alternative medicine. HMSO, London

Huang Q, Iwamoto M 1991 Anti-5-hydroxytryptamine3 effect galanacton, a diterpenoid isolated from ginger. Chemical and Pharmacological Bulletin (Tokyo) 39: 397-399

Hudson R, Distel H 1999 The flavour of life: perinatal development of odor and taste preferences. Schweizerische Medizinische Wochenschrift 129 (5): 176-181

Inoue T, Sugimoto Y, Masuda H et al 2001 Effects of peppermint (Mentha piperita L.) extracts on experimental allergic rhinitis in rats. Biological and Pharmacological Bulletin 24 (1): 92-95

International School of Aromatherapy 1993 A safety guide on the use of essential oils. Natural by Nature, London

Irikura B, Kennelly E J 1999 Blue cohosh: a word of caution. Alternative Therapies in Women's Health 1: 81-83

Jailwala J, Imperiale T F, Kroenenke K 2000 Pharmacologic treatment of the irritable bowel syndrome: a systematic review of randomised controlled trials. Annals of Internal Medicine 133 (2): 136-147

Janssen P L et al 1996 Consumption of ginger (Zingiber officinale) does not affect in vivo platelet thromboxane production in humans. European Journal of Clinical Nutrition 50: 772-774

Jensen-Jarolim E, Reder N, Fritsch R et al 1998 Fatal outcome of anaphylaxis to camomile-containing enema during labor: a case study. Journal of Allergy and Clinical Immunology 102 (6 Pt 1): 1041-1042

Jewell D, Young G 2000 Interventions for nausea and vomiting in early pregnancy. Cochrane Database (2) CD000145. Cochrane Review, Cochrane Library. Update Software, Oxford

Johanns E S, van der Kolk L E, van Gemert H M et al 2002 An epidemic of epileptic seizures after consumption of herbal tea. Nederlands Tijdschrift Geneeskunde 146 (17): 813-816

Johne A, Brockmoller J, Bauer S 1999 Pharmacokinetic interaction of digoxin with an herbal extract from St John's wort (Hypercium perforatum). Clinical Pharmacology and Therapeutics 66 (4): 338-345

Jones T K, Lawson B M 1998 Profound neonatal congestive heart failure caused by maternal consumption of blue cohosh herbal medication. Journal of Pediatrics 132: 550-2

Kajiyama Y, Fujii K, Takeuchi H et al 2002 Ginkgo seed poisoning. Pediatrics 109(2): 325-327

Kalb R, Trautman-Sponsel R D, Kieser M 2001 Efficacy and tolerability of hypericum extract WS 5572 versus placebo in mildly to moderately depressed patients. A randomised double-blind multicenter clinical trial. Pharmacopsychiatry 34(3): 96-103

Karamat E, Imberger J, Buchbauer G et al 1992 Excitory and sedative effects of essential oils on human reaction time performance. Chemical Senses 17 (4): 847

Katikova O I U, Kostin I A V, Iagudina R I et al 2001 Effect of plant preparations on lipid peroxidation parameters in acute toxic hepatitis (article in Russian) Vopr Med Khim 47 (6): 593-598 accessed via Pubmed on www.nccam.nih.gov September 2002

Keating A, Chez R A 2002 Ginger syrup as an antiemetic in early pregnancy. Alternative Therapies in Health and Medicine 8 (5): 89-91

Keeler R F 1988 Livestock models of human birth defects reviewed in relation to poisonous plants. Journal of Animal Science 66: 2414-2427

Kelly J 2002 Toxicity and adverse effects of herbal complementary therapy. Professional Nurse 17 (9): 562-565

Kenner D, Requena Y 1996 Botanical medicine : a European professional perspective. Paradigm Publications, Brookline, Massachusetts

Kikuchi A, Tanida M, Uenoyama S et al 1991 Effect of odors on cardiac response patterns in a reaction time task. Chemical Senses 16 (1): 183

Klepser T B, Klepser M E 1999 Unsafe and potentially safe herbal therapies. American Journal of Health System Pharmacy 56 (2): 125-138

Klier C M, Schafer M R, Schmid-Siegel B et al 2002 St John's wort (Hypericum perforatum) – is it safe during breastfeeding? Pharmacopsychiatry 35 (1): 29-30

Kline J P, Blackhart G C, Woodward K M 2000 Anterior electroencephalographic asymmetry: changes in elderly women in response to a pleasant and an unpleasant odor. Biological Psychology 52 (3): 241-250

Kline R M, Kline J J, Di Palma J et al 2001 Enteric-coated pH-dependent peppermint oil capsules for the treatment of irritable bowel syndrome in children. Journal of Pediatrics 138 (1): 125-128

Knasko S C 1992 Ambient odor's effect on creativity, mood and perceived health. Chemical Senses 17 (1): 27-35

Kobal G et al 1992 Differences in human chemosensory evoked potentials to olfactory and somatosensory chemical stimuli presented to left and right nostrils. Chemical Senses 17 (3): 233-244

Krone D, Mannel M, Pauli E et al 2001 Qualitative and quantitative olfactometric evaluation of different concentrations of ethanol peppermint oil solutions. Phytotherapy Research 15 (2): 135-138

Kuhn M A 2002 Herbal remedies: drug-herb interactions. Critical Care Nursing 22 (2): 22-28

Laing D G, Clark P J 1983 Puberty and olfactory preferences of males. Physiology and Behaviour 30 (4): 591-597

Langmead L, Rampton D S 2001 Review article: herbal treatment in gastrointestinal and liver disease – benefits and dangers. Alimentary Pharmacology 15 (9): 1239-1252

Li C, Homma M, Oka K 1998 Characteristics of delayed excretion of flavonoids in human urine after administration of Shosaiko-to, a herbal medicine. Biological and Pharmaceutical Bulletin 21 (12): 1251-1257

Lorig T S et al 1993 Visual event-related potentials during odour labelling. Chemical Senses 18 (4): 379-387

Lumb A 1994 Effect of dried ginger on human platelet function. Thrombosis and Haemostasis 71: 110-111

Lupien S, Karp F, Wildung M et al 1999 Regiospecific cytochrome P450 limonene hydroxylases from mint (Mentha) species: cDNA isolation, characterisation and functional expression of 4S-limonene-3-hydroxylase and 4S-limonene-6-hydroxylase. Archives of Biochemistry and Biophysics 368 (1): 181-192

Mabina M H et al 1997 The effect of traditional herbal medicines on pregnancy outcome: The King Edward VIII Hospital experience. South African Medical Journal 87: 1008-1010

Madisch A, Melderis H, Mayr G et al 2001 A plant extract and its modified preparation in functional dyspepsia. Results of a double-blind placebo-controlled comparative study. Zeitschrift fur Gastroenterologie 3997: 511-517

Madisch A, Heydenreich C J, Wieland V et al 1999 Treatment of functional dyspepsia with a fixed peppermint oil and caraway oil combination preparation as compared to cisapride. A multicenter, reference-controlled double-blind equivalence study. Arzneimittelforschung 49 (11): 925-932

Maliakal P P, Wanwimolruk S 2001 Effect of herbal teas on hepatic drug metabolizing enzymes in rats. Journal of Pharmacy and Pharmacology 53 (10): 1323-1329

Manley C H 1993 Psychophysiological effect of odour. Critical Reviews in Food Science and Nutrition 33 (1): 57-62

Masago R, Matsuda T, Kikuchi Y et al 2000 Effects of inhalation of essential oils in EEG activity and sensory evaluation. Journal of Physiological Anthropology and Applied Human Science 19 (1): 335-342

Mascher H, Kikuta C, Schiel H 2001 Pharmacokinetics of menthol and carvone after administration of an enteric coated formulation containing peppermint oil and caraway oil. Arzneimittelforschung 51 (6): 465-469

Marlier L, Schaal B, Soussignan R 1998 Bottle-fed neonates prefer an odor experienced in utero to an odor experienced postnatally in the feeding context. Developmental Psychobiology 33 (2): 133-145

May B, Kohler S, Schneider B 2000 Efficacy and tolerability of a fixed combination of peppermint oil and caraway oil in patients suffering from functional dyspepsia. Alimentary Pharmacology 14 (12): 1671-1677

McFarlin B L 1999 A national survey of herbal preparation use by nurse-midwives for labor stimulation. Review of the literature and recommendations for practice. Journal of Nurse-Midwifery 44: 205-216

McGeorge B C, Steele M C 1991 Allergic contact dermatitis of the nipple from Roman camomile ointment. Contact Dermatitis 24 (2): 139-140

McIntyre M 2001 Traditional medicine and childbirth. Paper presented at the Forum on Maternity and Newborn Conference on Complementary Therapies for Mothers and Babies, Royal Society of Medicine, London November 2001

Micklefield G H, Greving I, May B 2000 Effects of peppermint oil and caraway oil on gastroduodenal motility. Phytotherapy Research 14(1):20-3

Miller L G 1998 Herbal medicinals: selected clinical considerations focusing on known or potential drug-herb interactions. Archives of Internal Medicine 158 (20): 2200-2211

Millet Y, Jouglard J, Steinmetz M D et al 1981 Toxicity of some essential plant oils. Clinical and experimental study. Clinical Toxicology 18 (2): 1485-1498

Millot J L, Brand G, Morand N 2002 Effects of ambient odors on reaction time in humans. Neuroscience Letters 322 (2): 79-82

Mowrey D B, Clayson D E 1982 Motion sickness, ginger and psychophysics. Lancet 1: 655-657

Nagabhushan M, Amonkar A 1987 Mutagenicity of gingerol and shogaol and antimutagenicity of zingerone in Salmonella/microsomal assay. Cancer Letters 36: 221-223

Naganuma M, Hirose S, Nakayama Y et al 1985 A study of the phototoxicity of lemon oil. Archives of Dermatological Research 278 (1): 31-36

Nair B 2001 Final report on the safety assessment of Mentha Peperita (Peppermint) oil, Mentha Piperita (Peppermint) leaf extract, Mentha Piperita (Peppermint) leaf and Mentha Piperita (Peppermint) leaf water. International Journal of Toxicology 20 (Suppl 3): 61-73

Nathan P J 1999 The experimental and clinical pharmacology of St John's wort (Hypericum perforatum). Molecular Psychiatry 4 (4): 333-338

Nolte D L, Provenza F D, Callan R et al 1992 Garlic in the ovine fetal environment. Physiology and Behaviour 52 (6): 1091-1093

O'Brien B, Relyea M J 1999 Use of indigenous explanations and remedies to further understand nausea and vomiting during pregnancy. Health Care Women International 20 (1): 49-61

Occhiuto F, Limardi F, Circosta C 1995 Effects of the non-volatile residue from the essential oil of citrus bergamia on the central nervous system. International Journal of Pharmacology 33 (3): 198-203

Olowe S A, Ransome-Kuti O 1980 The risk of jaundice in glucose-6 phosphate dehydrogenase deficient babies exposed to menthol. Acta Paediatrica Scandinavica 69 (3): 341-345

Olsen P, Thorup I 1984 Neurotoxicity in rats dosed with peppermint oil and pulegone. Archives of Toxicology Suppl 7: 408-409

O'Mullane N M et al 1982 Adverse CNS effects of menthol-containing olbas oil. Lancet 1: 1121

Ondrizek R R, Chan P J, Patton W C et al 1999a An alternative medicine study of herbal effects on the penetration of zone-free hamster oocytes and the integrity of sperm deoxyribonucleic acid. Fertility and Sterility 71 (3): 517-522

Ondrizek R R, Chan P J, Patton W C et al 1999b Inhibition of human sperm motility by specific herbs used in alternative medicine. Journal of Assisted Reproduction and Genetics 16 (2): 87-91

Ortega J A, Lazerson J 1987 Anagyrine-induced red blood cell aplasia, vascular anomaly and skeletal dysplasia. Journal of Pediatrics 111: 87-89

Pages N, Fournier G, Baduel C et al 1990 Sabinyl acetate, the main component of Juniperus Sabina L'Herit essential oil, is responsible for anti-implantation effect Phytotherapy Research 10 (7): 438-440

Parsons M, Simpson M, Ponton T 1999 Raspberry leaf and its effect on labour: safety and efficacy. Journal of the Australian College of Midwives 12 (3): 20-25

Petty H R, Fernando M, Kindzelskii A L et al 2001 Identification of colchinine in placental blood from patients using herbal medicines. Chemical Research and Toxicology 14 (9): 1254-1258

Phillips S, Hutchinson S, Ruggier R 1993 Zingiber officinale does not affect gastric emptying rate. A randomised placebo-controlled crossover trial. Anaesthesia 48 (5): 393-395

Phillips S, Ruggier R, Hutchinson S E 1993 Zingiber officinale (ginger) – an antiemetic for day case surgery. Anaesthesia 48 (8): 715-717

Pimentel M, Bonorris G G, Chow E J et al 2001 Peppermint oil improves the manometric findings in diffuse esophageal spasm. Journal of Clinical Gastroenterology 33 (1): 27-31

Pinn G 2001 Herbs used in obstetrics and gynaecology. Australian Family Physician 30 (4): 351-354

Pinn G, Pallett L 2002 Herbal medicine in pregnancy. Complementary Therapies in Nursing and Midwifery 8 (2): 77-80

Power M L, Holzman G B, Schulkin J 2001 A survey on the management of nausea an vomiting in pregnancy by obstetricians/gynecologists. Primary Care Update in Obstetrics and Gynecology 8 (2): 69-72

Pradeepkumar V K, Tan K W, Ivy N G 1996 Is 'herbal health tonic' safe in pregnancy: fetal alcohol syndrome revisited. Australian and New Zealand Journal of Obstetrics and Gynaecology 36 (4): 420-423

Punnonen R, Lukola A 1980 Oestrogen-like effects of ginseng. British Medical Journal 281 (6248): 1110

Quian D S, Liu Z S 1992 Pharmacologic studies of antimotion sickness actions of ginger. Chung Kuo Chung His Chieh Ho Tsa Chih 12: 95-98

Rakieten N, Rakieten M L 1957 The effect of l-menthol on the systemic blood pressure. Journal of the American Pharmaceutical Association 46 (2): 82-84

Ratz A E, von Moos M, Drewe J 2001 St John's wort: a pharmaceutical with potentially dangerous interactions. Schweiz Rundschau-fur-Medizin und Praxis 90 (19): 843-849

Rayburn W F et al 2001 Effect of prenatally administered hypericum (St John's wort) on growth and physical maturation of mouse offspring. American Journal of Obstetrics and Gynecology 184: 191-195

Rayburn W F, Christensen H D, Gonzalez C L 2000 Effect of antental exposure to Saint John's wort (Hypericum) on neurobehaviour of developing mice. American Journal of Obstetrics and Gynecology 183 (5): 1225-1231

Recsan Z, Pagliuci G, Piretti M V et al 1997 Effect of essential oils on the lipids of the retina in the ageing rat: a possible therapeutic use. Journal of Essential Oil Research 9: 53-56

Rees W D, Evans B K, Rhodes J 1979 Treating irritable bowel syndrome with peppermint oil. British Medical Journal 2 (6194): 835-836

Reider N, Sepp N, Fritsch P et al 2000 Anaphylaxis to camomile: clinical features and allergen cross-reactivity. Clinical and Experimental Allergy 30 (10): 1436-1443

Reynolds J E F 1993 Martindale: the extra pharmacopoeia. The Pharmaceutical Press, London

Rosenberg Zand R S, Jenkins D J, Diamandis E P 2001 Effects of natural products and nutraceuticals on steroid hormone-regulated gene expression. Clin Chim Acta 312 (1-2): 213-219

Rudman D, Williams P J 1983 Megadose vitamins: use and misuse. New England Journal of Medicine 309 (8): 488-490

Santos F A, Rao V S N, Silveira E R 1996 Studies on the neuropharamcological effects of Psidium guyanensis and Psydium pohlianum essential oils. Phytotherapy Research 10: 655-658

Schempp C M, Schopf E, Simon J C 2002 Plant-induced toxic and allergic dermatitis (phytodermatitis). Hautarzt 53 (2): 93-97

Schrader E 2000 Equivalence of St John's wort extract (Ze 117) and fluoxetine: a randomised controlled study in mild-moderate depression. International Journal of Clinical Psychopharmacology 15 (2): 61-68

Schulten B, Bulitta M, Ballering-Bruhl B et al 2001 Efficacy of Echinacea purpurea in patients with a common cold. A placebo-controlled randomised double-blind clinical trial. Arzneimittelforschung 51 (7): 563-568

Scialli A, Fugh-Berman A 2001 Hot topics in healthcare: herbs and pregnancy http://www.ahcpub.com accessed 9.1.02

Scott G N, Elmer G W 2002 Update on natural product-drug interactions. American Journal of Health System Pharmacy 59 (4): 339-347

Shaw D 1997 Remedy or risk: guide to possible interactions and side-effects of herbal remedies. Pulse, 22 February

Shelton R C, Keller M B, Gelenberg A et al 2001 Effectiveness of St John's Wort in major depression: a randomised controlled trial. Journal of the American Medical Association 285 (15): 1978-1986

Simpson M, Parsons M, Greenwood J et al 2001 Raspberry leaf in pregnancy: its safety and efficacy in labor. Journal of Midwifery and Women's Health 46 (2): 51-59

Singer A, Wonnemann M, Muller W E 1999 Hyperforin, a major antidepressant constituent of St John's wort, inhibits serotonin uptake by elevating free intracellular Na+. Journal of Pharmacology and Experimental Therapeutics 290 (3): 1363-1368

Southwell I A, Markham C, Mann C 1997 Skin irritancy of tea tree oil. Journal of Essential Oil Research 9: 47-52

Spirling L I, Daniels I R 2001 Botanical perspectives on health peppermint: more than just an after-dinner mint. Journal of the Royal Society of Health 121 (1): 62-63

Spoerke D G, Vandenburg S A, Smolinske S C et al 1989 Eucalyptus oils: 14 cases of exposure. Veterinary and Human Toxicology 31 (2): 166-168

Stevinson C, Ernst E 2000 A pilot study of Hypericum perforatum for the treatment of premenstrual syndrome. British Journal of Obstetrics and Gynaecology 107 (7): 870-876

Stewart J J, Wood M J, Mims M E 1991 Effects of ginger on motion sickness susceptibility and gastric function.

Pharmacology 42: 111-120

Tate S 1997 Peppermint oil: a treatment for postoperative nausea. Journal of Advanced Nursing 26 (3): 543-549

Thorup I et al 1983 Short-term toxicity study in rats dosed with pulegone and menthol. Toxicology Letters 19 (3): 207-210

Tiran D 2000 Clinical aromatherapy for pregnancy and childbirth, 2nd edn. Harcourt, London

Tiran D 2001 Complementary strategies in antenatal care. Complementary Therapies in Nursing and Midwifery 7 (1): 19-24

Tisserand R, Balacs T 1995 Essential oil safety: a guide for health professionals. Churchill Livingstone, Edinburgh

Trabace L, Avato P, Mazzoccoli M et al 1992 Choleretic activity of some typical components of essential oils. Planta Medica 58 (suppl 1a): 650-651

Tsui B, Dennehy C E, Tsourounis C 2001 A survey of dietary supplement use during pregnancy at an academic medical center. American Journal of Obstetrics and Gynecology 185 (2): 433-437

Umezu T, Sakata A, Ito H 2001 Ambulation-promoting effect of peppermint oil and identification of its active constituents. Pharmacology and Biochemical Behaviour 69 (3-4): 383-390

Unnikrishan M, Kuttan R 1988 Cytotoxicity of extracts of spices to cultured cells. Nutrition in Cancer 11: 251-257

Vaes L P, Chyka P A 2000 Interactions of warfarin with garlic, ginger, ginkgo or ginseng: nature of the evidence. Annals of Pharmacology 34 (12): 1478-1482

Vale S 1998 Subarachnoid haemorrhage associated with ginkgo biloba. Lancet 352 (9121): 36

Valli G, Giardina E G 2002 Benefits, adverse effects and drug interactions of herbal therapies with cardiovascular effects. Journal of the American College of Cardiologists 39 (7): 1083-1095

Van Ketel W G 1981 Allergy to Matricaria chamomilla. Contact Dermatitis 8 (2): 143

Verma S et al 1993 Effect of ginger on platelet aggregation in man. Indian Journal of Medical Research 98: 240-242

Viollon C, Mandin D, Chaumont J P 1996 Antagonistic activities in vitro of some essential oils and natural volatile compounds in relation to the growth of Trichomonas vaginalis. Fitoterapia 67 (3): 279-280

Visalyaputra S, Petchpaisit N, Somcharoen K et al 1998 The efficacy of ginger root in the prevention of postoperative nausea and vomiting after outpatient gynaecological laparoscopy. Anaesthesia 53: 506-510

Vonau B, Chard S, Mandalia S et al 2001 Does the extract of the plant Echinacea purpurea influence the clinical course of recurrent genital herpes? International Journal of Sexually Transmitted Disease 12 (3): 145-148; Journal of Family Practice 48 (8): 615-619

Vutyavanich T, Kraisarin T, Ruangsri R 2001 Ginger for nausea and vomiting in pregnancy: randomized double-masked, placebo-controlled trial. Obstetrics and Gynecology 97 (4): 577-582

Wagner P J, Jester D, LeClair B et al 1999 Taking the edge off: why patients choose St John's wort . Journal of Family Practice 48 (8): 615-619

Wargovich M J, Woods C, Hollis D M et al 2001 Herbals, cancer prevention and health. Journal of Nutrition 131 (1 Suppl): 3034S-30346S

Webb N J A, Pitt W R 1993 Eucalyptus oil poisoning in childhood: 41 cases in southeast Queensland. Journal of Paediatrics and Child Health 29: 368-371

Weidner M S, Sigwart K 2001 Investigation of the teratogenic potential of a zingiber officinale extract in the rat. Reproductive Toxicology 15 (1): 75-80

West Z 2001 Acupuncture in pregnancy and childbirth. Churchill Livingstone, Edinburgh

Wiebe E 2000 A randomised trial of aromatherapy to reduce anxiety before abortion. Effective Clinical Practice 3 (4): 166-169

Wilkinson J M 2000 What do we know about herbal morning sickness treatments? A literature survey. Midwifery 16 (3): 224-228

Wilkinson K M 2000 Effect of ginger tea on the fetal development of Sprague-Dawley rats. Reproductive Toxicology 14 (6): 507-512

Winship K A 1991 Toxicity of comfrey. Adverse Drug Reactions and Toxicological Reviews 10: 47-59

Wood C D, Manno J E, Wood M J et al 1988 Comparison of efficacy of ginger with various antimotion sickness drugs. Clinical Research Practices and Drug Regulatory Affairs 6 (2): 129-136

Wysocki C J, Pelchat M L 1993 The effects of aging on the human sense of smell and its relationship to food choice. Critical Reviews in Food Science and Nutrition 33 (1): 63-82

Yamada K, Mimaki Y, Sashida Y 1994 Anticonvulsive effects of inhaling lavender oil vapour. Biological and Pharmaceutical Bulletin 17 (2): 359-360

Yarnell E 1997 Botanical medicine in pregnancy and lactation. Alternative and Complementary Therapies 3 (2): 93-100

6

The homeopathic approach

This chapter begins with a brief history of homeopathy in order to explore the differences between homeopathic and conventional pharmaceutical prescribing. There follows an examination of some of the evidence for its safety and efficacy. Various 'prescriptions' of appropriate homeopathic remedies for specific symptom pictures of gestational nausea and vomiting are presented.

HISTORICAL PERSPECTIVES

Homeopathy is a complete system of complementary healthcare, founded by the German doctor Samuel Hahnemann in the late 18th century. At that time disease was viewed as an invasion on the body which had to be fought by chemical or other means such as purging with emetics and blood letting with leeches. Toxic chemicals including arsenic and mercury were used in attempts to rid the body of disease. Hahnemann became increasingly disillusioned with conventional medicine and finally withdrew from practice. He also challenged the apothecaries of the day who frequently used complex combinations of drugs, which were often adulterated and for which high prices were charged to the public, and began using ever-decreasing doses of medications for his own patients. Having originally practised in Germany he eventually moved to Paris on his second marriage and continued to see patients from all over Europe until well into his eighties.

Unlike conventional medicine which suppresses symptoms by treating with opposites, homeopathy works on the principle of treating like with like, or *similia similibus curentur*. An example of this is the condition of constipation, for which conventional medicine would use laxatives to induce diarrhoea, whereas homeopaths would use a minute amount of a substance known to cause constipation. Hahnemann's theories developed from his questioning of malaria treatment with cinchona bark, thought to be effective due to its bitterness. He experimented by taking the substance himself and found that he was able to induce the physical and mental symptoms of malaria, although he was essentially healthy. He investigated further, which confirmed the *Law of Similars* from which the term 'homeopathy' originated, derived from the Greek *homios* (similar) and *pathos* (suffering or disease). This work with cinchona – now more commonly called China – is the process of 'proving', in which healthy volunteers are given doses of the test substance in order to elicit a symptom picture of the proposed remedy, and is still in use today. Easily comprehended examples in modern use are the administration of homeopathic doses of coffea (from the green coffee bean) to treat insomnia and of apis (from the bee) to relieve stings and histamine-type reactions.

Hahnemann had previously noted the effectiveness of mercury in treating syphilis, but his theory was based not on the popular idea that mercury caused purging in the form of increased salivation, perspiration, diuresis and diarrhoea, but because it triggered 'mercurial fever' with symptoms similar to those it was attempting to cure. In essence, this was a proving for mercury. His discovery of the phenomenon of the ability of substances to produce symptoms of a disease as well as to cure it was the fledgling *Law of Cure* which is a component of modern homeopathic practice. His theory was, in fact, similar to those of Hippocrates in the 4th century, who advocated treating vomiting with emetics, and of Paracelsus in the 15th century, who successfully treated plague victims by administering a tablet of bread mixed

with a minute amount of the patient's own excreta (Kayne 1997:23). Unfortunately, a 2001 attempt to demonstrate a 'proving' in a randomised double-blind placebo-controlled administration of homeopathic mercury to volunteers failed to produce any significant evidence that the mercury produced more symptoms than the placebo (Vickers et al 2001).

Hahnemann began to use this theory in his medical practice but found that undesirable side-effects occurred from continual use of the crude substances, so he experimented with increasingly small doses, eventually diluting the doses to the extent where nothing therapeutic happened. He then introduced the practice of vigorously shaking, or *succussing*, the remedies as they were prepared, which appeared to potentise them, making them more effective and with fewer unwanted side-effects.

Many of Hahnemann's conventional medical colleagues were sceptical until a fatal epidemic of scarlet fever in 1812 prompted them to test, with good effect, his theory that the symptoms of Belladonna toxicity reflected the symptom picture of this childhood illness. Over the following years Hahnemann tested a range of active substances on himself, his family and healthy volunteers to accumulate evidence and elicit the provings for other remedies. In contemporary homeopathy, provings may be undertaken in a comparable, experimental manner, or may be discovered as a result of acute, chronic, voluntary or accidental clinical toxicological effects. Clinical therapeutic observation also plays a part. The comprehensive drug/remedy pictures are then collated into *Materia Medica*, of which there are many different formats, with several now being computerised for more speedy, comprehensive and accurate homeopathic prescribing.

The first British homeopath is considered to have been Dr Frederick Hervey Foster Quin, who founded the London Homeopathic Hospital in 1850. The rise in popularity of homeopathy occurred initially as a result of an acknowledgement of the different mortality rates of cholera patients treated with homeopathy compared with conventional medicine, although this may also have been due in part to the withdrawal of conventional treatments which in themselves were potentially fatal. Other notable British homeopaths included the Liverpool-based Dr Dudgeon, who is also widely known for his construction of the first sphygmomanometer, and several Glasgow-based doctors in the 20th century including Dr Margery Blackie, the first woman to be appointed as Royal Physician.

American homeopathy began in 1825 when the Danish Dr Gram emigrated to New York, followed shortly afterwards by several German physicians, including Dr Constantine Hering, who practised homeopathy within the German communities. By the 1880s there were over 20 homeopathic medical educational establishments but there appeared to be a gradual move away from the original holistic teachings of Hahnemann. It was Dr James Tyler Kent, practising in St Louis, who became one of the most prominent teachers and practitioners of homeopathy in the late 19th century and who is credited with a return to the Hahnemann philosophy of homeopathic practice. The mid-20th century all but saw the demise of the system in the USA but a worldwide resurgence in complementary medicine appears to have arrested this decline. Homeopathy has been embraced by many other countries, including Australia, New Zealand, India, Canada, South Africa and several other areas of Europe.

Homeopathic prescribing is something of an alien concept to healthcare professionals trained in conventional methods, as appropriate selection of treatment is based on matching the precise nature of the patient's symptoms to a specific remedy, rather than identification of a condition which demands a particular drug. Furthermore, the patient's moods and personality are taken into account, together with *all* other factors, however apparently insignificant. Despite this difference, homeopathy was the only aspect of complementary and alternative medicine to be included at the inception of the British National Health Service in 1948, with five NHS hospitals designated as centres for both conventional and homeopathic medicine. In contemporary healthcare many general practitioners incorporate homeopathy into their normal practice, selecting whichever modality best suits the patient's needs. Homeopathy is now classified as one of the 'Big Five' complementary therapies, a discrete system of medicine in its own right (BMA 1993; FIM 1997; House of Lords 2000).

RESEARCH IN HOMEOPATHY

Although there is a growing body of evidence regarding the efficacy of homeopathic remedies, the acceptance of such research has been limited because the medical profession demands rigor in the form of the standard randomised double-blind controlled trial. However this is at variance with the way in which homeopathic prescribing is undertaken, individualising to each patient and taking into account every nuance of the person's condition. This often means that two people with the same disease 'label' (in conventional terms) but with different manifestations of the condition will require different homeopathic remedies. This can easily be seen in the debate later in this chapter on prescribing remedies for women with gestational sickness, in which every factor is considered relevant to the choice of prescription.

It is therefore problematic, when undertaking homeopathic research, to select two comparable groups, one for the test substance and one as control, to receive either a placebo or conventional treatment or none. One answer to this is to accumulate very large numbers, or to select a group of test subjects to receive a constitutional remedy (see above). Merrell and Shalts (2002) identify the difficulty of this 'differential therapeutics', which is an essential requirement for successful homeopathic practice, and one which only well-trained homeopathic practitioners are able to undertake. They suggest that remedies used in combination, individualised to one patient, cannot be appropriately applied to all subjects in a study exploring a specified condition, because the manifestation of the condition will be different in each person. Furthermore, the success of homeopathy cannot adequately be assessed by the collation of data from trials of one condition.

Preparation of the remedies is not standardised between producers or across countries, and although several brands of a specific remedy of a specific potency are likely to be sufficiently similar to be equally homeopathically effective, the differences have been challenged by orthodox medical researchers. Measurement of test parameters is also more difficult to define in homeopathic research because standard pharmaceutical research focuses on studying the potent and toxic effects of chemical preparations. This does not take account of the way in which homeopathy works by facilitating the body's own innate healing capacity without disturbing the functioning of the body, unlike drugs which may inhibit a disease process yet trigger other unpleasant symptoms. Additionally, it is difficult to eliminate the placebo response as accurate homeopathic prescribing is dependent on acquiring a lengthy case history which may, in itself, have a therapeutic effect. Finally, there may be 'publishing bias' (Kayne 1997:166), with positive results being published in journals of complementary medicine, which are more elusive to practitioners of orthodox medicine. 'Editorial censorship' (Schiff 1995) also features, in which work is rejected on supposed technicalities of the research methodology as a way of preventing new ideas from being publicised.

There is even less evidence available to demonstrate the mechanism by which homeopathy works and Ernst et al (2001:54) state that 'there is no scientific rationale for assuming that remedies devoid of pharmacologically active molecules can produce clinical effects'. However, these reviewers fail to acknowledge here that homeopathy does not, and never has, presumed to work pharmacologically, but instead is considered a form of 'energy' or vibrational medicine. What exactly this energy medicine constitutes remains under debate, but scientists should not dismiss a concept simply because they are unable to define it in contemporary terms. Ernst et al (2001:54) cite a scientific evaluation of homeopathy undertaken in Nazi Germany in the 1930s which, although unpublished, did not reveal any evidence in its favour, yet they do not debate the factors contributing

to the apparent success of homeopathic medicines in many recent trials. Its effectiveness cannot be wholly attributed to the placebo effect as veterinary homeopathy is frequently shown to have therapeutic benefits.

Investigations into the actions of homeopathic remedies have been undertaken by Boyd (1941), who demonstrated statistically significant effects of microdoses of mercuric chloride on the diastase activity of germinating seeds. It is often difficult for those working in conventional healthcare to understand how so minute a dose of the original substance can be increasingly more effective the more it is diluted, when modern pharmaceuticals depend on increasing the dose to maintain a therapeutic effect, yet at the risk of increasing the incidence of side-effects.

The most notable study was conducted by Benveniste, an immunologist, and his colleagues (Davenas et al 1988), who tested highly diluted doses of an antibody on human basophils with IgE on the surface. When exposed to anti-IgE antibodies the basophils release histamine from the intracellular granules and their staining properties are altered. In this investigation, increasingly diluted and succussed anti-IgE antibody solutions were prepared until there were theoretically no molecules left, yet the solution continued to produce a staining alteration from the immune cells, down to a dilution of 10^{-120}, equivalent to a homeopathic potency of 60C. The work of Benveniste and his colleagues appeared, at the time, to come closest to determining exactly how homeopathy works, with the theory that water molecules retained the 'memory' of a substance which had been diluted in it, even when there was little likelihood of a single molecule of the original substance remaining within the highly diluted preparation.

Unfortunately, although the work was published in the prestigious scientific journal *Nature*, after a three year delay, sceptical and disapproving colleagues sought to disprove the findings and discredit the research team. A concurrent disclaimer was included in the same issue of the journal expressing incredulity about the theory, and subsequently a team was sent to evaluate the results. Despite further attempts to replicate the findings, the credibility of the studies was again questioned and eventually funding for Benveniste's team was withdrawn. No other work since has yet reached any conclusions regarding the mode of action of homeopathy, although quantum physicists continue to investigate the subject.

A meta-analysis of 107 clinical trials by three professors of medicine who were not homeopaths (Kleijnen et al 1991) found that the remedies used were effective in 81 of the trials, ineffective in 24 and inconclusive in two, although they found only 22 in which the methodology was 'acceptable', of which 15 demonstrated that homeopathy was effective. A 1997 meta-analysis (Linde et al 1997) showed that homeopathy was 2.45 times more likely than placebo to initiate clinical improvements, although the report was much criticised for its assumptions. Other systematic reviews have failed to concur with such positive results (Ernst & Pittler 1998; Ernst & Barnes 1998; Ernst 1999).

Jonas et al (2001) conducted a systematic review of all English publications of homeopathic research between 1945 and 1995, of which 59 studies met the inclusion criteria for the review. Most studies were small, single-site, non-replicated investigations. Methodology was considered to be weak when compared to trials of conventional medicine, with 86% of research teams failing to identify confounding variables. Almost half of the studies failed to use random selection, less than one third had a placebo control group and only 79% were published in peer-reviewed journals. Gradual improvements were seen in more recent investigations, but the authors of the review stress the need for further development in methodology in order to improve the credibility of trials of homeopathic medicines.

Similar criticism of methodology was made in the systematic review to evaluate the safety of homeopathic remedies by exploring reports of adverse effects (Dantas & Rampes 2000). While the mean incidence of adverse effects was greater in the homeopathic group than placebo, only short-term, minor effects were reported and there appear to be very few accounts of complications and side-effects published in homeopathic journals, many of which are not well documented. Those available seem to report aggravation of current symptoms, or pathogenetic effects in healthy volunteers, but these are very much in keeping with homeopathic theoretical principles. It was pointed out that reports of adverse reactions were published in conventional medical journals, but occasionally these related to mislabelled homeopathic products rather than to true homeopathic remedies.

Investigations into specific uses of homeopathic remedies are increasing, many of which are undertaken by homeopaths who are also medically qualified doctors. For example, Reilly et al (1989) questioned the placebo effect in using homeopathy for hayfever symptoms, using a randomised, double-blind, placebo-controlled system and taking great care to emphasise the rigour of their methododology. They concluded that the beneficial effects of homeopathic remedies were greater than simply a placebo response. Davidson et al (1997) described the case of a woman apparently treated successfully with homeopathy in combination with fluoxetine for depression and anxiety, but single case reports are of limited value in convincing sceptics who practise conventional medicine, even though they add to the overall body of evidence. Fisher and Scott (2001), however, found no evidence that rheumatoid arthritis symptoms were improved with homeopathic medicines when compared to placebo.

Large case-reporting of efficacy of homeopathic medicines for chronic illness in patients for whom conventional treatment is ineffective, short-term or contraindicated, may be of value in partially excluding the placebo effect. An audit of 829 consecutive patients treated with homeopathic medicines showed that 61% had a sustained improvement, from 'good' (18%) to 'excellent' (43%), while only 0.8% found their condition worsened (Sevar 2000).

USE OF HOMEOPATHY FOR WOMEN'S REPRODUCTIVE HEALTH

Within general healthcare, Astin et al (1998) found that Californian physicians were more likely to recommend or refer for acupuncture (43%) or chiropractic (40%) than for homeopathy (9%), which corresponded to their beliefs in the efficacy of the different modalities (chiropractic 53%; acupuncture 51%; homeopathy 26%). Pirotta et al (2000) surveyed 488 Australian GPs (a 64% response rate from an initial 800 contacts) to determine their attitudes towards complementary therapies. They found that over 80% had referred to complementary practitioners; 23% practised acupuncture but only 5% used homeopathy. Somewhat surprisingly, Perry and Dowrick (2000) found that UK GPs had mixed feelings about the use of homeopathy compared to other complementary therapies but rated the therapy, together with acupuncture, as those in which they would most like to train. The difference in approach between the patient-centred focus of homeopathy and the disease-orientated approach of conventional healthcare puts GPs, in particular, at risk of demanding scientific evidence for a system which they do not comprehend, at the expense of appreciating the needs and expectations of patients (Calderon 1998).

Although many UK general practitioners use homeopathy alongside their normal therapeutic regimens, its use for pregnant and childbearing women does not appear to be as widespread as other therapies such as acupuncture or herbal remedies. Indeed, it may be the lack of understanding about its mechanism of action that inhibits its use or recommendation for expectant mothers. To this may be added the impact of the UK maternity care system, in which women without pregnancy complications are normally attended by midwives, whilst those requiring treatment for complications are seen by obstetricians, with the GP's role positioned uneasily and somewhat ill-defined between the two.

A limited number of midwives may utilise homeopathic medicines within their practice but the very fact of *prescribing* an oral remedy may conflict with hospital pharmacy dispensing regulations which require a doctor's signature. Some midwives *recommend* homeopathic remedies for women to purchase for themselves, but this leads to an inequitable service, especially when women in Britain are entitled to free (drug) prescriptions during pregnancy and for up to a year afterwards. Midwives working in independent practice may be in a more autonomous position to incorporate homeopathy alongside conventional antenatal care. A survey of US nurse-midwives in North Carolina showed that 94% recommended complementary therapies, with herbal medicines being the most prevalent (73%) and homeopathy being recommended by only 30% (Allaire et al 2000). This survey does not, however, identify whether or not the midwives were qualified homeopaths, had received appropriate education or were merely interested in alternatives to drugs.

The UK Complementary Maternity Forum (see Useful Addresses) notes only three midwives qualified in homeopathy, two of whom work independently, whilst the other, an NHS community midwife, is prohibited by her midwifery manager from prescribing remedies to the women in her care. Of more concern is the fact that, if she *recommends* remedies to women she is *not allowed* to record it in the maternity notes – effectively preventing her from promoting any natural therapeutics to her patients. More worryingly still, if expectant mothers *request information* on homeopathic medicines, this midwife, although qualified, is required by her managers to refer women to their local health food stores, where it is highly probable that inadequately trained but enthusiastic sales assistants will offer inaccurate or incomplete advice about the use of homeopathic remedies (personal communication 2002).

Pregnant women in Britain are therefore more likely to seek information on homeopathy from a complementary practitioner, who may or may not also be medically qualified. Alternatively they may have *self-administered* remedies prior to pregnancy and wish to continue to do so during the antenatal, intrapartum and postnatal periods. It is however important that pregnant women use the remedies as safely as contemporary knowledge permits (see homeopathic prescribing, below).

On the other hand, it is difficult, when *recommending* homeopathic remedies to pregnant women, in whom the avoidance of drugs has been ingrained by doctors, midwives and the media, to persuade some women that, as far as is known, homeopathic remedies (tablets) seem safe to use. Homeopathy does not appear to work chemically or biophysically but is defined as a form of energy or vibrational medicine. The use of infinitesimally small doses of the original substance has led some practitioners of conventional medicine to dismiss homeopathy as nothing more than a placebo, although if this is so, theoretically the remedy should therefore be safe. Conversely, *if* the homeopathic preparation appears to have any biophysical effect at all, this may be either beneficial or harmful and the remedies must therefore be used correctly to avoid detrimental effects.

In gynaecology, a proprietary homeopathic preparation, Feminon N, was administered to 20 postmenopausal women for six months, in a randomised, controlled study by Warenik-Szymakiewicz et al (1997) in Poland. Significant reductions in menopausal symptoms and in serum follicle stimulating hormone levels were recorded in the test group, but there were no significant alterations in the oestrodiol levels. Some interesting findings also arose from Bergmann et al's study (2000) of a homeopathic remedy for hormone-related sterility. The authors concluded that the remedy could safely be given to women with oligomenorrhoeic infertility for up to six months and demonstrated an increase in luteal progesterone levels, earlier ovulation and shortening of the cycle length, although the incidence of successful pregnancy outcomes did not appear to be statistically significant.

Hart et al (1997) conducted a randomised, double-blind placebo-controlled investigation using homeopathic arnica 30C for pain and infection in women who had undergone total abdominal hysterectomy. Arnica is a universally accepted homeopathic remedy considered to prevent or relieve bruising and shock following accidental or deliberate trauma such as surgery. However, this study of 73 postoperative women failed to provide any conclusive evidence for the beneficial effects of arnica, although the authors acknowledged a variety of factors which may have contributed to the negative results, including the number of subjects, chosen dose of the remedy and the possibility of initial homeopathic aggravation of symptoms. Similar findings, using arnica for muscle soreness in long distance runners, were published by Vickers et al (1998) and other trials investigating arnica in trauma have also been inconclusive (Hofmeyr et al 1990; Savage & Roe 1977), leaving unanswered the question of whether or not arnica is of value, despite the fact that many people, even those who do not regularly use homeopathic medicines, advocate arnica following physical or mental trauma.

Within obstetrics, Smith's review for the Cochrane database (2001) found insufficient evidence to suggest that homeopathic caulophyllum was effective for cervical ripening or induction of labour. However, only one trial of 40 women met the review criteria and, despite being placebo-controlled and double-blind, methodology was not considered to be of good quality. Caulophyllum is a remedy frequently used by women who are past their due date, yet inappropriate administration appears to trigger prostin-like hypertonic contractions which fail to dilate the cervix.

Medical practitioners seeking to discredit homeopathy might consider this review to be definitive in showing the ineffectiveness of caulophyllum, but must acknowledge the need for further studies and appreciate the differences in prescribing practices. On the other hand, the review could also be used to demonstrate to women that there is, as yet, no real evidence of either effectiveness or safety – and perhaps to dissuade them from 'jumping on the bandwagon' of injudicious self-administration in order to expedite the onset of labour. This author has long held that giving women a specific Expected

---

Practice point

Homeopathic remedies do *not* potentiate or inactivate pharmacological drugs, but may be inactivated by them.

Box 6.1 The principles of homeopathic prescribing

'Like cures like'	Minimal doses: dilution and succussion
Provings	Single remedy

Date of Delivery (EDD) is clinically inappropriate, physiologically incorrect and psychosocially disruptive, with the 'knee-jerk' reaction of obstetricians to force a woman's body into labour within ten to fourteen days of that date being potentially pathologically harmful. The use of caulophyllum may be an example of one of the reasons why women resort to natural remedies, since it empowers them to take control of their bodies and may avoid the need for medical induction, simply because they are post-dates, without understanding that the onset of labour occurs when fetomaternal factors are optimal.

Berrebi et al (2001), in France, administered homeopathic apis and bryonia in combination to postpartum women suppressing lactation and found significant improvements in lactation pain, breast tenderness and reduction in spontaneous milk flow. They suggested that the remedies could be incorporated into conventional management, although lactation inhibition in women in the UK is usually achieved without recourse to pharmaceuticals. The very fact that homeopathy is used alongside conventional medicines in France, coupled with the normal practice of artificially suppressing lactation, may have added an element of psychological bias which may not have occurred in Britain.

Hochstrasser and Mattman (1999) challenged the adequacy of questionnaires designed to compare conventional and homeopathic maternity care services in Germany, given the dissimilarities in the philosophies and practices of the two systems. It is difficult to compare two different patient populations when homeopathy is not comprehensively used within the orthodox maternity services, leading to a self-selected group of generally low-risk mothers using homeopathy. UK NHS maternity services do not offer women the alternative option of a homeopathic approach, thus it can be assumed that virtually *all* pregnant women using homeopathy to relieve discomforts and physiological disorders will be self-selected, and presumably low-risk, particularly those requesting natural childbirth practices or home birth.

HOMEOPATHIC PRESCRIBING

Pregnancy and childbearing are seen, in homeopathic terms, to represent an 'acute' episode which can readily be supported by homeopathic medicines when needed, whether prescribed by a registered practitioner, recommended by a conventional health professional or self-administered by the woman. Using homeopathic remedies to treat gestational nausea and vomiting is a prime example of how an holistic system of medicine can address the complex nature of a single symptom. Like other methods of complementary and alternative medicine, homeopathic practice focuses on 'teasing out' the details of the symptoms to give an overall picture of their precise nature. Thus, two women presenting with 'morning sickness' may, in fact, have completely different manifestations of the condition, requiring completely different treatments. Often the indicated remedy can be discerned simply by determining exactly what factors exacerbate or improve the symptoms; Box 6.2 identifies suitable questions to ask the woman about these factors.

All of the currently available research findings on homeopathy focus on the effectiveness or action of various remedies, and there does not appear to be any comprehensive work on safety or adverse events. Although most homeopathic medicines are taken in the form of small oral tablets or pillules (tiny seed-like pills), they do not work pharmacologically, i.e. they are not absorbed, metabolised, utilised and excreted via the same biophysical pathways as drugs. However it is also important to recognise that homeopathic remedies, whilst being gentle and non-

Box 6.2 Homeopathic history taking for pregnancy sickness	
Exact time of day when nausea and vomiting are worst Impact on appetite for food and drink Effect of smell of food and other odours Effects of eating and drinking Is nausea relieved by vomiting or not? Effect of motion or noise	Which position relieves or provokes the symptoms? Nature of the vomit, including amount of saliva Accompanying symptoms e.g. bowel changes, headaches Emotional state

toxic from a pharmacological viewpoint, are powerful substances which are harmless *only when used appropriately*. Generally, if an incorrect remedy is used, no response will be witnessed, which is deemed to be due to incorrect prescribing, but continual use or abuse of the remedy may detrimentally upset the balance of health and trigger a *reverse proving*, actually provoking the symptoms that the wrongly-used remedy is designed to treat. It is worth remembering also that, as the remedies do not work pharmacologically, they cannot interact with conventional drugs, but the lack of knowledge of medical staff may cause them concern (see Case 6.2).

Occasionally the woman may experience a temporary exacerbation of symptoms on first taking the remedy, which is generally an indication of selection of the most appropriate remedy. This aggravation may take one of three forms: the person may feel better despite an increase in symptoms; she may develop a new symptom characteristic of the prescribed remedy; or there is no improvement in the condition, which eventually worsens because, in effect, no treatment has been given. This latter is seen by Ernst et al (2001) as an indirect risk of homeopathy or any other ineffective complementary therapy. The exacerbation may be dealt with by reducing the frequency of administration of the chosen remedy. Unfortunately, however, it is

---

Practice point

Homeopathy is a powerful system of energy medicine and if used inappropriately has risk potential, usually by failing to treat the presenting symptom but also by triggering new symptoms in a 'reverse proving'.

---

this 'healing crisis', which not only occurs with homeopathic remedies, but with other complementary therapies, which causes sceptical medical practitioners to deride their value, claiming that they 'make the patient worse'. Indeed, Freer (1985) expressed concern that GPs are sometimes confronted with a patient undergoing a healing crisis, whose condition has apparently deteriorated as a result of a course of independent complementary treatment which has not been completed, perhaps due to lack of faith in its action, or to a lack of funds to continue private consultations, and that the doctors are then left to 'pick up the pieces'. It is important that the mother is informed of the likelihood of a healing crisis occurring when she first starts taking the homeopathic remedy; a strong reaction is, in fact, often a good indication of the correctly selected remedy.

Homeopathic remedies are made in varying potencies (strengths), indicated by a number and a letter eg 6C, 200X. The number represents the number of times the original substance has been diluted and succussed, while the letter denotes the dilution scale (C = 1:100; X = 1:10). Thus remedies such as commercially available arnica 6C have been diluted one part arnica to 99 parts water and the process of diluting and succussing has been repeated six times. The higher the number, the more dilute the original substance becomes but the more powerful a homeopathic remedy it is. Conversely, a lower number indicates that there is more of the original substance in the remedy. One of the problems for practitioners of conventional medicine is that they do not know what the mother is taking when she self-administers homeopathic remedies. This is even more of a problem with homeopathy than with herbal medicines or aromatherapy oils,

---

Case 6.1

A multiparous mother developed chest pain and cardiac arrhythmias within a few hours of Caesarean section. It was discovered that she had been taking homeopathic arnica (for bruising, shock and trauma) and hypericum (for wound healing) on the advice of the CT midwife. The junior obstetrician, aware of the Department of Health guidelines regarding St John's wort (Hypericum perforatum, see Chapter 5) was concerned about the impact which these remedies may have had on the mother and queried the potential risk of interactions if she required medication to correct the cardiac abnormalities. However, the doctor had failed to understand that homeopathic hypericum, whilst from the same plant, was in a much diluted form, that homeopathic remedies do not act pharmacologically, and that they do not potentiate or inhibit the actions of prescribed drugs. He was reassured when the differences between the two systems of homeopathy and herbal medicine were explained.

Case 6.2

A mother booked for homebirth had a rapid labour, and only one midwife had arrived by the second stage, although the independent homeopath was in attendance. The baby's Apgar score was, unexpectedly, only 2, and the midwife commenced resuscitation with little effect. After a few minutes the homeopath pushed the midwife out of the way and gave the baby a white powder sublingually, which she called the 'death remedy'; the baby's condition immediately began to improve. It is not possible to determine whether the remedy (which was possibly Arsenicum, see below) was responsible for the baby's recovery, whether simply putting a powder under his tongue caused a reactive inspiration or whether the resuscitative measures employed by the midwife had been effective. However, the midwife was concerned as she did not know what the baby had been given, and a full review of the relationship between the midwife, who was legally responsible for the care, and that of independent complementary practitioners was undertaken, with subsequent policies and protocols being drawn up to avoid conflict in future cases.

---

which can at least be explained in terms of their pharmacological action. Added to this is the fact that, if a midwife or doctor is aware of the plant or other substance from which the remedy is originally derived, they may be unwilling to sanction the administration of something known, in large doses, to be toxic. Pregnant women should, therefore, be advised to use a higher homeopathic potency (e.g. 30C) which will have less of the original substance in it. Remedies of the 6C and 6X potency are beneficial for minor physical complaints, whereas those of higher potencies such as 200C or 1M (diluted 1:1000) should only be prescribed by a registered homeopathic practitioner. Guidelines for appropriate administration are given in Box 6.3.

Given that pregnancy sickness is physiological and therefore considered normal and of little concern to obstetricians until it becomes more severe, there may a greater willingness to 'allow' women to 'experiment' with natural remedies. However, in the event of a pathological deterioration in a mother's condition, necessitating hospitalisation, it is less likely that homeopathic remedies will be encouraged, since the care of the woman is now the responsibility of the obstetrician. This is particularly pertinent in the case of an obstetric emergency (see Case 6.2).

The delicate nature of homeopathic remedies is based on their ability to stimulate a person's self-healing capacity, but other stimulants capable of effecting a change in the person's energy may counteract the action of the remedies. Certain specific homeopathic remedies are also thought to antidote each other, but this can be avoided by adhering to the principle of using a single remedy. The only problem may arise if a woman is advised to take one remedy for her nausea and vomiting and another for a different symptom. However, more careful selection will probably direct the prescriber to one remedy which is capable of treating both symptoms, the one being a part of the overall symptom picture for the other. Various possible antidotes are identified in Boxes 6.4 and 6.5.

Homeopathic prescribing is undertaken in two

Box 6.3 Guidelines for administration of homeopathic remedies

- Only *one* remedy should be given at a time
- Increased doses are achieved by increasing the *frequency* of administration, *not* by giving more tablets/pillules on one occasion
- The *smallest possible* dose should be given to gain a beneficial effect
- The patient should not eat, drink, smoke or clean the teeth for 15 minutes *before and after* taking each remedy

- The tablets/pillules should be *handled* only by the patient
- Remedies should not be administered on *metallic* spoons but *tipped directly* from the lid of the bottle into the mouth or hand of the patient
- Remedies should be allowed to *dissolve under the tongue* before swallowing

---

Box 6.4 Substances which may potentially antidote or inactivate homeopathic remedies

Analgesics, including aspirin and Calpol
Antacids
Antibiotics, antifungals
Anticoagulants
Coffee
Cough medicines and throat lozenges
Deodorants and antiperspirants
Decongestants including Karvol capsules, Olbas oil, Vicks vapour rub, Tiger balm and vaporisers
Electromagnetic sources such as televisions and microwaves
Essential oils of camphor, clove, eucalyptus, frankincense, peppermint, spearmint and other mint oils

Handling by anyone other than the person for whom the remedy is intended
Incense and moxa sticks
Medicated creams and liniments including Deep Heat, wintergreen
Mothballs
Peppermint, menthol, eucalyptus and camphor including toothpaste
Perfumes and other fragrant substances
Recreational drugs
Sunlight and extreme heat

(adapted from Geraghty 1997:17)

Box 6.5 Homeopathic remedies which may be antidoted by others

Aconite – coffea, nux vomica, rhus tox, sepia
Antim tart – sepia
Arsenicum – nat mur
Ipecacuanha – allium cepa

Phosphorus – natrum mur, nux vomica
Pulsatilla – chamomilla, coffea, nux vomica
Sepia – aconite, rhus tox, sulphur
Sulphur – china, sepia

---

ways: the person may generally exhibit the characteristics of a particular remedy (constitutional type) or the precise nature of their symptoms of nausea and vomiting may suggest a specific remedy. 'Constitution' refers to a symptom pattern which appears to apply to a group of people with common physical and mental characteristics, such as hair colour, weight, height, skin type, or a tendency to suffer from similar conditions e.g. premenstrual tension. A 'constitutional type' remedy is one to which a person reacts especially strongly, with people being described as, for example, a 'pulsatilla personality' or a 'phosphorus type'. In the following section, remedy pictures are preceded by general information which

is representative of the constitutional type of each remedy, with those discussed being specifically for gestational nausea and vomiting. Symptom pictures are based on accepted contemporary homeopathic theory, extrapolated from a variety of sources, but not based on recent research.

SPECIFIC HOMEOPATHIC REMEDIES FOR NAUSEA AND VOMITING IN PREGNANCY

Nux vomica

The seeds of the poison nut, or *Strychnos nux*

Case 6.3

A 39-year-old gravida five was referred to the complementary therapy (CT) midwife for nausea and vomiting at nine weeks' gestation. Her first son was three years old and she had experienced no sickness during that pregnancy but had been unwell soon after delivery. She had subsequently received a diagnosis of antiphospholipid syndrome. Three further pregnancies had resulted in miscarriage. The woman's history showed a previous lower back injury which seemed ordinarily to indicate that reflexology might have been effective (see Chapter 7). However as the midwife did not have a sufficiently in-depth understanding of the antiphospholipid syndrome she was unwilling to use

reflexology techniques which could have interfered with the pathology. The mother's symptom picture suggested that the sickness may respond to homeopathic sepia although the fact that she required anticoagulant therapy for her antiphospholipid syndrome suggested that the remedies might be inactivated by the drugs. However, she returned the following week to report a significant reduction in both the severity of nausea and frequency of vomiting; she continued to use the remedy with good effect for a further three weeks when the symptoms subsided. Whether or not this was due to the homeopathic remedy or simply an opportunity to talk and to have her symptoms validated is not known.

Box 6.6 Symptom picture for nux vomica

Nausea – constant, but **particularly in the morning**; exacerbated by tobacco smoke and perspiration; **worse after eating**, better after vomiting; accompanied by desire to open bowels
Vomiting – bile and mucus, bitter and odorous, with much retching
Mouth – bitter, sour taste, worst in morning, copious saliva, brown tongue
Mood – irritable, angry, violent, sensitive to cold,

workaholic, may hit out
Appetite – ravenously hungry, **craves stimulants** e.g. alcohol, cigarettes
Abdomen – feels as if heavy weight after eating; sensitive to pressure, cramping stomach pains; heartburn; **may have constipation**

N.B. Can be alternated with Ipecacuanha if heartburn and flatulence are features

---

vomica, are the source of this homeopathic remedy, a plant which is rich in strychnine, which, in overdose, can initiate convulsions as a result of nervous stimulation. Thus a woman for whom nux vomica is suitable may be subject to a degree of nervous hyperstimulation, being seen as an overbearing 'workaholic', who overdoes everything, including working too hard, staying out late, overeating and drinking, especially coffee and alcohol, the typical type A personality. Thin, nervous and irritable, she frequently suffers from gastrointestinal symptoms, especially constipation associated with painful urging of a hard stool against spasm of the anal sphincter. Any symptoms may be aggravated by lack of sleep and relieved by a normal bowel movement. She may be frenetic or aggressive, impatient and irritable, with little tolerance of others, particularly when contradicted. She expects high standards from those around her and does not 'suffer fools gladly'. This remedy

is particularly effective for the woman who abuses alcohol, cigarettes or drugs, although she may be sensitive to or intolerant of them. 'Burnout' may occasionally manifest as a means of enabling her overstimulated and exhausted nervous system to 'recharge'.

Ipecacuanha

Ipecacuanha is prepared from the tincture of the dried root, *Cephaelis ipecacuanha*, from South America, and in conventional medicine may be used to induce vomiting after accidental or deliberate ingestion of poison, or drug overdose. It is particularly useful for the woman whose gestational sickness is severe enough to warrant hospitalisation and intravenous fluid replacement, or in the case where another more specific remedy is ineffective. Profuse salivation is often a feature of the mother's condition. The woman best suited to ipecacuanha is notably

---

Box 6.7 Symptom picture for ipecacuanha

Nausea – constant, **not relieved by vomiting**, any time of day or night; worse after eating or vomiting; exacerbated by rich food, ice cream, **smell of food** or tobacco, **bending down, lying down, movement**, coughing, warmth; better in the open air or after drinking cold fluids
Vomiting – bile, undigested food, mucus, occasionally blood
Mouth – moist, **excessive saliva**, clean tongue
Face – pale, with bluish tinge, especially beneath eyes

Mood – anxious, irritable, frustrated, headaches
Appetite – disgust for food and drink, not thirsty
Abdomen – feels as if stomach is hanging down
Looks pale, short of breath, cold perspiration
N.B. If nausea pronounced on waking, take ipecacuanha before rising
N.B. May be effective in cases where woman is hospitalised for fluid replacement in **hyperemesis gravidarum**

Box 6.8 Symptom picture for sepia

Nausea – intermittent, with gnawing pains, worse in morning, before breakfast and after **1700 hours until retiring**; temporarily better after eating; exacerbated when lying on side, **smell or thought of foods previously enjoyed**, especially meat; sensitive to perfumes
Vomiting – often vomits after eating, bile, malodorous
Mouth – bitter, sour, bad taste
Face – **yellow**, pale, marked yellowness across fleshy part of nose, chloasma

Mood – snappy, indifferent, exhausted, depressed, weepy; **wants to be left alone**, ambivalence towards pregnancy and friends; dislikes being touched
Appetite – may be insatiably hungry, **craves vinegar**, sour and acidic foods and pickles; **dislikes bread**, milk, fatty foods
Abdomen – bloated, dragging, empty feeling, sensation that uterus is falling out, fears she will have a miscarriage whilst vomiting, feels need to cross legs
Accompanied by backache

---

one who readily becomes nauseated, with sickness accompanying almost all complaints, even when not pregnant. She may experience hot or cold sweating, which makes her feel cold externally and hot internally.

Sepia

The remedy is prepared from the ink of *Sepia officinalis*, the cuttlefish, which discharges it to cover its retreat when attacked or alarmed. It is most appropriate for the woman who is recognisable from her desire, during illness, to detach herself from loved ones, including the spouse and children, and to be alone. There is frequently an ambivalence towards the pregnancy/baby, but this leads to a feeling of tremendous guilt, especially as she may be over-conscientious towards her family responsibilities. She is depressed, lacks enthusiasm and the ability to think clearly, and has a low or absent libido. In appearance she may be **tall, slim and dark** with a waxy complexion. She often feels exhausted, is sensitive to cold, lacks muscle tone, and experiences a sensation as if there is something heavy and dragging inside her, making this a suitable remedy for a woman with a retroverted uterus (or, in later life, for the woman who suffers a uterine prolapse). There may be a history of bearing-down pains experienced premenstrually, and dyspareunia before pregnancy. Taking time for herself, especially exercise, helps to make her feel better.

Pulsatilla

This remedy is prepared from a tincture of the complete fresh plant, *Pulsatilla nigricans*, or European windflower. Almost the opposite of sepia, this woman is **feminine, fair, warm-hearted**, with a **changeable** nature, characteristic of the wind flower. She has a tendency to weep easily but is also likeable, cheerful and easy going. She readily accommodates to the demands of others, often to the detriment of her own self esteem. She is restless and constantly

---

Box 6.9 Symptom picture for pulsatilla

Nausea – constant, but worst in **late afternoon and evening**; worse after eating, sometimes **several hours afterwards**; exacerbated by hot foods, ice cream, fruit, rich fatty foods; better when in cool fresh air and after drinking cold fluids
Vomiting – does not relive nausea, bitter
Mouth – bitter, worse in morning, taste often remains in mouth and triggers belching; complains she has lost her taste for food; moist white tongue

Mood – **weepy, or may easily be moved to laughter,** needs a lot of comfort; easily hurt; **fears she may not be a good mother** and that something will happen to the baby
Appetite – aversion to spicy, fatty rich foods (although may crave the latter); craves things she cannot identify; thirstless
Abdomen – sensitive to overeating; intestinal gas with heartburn

---

Box 6.10 Symptom picture for colchicum

Nausea – may be continuous throughout the day or just in the morning; notably worse when faced with the **smell** or even the **thought of food**, especially **eggs**; extremely sensitive to any **odour**, including perfumes, tobacco, exhaust fumes, paint; condition exacerbated by even the slightest **motion**
Vomiting – gagging, retching and vomiting even when only thinking of food or seeing it at a distance e.g. on

television; especially pronounced in the evening
Appetite – may have unquenchable thirst, particularly for effervescent fluids; may have **intense cravings but unable to eat or drink them** without becoming nauseated or vomiting
Abdomen – distended, tendency to **diarrhoea** containing mucus; draws up knees to abdomen as lying, standing or stretching out legs triggers nausea

---

trying to keep busy. This remedy is especially effective for problems of the female reproductive tract in the absence of any more specific symptom picture, including menstrual and menopausal symptoms, fertility problems and deviations from the norm during pregnancy and childbirth, notably cephalic version and inhibition of lactation.

Colchicum

Colchicum autumnale, the meadow saffron, provides the tincture for this remedy, which is also a source of colchicine, often used for gout, and in homeopathic terms, suits the woman whose condition is exacerbated by movement of any type, such as walking or even just turning the head, often with accompanying joint pains, headache and mucus-like diarrhoea. She will have an acute sense of smell, particularly to things such as food, tobacco, car exhaust fumes, perfumes, babies' napkins etc. and will seek a place where she can sit or lie motionless as far away as possible from the source of any strong odours. She is sensitive to cold and damp and any symptoms are worse at night.

Antimonium tartaricum

The remedy is made from potassium antimony tartrate, or tartar emetic, and is of particular benefit for those suffering with excess fluid accumulation, such as mucus and bile. (It is also claimed to be suitable for babies with meconium aspiration or respiratory distress syndrome, the 'rattling lungs' being characteristic of the remedy.)

Sulphur

The remedy is made from elemental sulphur, or brimstone, and, in Yin and Yang terms, is related to heat and excess energy (see Chapter 4). Thus, a woman who benefits from sulphur is generally overheated, and does not tolerate heat well, often removing clothes in winter, but conversely, may be a source of heat, energy and support to those around her. She may report needing to stick her feet out of the bed at night to keep cool. She is a natural leader, but has an ebullient, controlling tendency, always keen to offer her own opinions and rarely taking 'no' for an answer. In appearance she may be solid,

---

Box 6.11 Symptom picture for antimonium tartaricum

Nausea – comes in waves, worse in evening, may be accompanied by collapse, exhaustion; exacerbated by lying down at night, drinking milk, coughing; better if lying on right side
Vomiting – difficult with ineffectual retching; undigested food with thick, stringy mucus and sour bile vomited immediately after eating; usually sudden, severe and spasmodic; worse if there is also a fever
Mouth – bitter, sour; thick white coating on tongue with reddened papillae and red edges

Face – pale, sunken eyes, lips may be bluish
Mood – clinging and **frightened of being alone** while vomiting, yet averse to consolation; fear that something is wrong; weak, apathetic, lethargic, exhausted
Appetite – **craves sips of cold water** but generally thirstless, **acid foods, apples**, other fruit, but sour tastes make symptoms worse; absolute aversion to **milk**
Abdomen – feels 'full of stones', diarrhoea
Whole body is cold and clammy with perspiration

Box 6.12 Symptom picture for sulphur

Mouth – red
Face – flushes easily, red
Mood – aggravated by heat; lacks energy especially around 11am; overactive imagination
Appetite – voracious, especially for carbohydrates and sweet, salty or spiced foods, thirsty

Abdomen – chronic constipation with pain on defaecation, odorous small, hard and knotty stool; worse at 5am
Also complains of internal and external burning and bleeding haemorrhoids and varicose veins aggravated by standing

---

heavily-set or stout, but not necessarily obese, and is dishevelled and grubby, with skin complaints and a dislike of water. This woman may be susceptible to developing pre-eclampsia in later pregnancy.

Arsenicum album

Derived from arsenious trioxide, or arsenic, which is poisonous to all living cells, in homeopathic medicine, it can be used to good effect to treat women whose symptoms are similar to food poisoning or other toxicity. Profound fatigue is typical, and the woman for whom arsenicum would be appropriate is often intelligent, restless and 'fussy', who becomes exhausted out of all proportion to any, even minimal, activity, such as minor exertion after a bowel movement. She is invariably cold, seeking overheated rooms and layers of clothing and benefits from hot drinks, water bottles or heat in any form. In keeping with the symptoms of arsenic overdose, the woman may feel she has been poisoned by something irresolvable which may trigger a deep anguish or a conscious fear of death. She fears being alone and may exhibit

excessive-compulsive behaviour, especially demanding constant reassurance. (Arsenicum is the first homeopathic remedy of choice for terminal illnesses such as metastatic carcinoma, and in neonates with life-threatening Apgar scores, with or without meconium aspiration, arsenicum is claimed to be lifesaving.)

Phosphorus

The homeopathic remedy contains a saturated solution of elemental phosphorus. Typically, the woman who would suit phosphorus is tall and slim, burns up food easily and therefore needs to eat frequently; she is also thirsty, needing cold drinks, especially milk. She bleeds easily and copiously, usually bright red blood, especially menstrual blood and nosebleeds. The phosphorus woman is affectionate and characteristically dislikes being alone, particularly at night and during thunderstorms. When unwell, she becomes debilitated, needing sympathy and responding well to touch and massage. Bearing in mind that symptoms of phosphorus poisoning include cellular hepatic necrosis, clotting disorders and haemorrhagic disease, this reme-

---

Box 6.12 Symptom picture for arsenicum album

Nausea – no real nausea, only retching, worse for smell of food
Vomiting – frequent, violent vomiting of watery malodorous bile and food, with no warning; often causes her to perspire and to **faint**; feels worse after vomiting; at most intense in the afternoon; better if warm

Mouth – bitter, red tongue
Mood – anxious, **extreme mental restlessness with fatigue**
Appetite – desire for sour things and for coffee; dislikes cold drinks, ice cream
Abdomen – burning pain in stomach; **diarrhoea**

Box 6.14 Symptom picture for phosphorus

Nausea – occurs about 15 minutes after ingesting food and drink, especially hot; **characteristically has total aversion to water** – sight, touch or taste of water triggers severe nausea and vomiting
Vomiting – violent vomiting of yellow, bitter mucus and bile
Mouth – sour, tongue is red-coated
Face – red, with spots, hot flushes; hair loss; sinus

congestion
Mood – gregarious but fearful; requires sympathy but easily comforted and reassured
Appetite – craving for ice cold drinks, salt; aversion to tea, coffee, meat or boiled milk
Heat and pain between shoulder blades; weakness
May even have to close eyes whilst washing or bathing

Box 6.15 Symptom picture for cocculus

Nausea – worse with any motion, travelling by road, rail, air or sea
Appetite – sensitive to smell and thought of food

Strongly affected by **loss of sleep**, especially from excessive worry or excitement

---

dy is particularly suited to patients with anaemia, antenatal or postpartum haemorrhage and deficiencies of prothrombin and other clotting factors. However, the acute nature of these problems in pregnancy make it unlikely that obstetricians would countenance its use in preference to, or simultaneously with, conventional drugs. Although its concomitant use will theoretically not interact with pharmacological drugs, indirect potentisation could occur, and with such serious conditions, it is preferable to administer conventional treatment which is known to work, without the risk of compromise from natural remedies.

Cocculus

The remedy is prepared from a tincture of the powdered seeds of *Cocculus indicus*, the Indian cockle, containing an alkaloid, picrotoxin, which can cause excitement of the central nerv-

ous system, resulting in convulsions. In homeopathic terms, cocculus has an affinity for the vestibular organ of the inner ear, so that it is useful for any disorders of neurological equilibrium, including headache, vertigo and nausea. It is the leading homeopathic remedy for simple motion sickness.

Kreosotum

As assumed from the name, this remedy is derived from the volatile oils of guaiacol and creosol, obtained from the distillation of beechwood tar, creosote.

Traditionally, creosote was used as a preservative in the smoking of fish and meat, as an aid to prevent putrefaction, and homeopathically is suitable for conditions which suggest infection with suppuration or discharge, such as excoriating vaginitis and discharge.

Box 6.16 Symptom picture for kreosotum

Nausea – worst several hours after eating, quickly followed by vomiting **Extreme salivation**, constantly swallowing saliva, which exacerbates nausea	Remedy particularly effective with threatened miscarriage 8-12 weeks, especially when triggered after intercourse

---

HOMEOPATHIC REMEDIES FOR SYMPTOMS ACCOMPANYING NAUSEA AND VOMITING

Occasionally it is appropriate to treat an accompanying symptom rather than selecting a remedy which is directly suited to the mother's nausea and vomiting. Homeopathy, more than any other therapy, places great emphasis on taking into account the whole person, without disregarding anything which the patient reports. Symptoms such as constipation, headaches or specific emotional moods can be equally as disrupting to the woman's daily life as the nausea, and by treating these, the nausea may also be alleviated. The following are a few examples, which indicate how one remedy can be useful for more than one symptom.

Constipation is a common problem in pregnancy, attributed to the reduced peristalsis as a result of progesterone relaxing the smooth muscle of the gastrointestinal tract. Haemorrhoids often occur for similar reasons, but are exacerbated by constipation. *Sepia* is viewed by many authorities as 'specific for gestational constipation', especially for women who are drained and worn out, perhaps by repeated childbearing, while *Lycopodium* is for those whose hepatic function is sluggish, with heartburn, flatulence and burping, abdominal distension and a tendency, even when not pregnant, to become constipated when away from home for any length of time. In keeping with its changeable nature, *Pulsatilla* is suited to the woman who may be constipated one month and not the next, such as someone who suffers from irritable bowel syndrome. Constipation with backache, an ineffectual urging to pass a stool and an 'unfinished feeling' may respond to *nux vomica* especially if

the mother needs stimulation, perhaps in the form of coffee, to start the day. If the constipation is accompanied by headaches, *Bryonia* is indicated.

Haemorrhoids may respond to *Pulsatilla*, particularly if accompanied by heartburn and varicose veins, or to *Hammamelis virginica* if they are external and tender to touch, and the mother has numerous leg varicosities and oedema which cause her great emotional distress.

Heartburn can be treated with *Nux vomica* if it occurs after eating, leaves a metallic taste in the mouth and is worse if the mother wears tight clothes, whereas *Pulsatilla* may be most appropriate for the woman whose heartburn is worse at night, leaves a slimy salty taste in the mouth and whose mood is changeable.

CONCLUSION

Homeopathy offers a gentle method of dealing with the range of symptoms associated with nausea and vomiting, and enables the mother to be in control of her own condition by self-administering the remedies. When used appropriately, it is considered safe to use in pregnancy, although mothers should endeavour to purchase the more dilute potencies as these contain less of the original ingredient. Although there is little research specific to homeopathic medicines for pregnancy sickness, and the randomisation and control of homeopathic trials is difficult, given the individualisation of the remedies, there is an increasing body of evidence to support its use. Women are best advised to consult a homeopath who is also a conventional healthcare professional or one who is experienced in treating pregnant and childbearing mothers.

Table 6.1 Summary of homeopathic remedies for gestational nausea & vomiting

REMEDY	CHARACTERISTICS	REMEDY	CHARACTERISTICS
Nux Vomica 30C	AM and after eating Ravenous Craves stimulants	Pulsatilla 30C	Constant esp late afternoon, evening
	Heartburn, constipation with backache		Not thirsty, sensitive to overeating
	Irritable, WORKAHOLIC		Cravings non-specific
			Averse to rich, spicy, warm food
Ipecacuanha 30C	Constant esp on waking		TEARFUL, needing comfort, CHANGEABLE
	No appetite / thirst	Colchicum 30C	Constant esp AM, evening
	Craves cold drinks		Thirsty – fizzy drinks
	V ++ immediately after eating, no effect on N		Intense cravings
	Heartburn, saliva+		Averse to any ODOURS
	ANXIOUS, frustrated	Cocculus 30C	Afternoon
Sepia 30C	Intermittent, AM, after 1700 with backache		Hunger, no appetite, metallic taste
	Hungry, N better after eating		Craves cold drinks
	Craves sour foods		Averse to many odours
	Averse to foods previously enjoyed		MOTION
	V bile soon after eating		
	Dragging bloated abdomen		
	Wants to be alone, may REGRET pregnancy, fears miscarriage		

REFERENCES

Allaire A D, Moos M K, Wells S R 2000 Complementary and alternative medicine in pregnancy: a survey of North Carolina certified nurse-midwives. Obstetrics and Gynecology 95 (1): 19-23

Astin J A, Marie A, Pelletier K R et al 1998 A review of the incorporation of complementary and alternative medicine by mainstream physicians. Archives of Internal Medicine 158 (21): 2303-2310

Bergman J, Luft B, Boehmann S 2000 The efficacy of the complex medication Phyto-Hypophyson-L in female hormone-related sterility. A randomised placebo-controlled clinical double-blind study. Forsch Komplementarmed Klass Naturheilkd 7 (4): 190-199

Berrebi A, Parant O, Ferval F et al 2001 Treatment of pain due to unwanted lactation with a homeopathic preparation given in the immediate postpartum period. Journal of Gynecology Obstetrics and Biological Reproduction 30 (4): 353-357

Boyd W E 1941 The action of microdoses of mercuric chloride on diastase. British Homeopathic Journal 31: 1-18 and 32: 106-111. Cited in Geraghty B 1997 Homeopathy for Midwives. Churchill Livingstone, Edinburgh

British Medical Association 1993 Complementary medicine: new approaches to good practice. Oxford University Press, Oxford

Calderon C 1998 Homeopathic and primary care doctors: how they see each other and how they see their patients: results of a qualitative investigation. Aten Primaria 21 (6): 367-375

Dantas F, Rampes H 2000 Do homeopathic medicines provoke adverse effects? A systematic review. British Homeopathic Journal 89 (Suppl 1): S35-38

Davenas E, Beauvais J, Amara J et al 1988 Human basophil degranulation triggered by very dilute antiserum against

IgE. Nature 333: 816-818

Davidson J et al 1997 Homeopathic treatment of depression and anxiety. Alternative Therapies 3 (1): 46

Ernst E, Pittler M H, Stevinson C et al 2001 The desktop guide to complementary and alternative medicine. Mosby, Edinburgh

Ernst E 1999 Homeopathic prophylaxis of headaches and migraine? A systematic review. Journal of Pain and Symptom Management 18: 353-357

Ernst E, Barnes J 1998 Are homeopathic remedies effective for delayed onset muscle soreness? A systematic review of placebo-controlled trials. Perfusion 11: 4-8

Ernst E, Pittler M H 1998 Efficacy of homeopathic arnica. A systematic review of placebo-controlled clinical trials. Archives of Surgery 133: 1187-1190

Fisher P, Scott D L 2001 A randomized controlled trial of homeopathy in rheumatoid arthritis. Rheumatology (Oxford) 40 (9): 1052-1055

Foundation for Integrated Medicine 1997 Integrated healthcare: a way forward for the next five years? FIM, London

Freer C 1985 What kind of alternative is alternative medicine? Journal of the Royal College of General Practitioners 10: 459-460

Geraghty B 1997 Homeopathy for midwives. Churchill Livingstone, London

Hart O, Mullee M A, Lewith G et al 1997 Double-blind placebo-controlled randomised clinical trial of homeopathic arnica C30 for pain and infection after total abdominal hysterectomy. Journal of the Royal Society of Medicine 90 (2): 73-78

Hochstrasser B, Mattman P 1999 Mainstream medicine versus complementary medicine (homeopathic) intervention: a critical methodology study of care in pregnancy. Forsch Komplementarmed 6 (Suppl 1): 20-22

Hofmeyr G J, Piccioni V, Blauhof P 1990 Postpartum homeopathic arnica montana: a potency finding pilot study. British Journal of Clinical Practice 4: 619-621

House of Lords Select Committee 2000 Sixth report on complementary and alternative medicine. HMSO, London

Jonas W B, Anderson R L, Crawford C C 2001 A systematic review of the quality of homeopathic clinical trials. Complementary and Alternative Medicine 1 (1): 12

Kayne S B 1997 Homeopathic pharmacy: an introduction and handbook. Churchill Livingstone, Edinburgh

Kleijnen J, Knipschild P, Riet G 1991 Clinical trials of homeopathy. British Medical Journal 302: 316-323

Linde K, Clausius N, Ramirez G et al 1997 Are the clinical effects of homeopathy placebo effects? A meta-analysis of placebo-controlled trials. Lancet 350: 834-843

Merrell W C, Shalts E 2002 Homeopathy. Medical Clinics of North America 86 (1): 47-62

Moskowitz R 1992 Homeopathic medicines for pregnancy and childbirth. North Atlantic Books, Berkeley, California

Perry R, Dowrick C F 2000 Complementary medicine and general practice: an urban perspective. Complementary Therapies in Medicine 8 (2): 71-75

Pirotta M V, Cohen M M, Kotsirilos V et al 2000 Complementary therapies: have they become accepted in general practice? Medical Journal of Australia 172 (3): 105-109

Reilly D et al 1986 Is homeopathy a placebo response? Controlled trial of homeopathic potency in hay fever as model. Lancet 2: 881

Savage J, Roe B 1977 A double blind trial to assess the benefit of arnica montana in acute stroke illness. British Homeopathic Journal 66: 207-220

Sevar R 2000 Audit of outcome in 829 consecutive patients treated with homeopathic medicines. British Homeopathic Journal 89 (4): 178-187

Schiff M 1995 The memory of water. Thorsons, London. Cited in Kayne S B 1997 Homeopathic pharmacy: an introduction and handbook. Churchill Livingstone, Edinburgh

Smith C A 2001 Homeopathy for induction of labour (Cochrane Review) Cochrane Database 4: CD 003399

Vickers A J, van Haselen R, Heger M 2001 Can homeopathically prepared mercury cause symptoms in healthy volunteers? A randomised double-blind placebo-controlled trial. Journal of Alternative and Complementary Medicine 7 (2): 141-148

Vickers A J, Fisher P, Smith C et al 1998 Homeopathic arnica 30x is ineffective for muscle soreness after long distance running; a randomized double-blind placebo-controlled trial. Clinical Journal of Pain 14 (3): 227-231

Warenik-Szymankiewicz A, Meczekalski B, Obrewobowska A 1997 Feminon N in the treatment of menopausal symptoms. Ginekol-Pol 68 (2): 89-9

FURTHER READING

Cummings B 2000 Homeopathy for pregnancy and childbirth. In: Tiran D, Mack S (eds) 2000 Complementary therapies for pregnancy and childbirth, 2nd edn. Bailliere Tindall, London

7

The structural approach

This chapter explores further the physiological processes involved in some aspects of nausea and vomiting in pregnancy and challenges the traditional view that the condition arises solely as a result of endocrine and other pregnancy-specific factors, by suggesting a relationship with the musculoskeletal structure of the body. Based on this inter-relationship, there follows a debate about the value of some complementary therapies which may be effective in relieving gestational sickness, including osteopathy and chiropractic and massage, and introduces the use of a precise reflexology technique which this author has devised and used successfully to treat pregnant women suffering from sickness.

INTRODUCTION

Within conventional medical practice the division of the body into 'systems' presents a somewhat artificial differentiation without any overt acknowledgement that one may interact with another. Thus gynaecologists focus on the reproductive and endocrine systems, gastroenterologists on the digestive tract and psychiatrists on the mind. When a patient develops a condition incidental to the primary presenting one, a different specialist team is required to deal with it, the emphasis being put on the *condition* rather than the *person*. An example of this would be the woman who develops appendicitis during pregnancy, whose hospitalisation predisposes her to clinical depression, whose care is then divided between obstetricians, general surgeons and psychiatrists.

Furthermore, orthodox medical diagnosis concentrates only on those detectable signs and reported symptoms which *seem* to be relevant – the decision about relevance being made arbitrarily by the doctor, based on conventional medical reductionism or on theories which can be easily comprehended. Therefore, normal breathlessness in pregnancy is viewed solely as a response to the physical pressure of the gravid uterus below the diaphragm, yet in Traditional Chinese Medicine (TCM), would be seen as weakened energy in the kidney meridian (see Chapter 4). An expectant mother presenting with sinus congestion will be considered as having symptoms totally incidental to the pregnancy, but a TCM practitioner would take it as further evidence of poor kidney energy. Working on the kidney meridian, which, in TCM, has strong links to the proper functioning of the lungs, would resolve both the sinus congestion and the breathlessness.

This concept may seem alien to practitioners of western or orthodox medicine, for complementary medicine encompasses the concept of holism which stresses the relationship between the body, mind and spirit. The philosophy of most complementary therapies is that no single part can be extricated from the whole – an individual consists of all these, and the practitioner takes into account *any* factor affecting the patient's health. In homeopathy, for example, there is an appreciation that many seemingly minor issues may have a bearing on the person's condition; in hypnotherapy, psychological and emotional wellbeing are recognised as impacting on physical health, and vice versa. The environment is known to influence recovery from illness, and alternative therapeutic interventions such as music and feng shui are gradually being used within healthcare settings (Savarimuthu & Bunnell 2002; Jeffreys 2000; Brewer 1998). Other therapies, such as reflexology, auricular acupuncture and diagnostic techniques such as iridology work on using one area of the body to represent a map of the whole, in miniature, or the 'homuncular reflex theory' (Suen et al 2001).

The Alexander technique is based on the relationship between the central axis of the body (the head, neck and back), the mechanism and control of posture, movement and coordination and the conscious and unconscious mental processes which affect them.

MANIPULATIVE THERAPIES

Osteopathy and chiropractic are related systems of healthcare, now considered in Britain to be professions supplementary to medicine, since the passing of the Osteopaths' Act in 1993 and the Chiropractors' Act in 1994. Both therapies are classified in Group 1 of the House of Lords Report (2000) and are statutorily regulated by the General Osteopaths' Council and the General Chiropractic Council, and debate is currently focusing on the increasing incorporation of manipulative therapies into the National Health Service (Langworthy et al 2002). In the USA, osteopaths have long enjoyed the distinction of being considered comparable to medical doctors, using conventional therapeutic interventions in conjunction with specialised osteopathic techniques.

Osteopathy was devised by Andrew Taylor Still, an American doctor in the late 19th century, and is based on the principle that the body should be unified, with a properly aligned and functioning musculoskeletal system, since every other part of the body is directly or indirectly attached to it. It is a manipulative therapy, aimed at restoring and maintaining neuro-musculoskeletal homeostasis through facilitating appropriate biomechanical functioning of the body, by preserving the balance between all the muscles, joints, ligaments and nerves. Osteopaths use long leverage techniques to release affected joints, using rotation and flexion or extension to lock the joint into position before applying a high velocity thrust to a single specific apophyseal joint. Often the treatment is preceded by soft tissue massage to aid mobility of the joint. The techniques used can be summarised as high velocity, low amplitude thrusts and counterstrain, muscle energy techniques, myofascial release, lymphatic pumping techniques and craniosacral manipulation, with craniosacral therapy now being a therapy in its own right.

Chiropractic is concerned more with the relative position of joints, particularly vertebral joints, and the relationship between the nervous system and the mechanical framework of the body. The word 'chiropractic' originated from the Greek *cheir* (hand) and *praktikos* (to do or to perform), but although some of the principles of the therapy can be traced back to the time of the ancient Greeks, modern chiropractic was devised by Daniel D Palmer in the United States, in the 1890s, partly as a result of a difference of opinion between groups of osteopaths and anatomists about the precise mechanisms by which the body functions and the optimum methods of treatment to correct imbalances. The fundamental principle is the belief that the nervous system is the primary determinant of health and that subluxation of the vertebral joints places undue pressure on the spinal nerves and on the alignment of connective tissue fibres through the joint. Manipulation, using high velocity low amplitude thrusts, focuses mainly on the spinal rather than the peripheral joints of the body. X-rays are often used to provide a diagnosis and confirmation of the effects of treatment, and have, on at least one occasion, revealed cervical vertebral fractures which have been missed in an accident and emergency department, with standard radiographic techniques (King et al 2002). The high velocity thrust techniques are applied locally to an affected joint, with little use of massage or soft tissue work. Mobilisation is also employed, using manual force applied to joints to extend them beyond the normal passive range of movement. Chiropractic is far more popular with both consumers and medical practitioners in the USA than in the UK, with over 50% of doctors in one Midwestern area referring patients for treatment, or wishing to offer chiropractic, amongst other complementary therapies, to their patients (Rooney et al 2001).

Reflexology, or reflex zone therapy, is a system of healthcare, derived originally from ancient Chinese, Indian and Egyptian techniques, and more recently developed from the observations of an American ear, nose and throat surgeon, William Fitzgerald, who discovered that native American Indians used a form of treatment focusing on the feet. It is based on the principle that the feet represent a map of the whole body, so that by working manually on the feet, distal areas of the body can be treated. The hands are also used as a functioning map, and less frequently, other areas such as the ear, as in auriculotherapy, a form of ear acupuncture (Turgeon 1994), or the tongue may be used (Wong et al 2002). The feet are divided into ten longitudinal and three transverse zones, with each section corresponding to an area of the whole body. Treatment is via a method of manual compression techniques, although this is not simply foot *massage*; perhaps more descriptive terms for the special techniques used are 'caterpillar crawling' (Wagner 1987) or 'thumb walking' (Enzer 2000). Like massage, reflexology is classified as one of the 'supportive therapies' in group 2 of the House of Lords report (2000).

There are many theories about how reflexology works, for undoubtedly it has a profound effect on recipients, but whether this is just a degree of relaxation or something physiologically more significant is difficult to confirm, even by experienced practitioners. In his early work Fitzgerald attributed the actions of the therapy to its analgesic, relaxing and nerve blocking effects (Crane 1997; Marquardt 2000), possibly in a similar way to the gate control theory (Melzack & Wall 1965), although the impact of therapeutic touch may be responsible for the release of endorphins and encephalins and the consequent relaxation which has been demonstrated by Ferrell Torry and Glick (1993) and others. One of the most popular theories supports the concept of meridians as used in Traditional Chinese Medicine (see Chapter 4), since many of the reflexology points correspond to known acupuncture tsubos (Lett 2000). Other more contemporary and controversial theories include that of electromagnetism, in tandem with Schuman resonance of the earth (Bliss & Bliss 1999) and a neural pathway relationship (Baldry 1998).

Massage is, simply, the applied use of touch, but there are various types and styles, including Swedish massage, lymphatic drainage, Indian head, Feldenkrais, rolfing, tuina and others (see Glossary). A range of manual techniques is used including stroking, friction, tapping and percussion to manipulate the soft tissues of the body, reducing muscle tension, enhancing circulation and aiding elimination processes. Massage is a discrete therapy in its own right but can also be incorporated into other therapies such as aromatherapy, shiatsu, Chinese, Indian Ayurvedic and other traditional systems of healthcare.

SAFETY OF MANIPULATIVE THERAPIES

Generally accepted contraindications to manipulative treatments such as osteopathy and chiropractic include advanced osteoporosis, coagulation disorders and people taking anticoagulant therapy, spinal malignancies, inflammatory or infectious disease, which would also be applicable to the practice of massage. (Ernst et al 2001:47, 60, 65). In addition, anyone who feels uncomfortable with close physical contact (closer than in therapies such as massage or reflexology) is probably not suited to osteopathy or chiropractic.

Schvartzman and Abelson (1988) expressed concern about the potential side-effects of chiropractic, noting that patients often feel worse after treatment, although this may be due to a healing crisis taking place and be a normal part of the progress of treatment. In more recent surveys, Leboeuf-Yde et al (1997) and Senstad et al (1997) suggest that these mild and transient reactions are common, usually arising and resolving shortly after spinal manipulation. Approximately two thirds of patients report discomfort local to the affected (i.e. treated) area of the body, with 10% complaining of fatigue and headache and less than 5% suffering nausea, dizziness or other reactions. However, more severe, but rare, complications include reports of cerebrovascular accident (Turgut 2002; Assendelft et al 1996) and brain stem dysfunction (O'Neill 1994; Mueller & Sahs 1976), arterial dissection and cauda equina (Fibio 1999).

Practice point

Osteopathy and chiropractic should not be recommended for women taking anticoagulants and care should be exercised in whether or not to recommend these therapies to potentially pre-eclamptic women taking prophylactic aspirin.

Marquardt (2000:28-9) suggests that conditions most appropriately treated with reflexology are those affecting the musculoskeletal, digestive and lymphatic systems, and aches and pains such as headache, sinus congestion and dysmenorrhoea, and identifies absolute contraindications as major problems including aneurysms, organ transplantation, thromboembolitic or acute inflammatory disorders or when foreign bodies lie in close proximity to vital organs, such as a cardiac pacemaker. Women with a history of kidney or gallstones should be treated with caution, especially when the pregnancy has triggered renal complications. Patients who are hyperpyrexial or have an infectious disease, as well as those with psychoses, should be treated with caution. Major conditions affecting the feet, such as gangrene or acute eczema are classified as 'relative' contraindications, since reflexology can be performed on the hands. Theoretically it is also possible to interfere with certain drugs, for example insulin, by over-stimulating the pancreas zone, and care should be taken with diabetic women or those with epilepsy.

Reflexology should be used with caution for pregnant women, preferably performed by a midwife or other conventional healthcare professional, and avoided in women with actual or potential antenatal complications such as threatened miscarriage, antepartum haemorrhage or fulminating pre-eclampsia. Reflexology will *not*, as is often presumed by novices, initiate spontaneous abortion, but extreme care should be exercised with women with a history of previous miscarriage or preterm labour, as women will look for reasons, should complications arise. As there is insufficient evidence to prove conclusively that reflexology does not cause or encourage miscarriage, therapy is best avoided in these women except where the practitioner is experienced in both reflexology *and* conventional maternity care (Tiran 2002). This is particularly pertinent to the care of women with pregnancy sickness which commences in the first trimester, when miscarriage also most commonly occurs.

Direct massage to areas of phlebitis or thrombosis, burns, scalds, skin infections, open wounds and eczema is contraindicated, as well as over areas of bony fractures or osteoporosis. There is some controversy about its use in patients with cancer as it was originally thought that massage could cause spread of localised tumour growth, but this has not been borne out in clinical practice and the majority of hospices now offer it as a means of relaxation. Massage is not contraindicated during pregnancy but care should be taken when treating women with current or previous obstetric problems. Deep kneading type massage is contraindicated on specific points of the body corresponding to acupuncture tsubos which may initiate labour (see Chapter 4). There are very few reports of adverse effects from Swedish-style massage, although Ernst et al (2001:60) claim that bone fractures and rupture of the liver have been published, but give no references for these.

RESEARCH EVIDENCE

Pittler (2000) expressed concern about the 'glaring lack' of rigorous clinical trials in osteopathy in Europe, and Shwerla et al (1999) found that, of 30 studies identified, only five were of a reasonably acceptable standard and only *one* could be classified as a randomised clinical trial. Much of the research currently available involves studies on the use of the therapies, primarily chiropractic, for conditions such as back pain, particularly comparing these techniques with either physiotherapy or conventional management (Bronfort 1999). For example, Hurwitz et al (2002) found comparable outcomes in relieving neck pain between spinal chiropractic manipulation and mobilisation, although some authorities are less convinced of the superiority of spinal manipulation over other treatments for low back pain (Andersson et al 1999; Cherkin et al 1998; Skargren & Oberg 1998). Hertzman Miller et al (2002) revealed that patients with back pain enjoyed better communication with chiropractors than with physicians, although Stano et al (2002) highlighted the increased costs to patients of accessing chiropractic which is, in the main, provided in the private sector. Similarly, Licciardone et al (2002) demonstrated that patients seeking osteopathic manipulation were generally satisfied with the efficacy of the treatment but less so with the costs incurred and the lack of availability of insurance cover for osteopathy. Headache and other types of pain appear to have responded encouragingly to chiropractic, although studies reviewed may not be of sufficiently high calibre methodology (Vernon 2000; Vernon et al 1999).

Although both osteopathy and chiropractic are traditionally used to treat or prevent specific musculoskeletal conditions, they can also be very effective in alleviating conditions affecting soft tissues, but treatment is still based on the principle that all internal organs are indirectly related to changes in the skeletal framework of the body. Bryner and Staerker (1996) identified that, during one month, almost half of patients consulting Australian chiropractors for back pain also complained of indigestion and heartburn, and 22% obtained relief from the oesophageal problem after treatment for the musculoskeletal condition. Chiropractic is the most commonly used form of complementary therapy in children (Loo 1999) and has been used to good effect to treat children with asthma (Donnelly et al 1985) and infants with colic (Klougart et al 1989; Nilsson 1985) although similarly, the impact of relaxation and human touch cannot be eliminated; its value in the treatment of allergic disease has not been confirmed (Watkins 1994). Proctor et al (2001) reviewed several studies of chiropractic for primary and secondary dysmenorrhoea but found no statistically significant differences in effectiveness between specific manipulative techniques and sham procedures. However, ongoing or recurrent problems, as is the nature of dysmenorrhoea, require repeated treatments, sometimes over many months, making realistic evaluations of any complementary therapy difficult, as other factors come into play such as dependence on the therapist.

There is a relative paucity of research findings in reflexology when compared to some other areas of complementary medicine, with the majority showing positive results, possibly because those with negative findings fail to be published in the relevant academic and professional journals (Graham 1999; Kristof et al 1997). Many authorities consequently suggest that there is no evidence for the efficacy of the therapy (Botting 1997; Ernst & Koder 1997), and Maier (1999) somewhat disparagingly attributes *any* therapeutic effects *solely* to the improved sense of wellbeing from human touch without any apparent understanding of the mode of action.

Of the clinical reflexology investigations, one of the earliest was a small (n=16) randomised controlled trial to assess the effect of reflexology on surgical stress in patients undergoing cholecystectomy, by measuring plasma cortisol levels, but no differences were found between the trial group and a control (Engwquist & Vibe Hansen 1977), although a later study by Thomas (1989) (n=9) reported a general (subjective) reduction in patient anxiety. Analgesic effects have been demonstrated in studies on people with multiple sclerosis (Joyce & Richardson 1997), headache (Lafuente et al 1990; Launso et al 1999) and following gynaecological surgery (Eichelberger 1993), but not significantly so for those with chronic low back pain (Poole et al 2001; Degan et al 2000). Some minor improvement in bronchial asthma symptoms has been shown by Petersen et al (1992), and alleviation of constipation may be possible (Eriksen 1992), although Tovey's small single-blind study (2002) found no evidence of its value for

patients with irritable bowel syndrome. Interesting findings from Kesselring's randomised study of women following abdominal surgery (1998) indicated that reflexology may have some effect in facilitating postoperative micturition, but those who received reflexology rather than foot/leg massage or having a nurse talk to them, did not sleep as well, which is surprising given the supposed relaxation effects of the therapy. Frankel (1997) monitored changes in baroreceptor reflex sensitivity, blood pressure and sinus arrhythmia, but found little difference between the reflexology group and a group who received foot massage. The possibility that reflexology impacts on blood flow was investigated by Mur et al (2001) who showed a positive correlation between specific reflexology and improved blood flow during treatment, whereas a group of subjects receiving non-specific reflexology had no corresponding improvement. Spasticity and urinary symptoms improved in a group of people with multiple sclerosis when compared with non-specific calf massage (n=71) (Siev-Ner et al 1997), and 15 women attending a mental health drop-in centre responded well to a course of reflexology, with increased energy levels and physical activity, but this latter study had no control group (Trousdell 1996).

In the area of women's health, Oleson and Flocco (1993) used hand, foot and ear reflexology to relieve the symptoms of premenstrual syndrome, although this study highlighted one of the problems of reflexology, as did the Trousdell (1996) study above, of the need for repeated treatments to be performed, bringing into question the issue of both the client-therapist relationship (Thorlby & Panton 2002) and that of touch as the therapeutic medium. A more recent randomised controlled study into the use of reflexology for menopausal psychological symptoms (Williamson et al 2002) provided a course of nine treatment sessions of reflexology compared to foot massage, but found no significant differences between the groups, although almost 50% of the control (foot massage) group believed they had not received true reflexology. This highlights the difficulties of researching a therapy which involves human touch rather than a pharmacological therapy such as aromatherapy.

Only two maternity-specific reflexology studies have been found, in both of which women had received treatment regularly throughout pregnancy and then reported easier and more efficient labour contractions (Feder et al 1993; Motha & McGrath 1993). Case reports of the use of reflexology for pregnancy-induced hypertension (Yongsheng & Xiaolian 1995), carpal tunnel syndrome (Tiran 2002:140) and nausea and vomiting (Tiran 2002:140) have also been published.

Massage has been used successfully in the treatment of constipation (Ernst 1999a), to alleviate premenstrual symptoms (Hernandez-Rief et al 2000) and for relaxation for intensive care unit patients (Hayes & Cox 2000) and elderly institutionalised patients (Fraser & Kerr 1993). Massage is frequently used in conjunction with aromatherapy essential oils, but it is difficult to make any conclusive judgement as to whether the massage or the essential oils – or both – are the therapeutic mechanism, since many of the aromatherapy studies incorporating massage revolve around relaxation or associated disorders such as insomnia (Stevenson 1994; Dunn et al 1995).

The analgesic benefits of massage have been demonstrated in people with low back pain (Ernst 1999b) and fibromyalgia (Brattberg 1999) and for pain control in cancer patients (Weinrich & Weinrich 1990), presumably due to the release of endorphins (Kaada & Torsteinbo 1989) and the gate control mechanism (Doehring 1989). This latter theory has been supported by more recent work by Drevets et al (1995) who demonstrated changes in cerebral blood flow using positron emission tomography. Reduction of ischaemia as a result of local circulatory stimulation and skeletal muscle relaxation via stimulation of the parasympathetic nervous system may also contribute to a decrease in pain levels (McKechnie et al 1983).

TOUCH AS A THERAPEUTIC INTERVENTION

Although the theoretical basis, rationale and application to care of women with pregnancy sickness differ for each of these therapies (osteopathy, chiropractic and reflexology), they are all manual therapies, and therefore the impact of human touch cannot be disregarded. The psychological causes, predisposing factors and issues which exacerbate nausea and vomiting are explored in Chapter 8, but it is reasonable to assume that facilitating psychological and physical relaxation, by whatever means, may contribute to a perceived improvement in the severity of symptoms for some women.

Touch as a therapeutic intervention has been explored by many researchers, and a specific system of Therapeutic Touch (TT), devised by nursing professor Dolores Krieger in the 1970s, is an inherent component of nursing practice in the USA (Krieger 1975; Quinn 1989; Heidt 1991). However, massage, in various forms, has long been known to aid relaxation, but may also have other effects which can more specifically be applied to the treatment of women with nausea and vomiting. Much of the research on the physiological effects of massage has been done with neonates, most notably by Tiffany Field's team at the Miami Research Centre in Florida. Massage has been shown to assist in the maintenance of body temperature (Johanson et al 1992), improve oxygen saturation levels and heart rate (de Roiste et al 1995; de Roiste and Bushnell 1995; Adamson-Macedo et al 1994; Harrison et al 1990), adrenocorticol function (Acolet et al 1993; Kuhn et al 1991) and enhance long-term intellectual prognosis (Adamson-Macedo et al 1993). Maturation and growth has improved in babies given regular light massage (Kuhn et al 1991) and Scafidi et al (1996) demonstrated its effects on weight gain, attributed to increased vagal activity (assessed by vagal tone monitor), which in turn increased insulin levels.

Increased vagal activity is associated with a decrease in stress hormones such as cortisol, with an associated improvement in immune function. Massage has been shown to reduce cortisol and norepinephrine (Field et al 1992) and increase serotonin 5-HIAA levels (Hernandez-Rief et al 1999; Ironson et al 1996; Field, Grizzle, Scafidi et al 1996). An immunological link to gestational sickness has already been postulated by Leylek et al (1999) (see Chapter 1), implying that any means of enhancing immune function may have beneficial effects on the severity of nausea and vomiting in pregnancy. Furthermore, when vomiting is excessive, the production of energy from sources other than food has been associated with increased cortisol levels, and higher levels linked to greater weight loss and depression (Turner & Shapiro 1992; Faustman et al 1990).

Pain relief with massage can be attributed in part to the production of endorphins (Ferrell Torry & Glick 1993). The analgesic effects of serotonin (Field, Ironson, Pickens et al 1996) and its possible implication in the aetiology of muscular contraction and vascular headaches (Marcus 1993) may mean that massage is beneficial for those women with accompanying headaches and migraine, as may also reflexology (Brendstrup et al 1997). Maternal coping mechanisms may be facilitated by the use of massage or other therapies which increase psychological relaxation and aid sleep, especially as insomnia is another commonly reported concern of pregnant women. The increased secretion of substance P when an individual is deprived of sleep is known to cause pain, but its secretion is inhibited by the production of somatostatin which occurs during deep sleep (Sunshine et al 1996), and it is possible that better quality sleep with less disturbance has a beneficial effect on the severity of first trimester headaches and other discomforts.

Some improvement in essential hypertension has been shown using chiropractic, although whether this is as a result of a physiological or psychological effect is difficult to assess (Yates et al 1998). Plaugher et al's (2002) study revealed positive results for hypertension but it was noted that there were methodological difficulties in comparing groups receiving manipulation, massage or no treatment, due to the ineligibility of many patients who were already taking anti-hypertensive medication. Reflexology has also been shown to cause a statistically significant reduction in systolic blood pressure, although the number of subjects in Dryden et al's study (1999) was relatively small (n=19).

Practice point

Manual therapies may not have a direct impact on the nausea and vomiting experienced by pregnant women, but could be used effectively to alleviate associated symptoms such as headache, migraine or constipation, or to improve the general sense of wellbeing by reducing anxiety and depression.

Plotkin et al (2001) achieved relief for 100% of women receiving osteopathy for newly-diagnosed depression, compared to 33% of the control (no treatment) group. All women, in both groups, were already receiving conventional antidepressant medication, but it is impossible to extrapolate the impact of human touch through manipulation on the osteopathy group, especially for a psychological condition.

THE STRUCTURE OF THE BODY AND GESTATIONAL SICKNESS

The bilateral symmetry of the physical body is normally in equilibrium, but injury, disease or posture to compensate for previous trauma may upset this balance and cause minor, generally unrecognised tensions in one part of the body. This can be likened to the pressure exerted on the corner of a square cardboard box, which causes it to become more diamond-shaped – it is still the same box, but has compensated for tension in one part by adapting its shape. It is, therefore, not difficult to appreciate that tensions on the human body may be compensated for by minor adjustments in posture, but that these changes may in turn trigger other problems. Davis (2000) debated the impact of road traffic accidents on the musculoskeletal system and on the surrounding soft tissues, and concluded that individuals react to a minor impact in different ways, depending on their position in the vehicle and their ligamentous tensile strength, collagen fibres, muscle activation or inhibition, excitability of the nervous system and the size of the spinal canals. Peripheral trauma affects the central nervous system and, where whiplash injuries are involved, the somatosensory system of the neck may affect control of the neck, limbs, eyes, respiratory muscles and some preganglionic sympathetic nerves. Whiplash injuries can also cause post-traumatic neck and headache, jaw fatigue and severe temporomandibular joint clicking (Friedman & Weisberg 2000). Any of these may in turn lead to other acute or chronic pathology. A clinical example of this principle would be a woman sustaining a cervical vertebral injury, causing her to develop torticollis, which in turn puts tension on the head and its contents, namely the brain, indirectly affecting output of pituitary hormones and ultimately leading to disordered menstrual function.

We have already seen that gestational sickness is not simply the first trimester nausea and vomiting so frequently dismissed by those not actually suffering from it, but is indeed a complex phenomenon in which symptoms such as heartburn, hypersalivation, headaches and constipation may co-exist, either as an associated problem, or incidental to it. The accepted conventional scientific theories regarding the aetiology of nausea and vomiting in pregnancy have been discussed in depth in Chapter 1, and revolve mainly around the influence of hormones and other chemical and metabolic processes within the body. However, given the proximity of the vagus nerve, the vestibular apparatus and the vomiting centre in the brain to the cervical vertebrae, of the stomach and cardiac sphincter to the thoracic vertebrae, and of the reproductive tract to the lumbosacral vertebrae, it is not beyond the realms of feasibility to consider a structural, i.e. physical, link between parts of the body directly involved in the emetic process and those which initially appear not to be related.

Proctor et al's work into chiropractic for dysmenorrhoea (2001) reviewed the theoretical basis of the techniques used. It is thought that mechanical dysfunction in the second to fourth sacral vertebrae and between the tenth thoracic and second lumbar vertebrae, which are in close proximity to the parasympathetic and sympathetic pelvic nerve pathways, could decrease spinal mobility, leading to impairment of the

sympathetic nerve supply to the blood vessels of the pelvic viscera and consequent vasoconstriction and menstrual pain. An alternative theory is that of dysmenorrhoea being referred pain from musculoskeletal structures sharing the same pelvic nerve pathways.

These theories give some insight into the possible link between the musculoskeletal frame and more severe nausea and vomiting in pregnancy, although no chiropractic or osteopathic research specific to gestational sickness could be found in the literature. Conway (2000:47) suggests that thoracic vertebral misalignment occurs as a result of constant retching and vomiting, although conversely, pre-existing spinal problems may exacerbate hormonally-induced nausea. The influence of progesterone and other circulating hormones on the musculoskeletal system are well known, as the body adapts in preparation for labour (Penna 1989; Fallon 1990) although the effects of relaxin are disputed (Petersen et al 1994; Hansen et al 1996; Schauberger et al 1996). Biomechanical effects, such as increased mobility of joint capsules, and spinal segmental motor units as well as an altered structure in the connective tissue occur, which, together with increasing weight, cause the mother to adapt her posture and adopt a more pronounced lumbar lordosis, with the centre of gravity moving posteriorly to compensate (Blankenship & Blankenship 1980; Fligg 1986; Chalker 1993), although Dumas et al (1995) and Moore et al (1990) found no real evidence of lordosis. However, when exaggerated lordosis does occur, a corresponding kyphosis may also develop in the thoracic vertebrae to compensate, compounded by the development in breast size and weight which increases forward rotation of the shoulders. Probably half of all pregnant women suffer some degree of lower back pain during the antenatal period (Ostgaard et al 1994) but instability in the thoracic vertebral joints and early changes in the angles of the ribs due to increasing respiratory demand may cause discomfort and pain in the sternal, diaphragmatic and inter-scapulae regions (Mens et al 1996; Fallon 1986). Effects on the spinal and intercostal nerves also refer pain anteriorly to the chest. Heartburn, triggered by hormonal relaxation of the cardiac sphincter, may also be exacerbated if the musculoskeletal misalignments are pronounced. The cervical vertebrae compensate for the impact on the thoracic spine by inclining forwards and the occiput may extend on top of the first cervical vertebra, leading to headaches, neck and shoulder pain. Conway (2000:48) postulates that the inability of a woman to adapt to the changing centre of gravity as the uterus enlarges to become an abdominal organ may, in some, be due to previous lumbar spine injury.

Chiropractic and osteopathy can be used effectively to improve maternal postural adaptations to the pregnancy, thus directly or indirectly reducing the severity or occurrence of nausea and vomiting, as well as other discomforts such as backache, sciatica and symphysis pubis diastasis, and associated impact on the knees, hips, shoulders etc. Manipulative therapies for antenatal back pain may decrease the tendency of the fetus to settle into an occipito-posterior position, thereby reducing back pain in labour (Diakow et al 1991). A specific technique, the Webster technique, has also been used effectively by chiropractors to turn a breech presentation to cephalic (Pistolese 2002; Ohm 2001).

The theoretical principles of osteopathy and chiropractic, that the musculoskeletal system is the main supportive framework of the body, can be applied to reflexology. The experience of this author suggests a strong correlation between more severe sickness in pregnancy and a history such as whiplash injury from a road accident or coccygeal trauma following a fall, although this has not been tested scientifically and no anecdotal reports by other writers have been found in the literature. Trauma to the temporomandibular bone and jaw may also affect the salivary glands, giving a possible explanation for more severe salivation in some pregnant women (see Case 7.3).

However, successful alleviation of nausea and vomiting has been achieved in many women with this type of history when treated with reflexology, working on the zones of the feet corresponding to the head, neck and spine, rather than the zones for the organs directly involved in the physiopathology of sickness (see Cases 7.1, 7.2). Over many years of working with pregnant women suffering sickness, treatment strategies have evolved, and whereas initially, four to five reflexology sessions of 30 minutes may have been necessary (during which time the symptoms may have resolved simply with the passage of time), effective reduction in the severity of nausea and frequency of vomiting can now usually be achieved with one ten-minute treatment. Often an immediate sense of relief is obtained by the mother, after manipulations of the feet which produce 'cracking' sounds and sensations, in the zones relating to the neck and ribs; these responses usually indicate a release of tensions in the relevant parts of the body. Any associated heartburn may also be relieved with this technique. If there has been no improvement in symptoms after three consecutive weeks, reflexology is deemed not to be appropriate and treatment is discontinued in favour of other complementary therapies. However, ad hoc, over-enthusiastic application of the relevant techniques by therapists who are not also midwives is actively discouraged as immediate, short-term side-effects can arise, such as extremes of temperature, exacerbation of nausea, fainting and dizziness and excessive fetal movements. More long-term complications are also possible, which require expert midwifery or obstetric management, although these should not occur if caution is exercised in the first instance.

A more controversial explanation of the effects of trauma on the body is that of 'energy medicine', relating the displacements caused by injury to gravitational pull within the body (Oschman 2000:160). Thus, physical trauma leads to physical displacements of the affected area, resulting in compensatory changes throughout the body, such as muscular contraction, circulatory and lymphatic flow impediment and alterations in neural activity. Even the habitual way in which a person holds the head in relation to gravity, frequently tipped forwards with the cervical spine bent, can trigger distal adaptations. The vertebral artery becomes

---

Practice point

Reflex zone therapy may be an appropriate technique to treat nausea and vomiting in women with a history of neck or back problems, but should not be attempted by inexperienced practitioners or those who do not have a comprehensive understanding of the pathophysiology of pregnancy.

Figures 7.1 – 7. 3 Reflex zone therapy techniques for treating pregnancy sickness in women with a history of neck or back problems

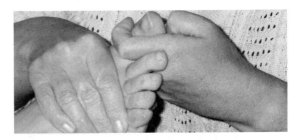

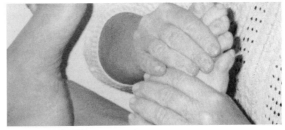

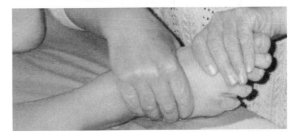

curved instead of straight, narrowing the lumen and restricting cervical circulation. This means that oxygenation and nourishment of the brain and sensory organs situated in the head are decreased, affecting the cerebral ventricles and the sympathetic-parasympathetic balance, leading to gastrointestinal conditions. Similarly, psychological upheaval may cause an individual to adopt a particular stance or pose (body language), precipitating contraction of flexor muscles and deviations from structural equilibrium, leading to tension and compensatory functional changes. Previous accidental or intentional traumas (e.g. from surgery) can thus have a bearing on current health status and in the case of gestational sickness may appear at first to be totally unrelated (see Case 7.2).

Reflexology should not normally be considered as a diagnostic tool in the conventional sense of the word, but most experienced therapists are able to deduce, from the feet, changing physiology and current, previous or impending pathology, although Mackereth (2001) views this as an adjunct to more traditional methods of diagnosis. One investigation of the potential of reflexology as a means of diagnosis (Baerheim et al 1998) found a tendency of therapists to *over*-diagnose, finding supposed pathology where none existed. Conversely, there are many anecdotal reports of practitioners detecting visual or palpable deviations from the expected norm which alerts them to abnormal conditions (see Cases 7.4, 7.5).

Case 7.1

A 32-year-old multigravid woman came to the CT clinic with severe sickness, worse than any she had experienced with her previous two pregnancies. On questioning her the CT midwife discovered that she had been in a road accident the year before when she suffered a whiplash injury which had left her with persistently recurring headaches and neck pain. The CT midwife performed a ten-minute treatment using osteopathic/chiropractic theory applied to reflexology

techniques, working on the foot zones related to the head, neck and spine. The woman returned the following week, and although she reported an exacerbation of the nausea and vomiting the day after the reflexology, which was probably a healing crisis, she had then improved and had not vomited once since then, nor had she suffered a headache. Although the nausea remained, the expectant mother now felt able to cope with her symptoms and no further treatment was required.

Case 7.2

A 21-year-old woman consulted the CT midwife for treatment of her nausea and vomiting. She also reported a preconceptional history of neck pain and headaches which had become more severe since becoming pregnant. The midwife asked to examine the woman's feet, from a reflexology perspective and was fascinated to find prominent scarring along the medial aspects of the large toes, suggestive of previous surgery to remove bunions, which the woman confirmed as having been undertaken at the age of ten. On closer questioning the woman identified the onset of her headaches at about the age of 11, shortly after the surgery, which, in reflexology terms, would explain the aetiology, as the large toes represent the zones for the head and neck. The midwife then performed reflexology techniques specifically on the large toes as she believed the pregnancy sickness to be exacerbated by the trauma in these areas. The following week the woman cancelled her appointment, reporting that she had experienced almost immediate relief of both her headaches and her vomiting, although a minor degree of nausea persisted.

Case 7.3

A 34-year-old West African woman in her second pregnancy came to the CT clinic with intractable hypersalivation; during the consultation she needed constantly to spit out the excess saliva and by the end of her appointment she had filled a small pot which she was obliged to carry with her. She was extremely distressed as she had suffered the symptom in her previous pregnancy which had ended in an intra-uterine death and she was anxious that the same would happen in this pregnancy. As she was a doctor, her professional knowledge added to her personal anxiety, but she was prepared to try anything which might help her. She also reported jaw ache, which seemed secondary to a previous fracture. The CT midwife performed a five-minute focused reflexology technique, working on the foot zones specifically for the mouth, jaw and neck. The following week the woman returned, looking much better and announced that she did not need further treatment as the hypersalivation was much reduced and she was now able to control it. The decrease in the physical problem had made her feel psychologically much better and her concerns for the prognosis of the pregnancy were also much more in perspective.

Case 7.4

A woman had suffered hyperemesis gravidarum in both her previous pregnancies but this time her condition was even worse. She vomited up to ten times daily and had already been admitted to hospital for rehydration seven times by the 16th week of her pregnancy. She attended the CT clinic accompanied by her mother who walked with a stick. The pregnant woman had a history of neck and back pain before pregnancy and was complaining of lower abdominal pain for which no cause could be found. On examining her feet, the CT midwife immediately noticed a brown pigmented area over the lower aspect of the inner ankle bone on the left foot, an area in reflexology terms corresponding to the symphysis pubis. On closer questioning it transpired that her abdominal' pain was, in fact, suprapubic, which from a midwifery perspective seemed to indicate symphysis pubis diastasis. The woman also felt tenderness when the midwife palpated the lower edge of the outer ankle bone on the same foot, the area related, in reflexology, to the hip and sacroiliac joint. The CT midwife intuitively asked the woman's mother the reason for her use of a stick and was told that she had been born with no acetabulum, a fact which was only discovered at the age of 31 when a pelvic X-ray was performed. The CT midwife returned to the patient's feet, working on the reflexology zones for the spine, neck, hip, sacroiliac joint and symphysis pubis zones. The woman could only tolerate a few minutes' work but reported feeling much better, less nauseated and relieved of much of the pain in her lower abdomen.

The following week the woman arrived looking dreadful and said she had been so severely sick that she had been readmitted to hospital five days after the reflexology. However she agreed to further treatment and again left the clinic feeling much more at ease, both physically and psychologically. On the third week the woman required virtually no reflexology treatment – the vomiting had decreased to just a couple of times a day and the perpetual nausea had ceased. She was delighted, needed no further treatment and progressed with her pregnancy with no other problems.

Following delivery, she underwent orthopaedic investigations and was found to have an acetabular problem similar to that of her mother, for which she was then able to have surgery.

(Tiran 2002:140)

Case 7.5

The complementary therapy (CT) midwife was asked to see a 31-year-old primigravida admitted to the gynaecology ward at 17 weeks' gestation for hyperemesis gravidarum, with vomiting six to seven times daily. The woman reported a history of back problems, prompting the midwife to consider reflexology as a possible treatment for the sickness (see Box 7.1). On inspection, the mother's feet showed a marked greyish tinge over the dorsal aspect of the large toes, at the junction with the foot, an area corresponding to the throat. Making an educated guess, based on her knowledge of the aetiology of hyperemesis gravidarum, the midwife suggested that there could be a thyroid implication in the woman's condition and advised the taking of blood samples, which later showed changes in the thyroid hormone levels, which were then treated with conventional thyroxine (see Chapter 1).

Box 7.1 Identification of women with pregnancy sickness for whom reflex zone therapy may be appropriate

- Pregnancy sickness or associated complaints unresponsive to other conventional or complementary strategies
- History of previous head, neck or back injury
- No antepartum haemorrhage, threatened miscarriage or preterm labour
- No current fulminating pre-eclampsia; not on prophylactic aspirin

- No hyper-pyrexia, infectious disease or problems directly affecting feet
- No cardiac illness/pacemaker in situ
- Caution with diabetics, epileptics, history of renal or gallstones
- Caution with women with thyroid conditions
- Avoid in women who reject foot-focused therapy

VESTIBULAR APPARATUS STIMULATION

Although stimulation of the vestibular apparatus as a means of relieving nausea and vomiting is not directly *structural*, it is based on the *neuro-anatomical* relationship between the vomiting centre and the balancing mechanism in the ear, and is dependent on a gravitational balance involving posture and the relative positioning of the head, neck and body. Changes in the position of the head cause an alteration in the force exerted on hairs of the maculae with consequent bending, leading to stimulation of dendrites in the vestibular neurons, with impulses transmitted via the vestibulocochlear nerve to the vestibular nuclei of the medulla. Exaggerated stimulation of the vestibular apparatus due to movement results in nausea and vomiting. It is also possible that previous neck or upper spinal injury or trauma, coupled with the relaxation effects of progesterone and relaxin, may in some pregnant women lead to increased susceptibility for over-stimulation of the vestibular apparatus, perhaps through a mechanism as yet not fully understood.

Treatments aimed at influencing the impact of the vestibular apparatus on nausea and vomiting are not new but neither are they well known nor recognised as being of value. The principle of interrupting neurological receptor chains with signals from the ear is borne out by an understanding of the processes involved in vomiting. Electrostimulation of the vestibular apparatus has been used to treat motion sickness, and, in one study of 26 women with hyperemesis gravidarum, was found to be effective in 89% of cases (Golaszewski et al 1995).

A vestibular apparatus self-help programme has been developed recently, in which an auditory tape using a range of specific frequencies, pulses and tones aims to intercept the impulses between the gut and the brain. Although the tape contains music, this is *not* a relaxation tape, nor does it contain hypnotherapeutic suggestions, but is precisely formulated with three distinct phases, the music only being used to make the tape more pleasant to use. The tape must be used via personal headphones in order that the pulsations can have a direct effect on the vestibular apparatus.

The first phase is an 'attention grabbing' phase, in which the vestibular apparatus is distracted from its preoccupation with balance and acoustics and forced to focus on the frequencies of the programme. The second phase provides the vestibular apparatus with tones, pulses and frequencies which prevent it from returning to its pre-treatment mode of maintaining balance and acoustics so that the passage of signals to the brain and digestive tract are different from signals which would normally trigger the emetic process, causing nausea and leading to vomiting. The final phase is critical and enables the vestibular apparatus to return to normal functioning by gradually reducing the tones and pulses until they are reconstituted with normal audio signals. The programme has been devised by a commercial company, originally to help people with motion sickness, but has since been piloted in various oncology units and at the Andover Birth Centre in Hampshire (Mayo 2001) with a 90% success rate in women with pregnancy sickness. There appear to be no reported side-effects and theoretically no dangers to either the mother or fetus.

CONCLUSION

This chapter has explored the theory that pregnancy sickness is not only a condition of endocrine aetiology, but may be initiated or exacerbated by misalignments in the musculoskeletal system which place tensions on the soft tissues. Osteopathic/chiropractic theory, in which all elements of disease or disorder within the body are considered to be due to postural and structural adaptations to compensate for habitual or traumatic effects on individual components of the body, has been applied to this author's practice of reflex zone therapy to treat successfully women with nausea and vomiting

and associated hypersalivation, heartburn, constipation and headaches.

The theoretical basis on which this practice is based has not yet been tested scientifically, but may offer an alternative perspective on sickness and other discomforts and disorders of pregnancy, which is worthy of further investigation. Despite wide searches of the literature, dissemination of ideas and networking at professional academic events, no other written or verbal confirmation has been obtained to sustain this theory, and this author has not learned of other practitioners employing specific reflexology techniques such as these, although osteopaths and chiropractors frequently use manipulative techniques to alleviate nausea and vomiting in pregnant women. It is therefore difficult to determine whether its effectiveness is due to the specific reflex zone technique, to the relaxation effects of a brief reflexology treatment, to the impact of human touch, or to the psychological benefits on the women of being able to talk over their condition with someone who has the time to validate it.

There could be a tendency to state that the placebo effect of being told that a precise technique may relieve the symptoms is the mechanism by which it works, and that, if it does no harm, it can be attempted in the hope that it may do some good. However, the repeated success of this treatment over many years, albeit by a single practitioner, offers, at the very least, a possibility for future studies. Although osteopathy and chiropractic require a fully qualified practitioner to perform any manipulations, applying their theories to reflexology may enable midwives to learn a precise, focused technique which takes very little time to perform, and to offer this to appropriately identified expectant mothers to assist in relieving the sickness.

REFERENCES

Acolet D, Modi N, Giannakoulopoulos X et al 1993 Changes in plasma cortisol and catecholamine concentrations in response to massage in preterm infants. Archives of Diseases in Childhood (Fetal & Neonatal Edition) 68 (1): 29-31

Adamson-Macedo E N, Dattani I, Wilson A et al 1993 Small sample follow-up study of children who received tactile stimulation after preterm birth: intelligence and achievements. Journal of Reproductive and Infant Psychology 11 (3): 165-168

Adamson-Macedo E N, de Roiste A, Wilson A et al 1994 TAC-TIC therapy: the importance of systematic stroking. British Journal of Midwifery 2 (6): 264, 266-269

Andersson G B J, Lipton J A, Leurgans S A 1999 A comparison of osteopathic spinal manipulation with standard care for patients with low back pain. New England Journal of Medicine 341: 1426-1431

Assendelft W J, Boulter L M, Knipschild P G 1996 Complications of spinal manipulation. Journal of Family Practice 42: 475-480

Baerheim A, Algroy R, Skogedal K R et al 1998 Fottene et diagnostic hjelpemiddel? Tidsskr Nor Laegeforen 5: 753-755

Baldry P E 1998 Trigger point acupuncture. In: Filshie J, White A (eds) 1998 Medical acupuncture: a Western scientific approach. Churchill Livingstone, New York

Blankenship T, Blankenship V G 1980 Biomechanics of back pain in the gravid female. American Chiropractic Association Journal of Chiropractic 1: 113-115

Bliss J, Bliss G 1999 How does reflexology work? Theories on why it does work. Reflexology Association of California www.reflexcal.org/article4.html (accessed 15 February 2000)

Botting D 1997 Review of the literature on the effectiveness of reflexology. Complementary Therapies in Nursing and Midwifery 3 (5): 123-130

Brattberg G 1999 Connective tissue massage in the treatment of fibromyalgia. European Journal of Pain 3: 235-245

Brendstrup E, Launso L, Eriksen L 1997 Headaches and reflexological treatment, 4th edn. Association of Reflexologists, London

Brewer J F 1998 Healing sounds. Complementary Therapies in Nursing and Midwifery 4 (1): 7-12

Bronfort G 1999 Spinal manipulation, current state of research and its indications. Neurological Clinics in North America 17: 91-111

Bryner P, Staerker P G 1996 Indigestion and heartburn: a descriptive study of prevalence in persons seeking care form chiropractors. Journal of Manipulative and Physiological Therapeutics 100 (7): 27-31

Cherkin D C, Deyo R A, Battie M et al 1998 A comparison of physical therapy, chiropractic manipulation and provision of an educational booklet for the treatment of patients with low back pain. New England Journal of Medicine 339: 1021-1029

Conway P 2000 Osteopathy during pregnancy. In: Tiran D, Mack S (eds) Complementary therapies for pregnancy and childbirth, 2nd edn. Bailliere Tindall, London

Crane B 1997 Reflexology: the definitive practitioner's manual. Element, Shaftesbury

Davis C G 2000 Injury threshold: whiplash-associated disorders. Journal of Manipulative and Physiological Therapeutics 23 (6): 420-427

Degan M, Fabris F, Vanin F et al 2000 The effectiveness of foot reflexotherapy on chronic pain associated with herniated disk. Professioni Infermieristiche 53 (2): 80-87

De Roiste A, Bushnell I W R 1995 The immediate gastric effects of a tactile stimulation programme on premature infants. Journal of Reproductive and Infant Psychology 13 (1): 57-62

De Roiste A, Bushnell I, Burns J 1995 TAC-TIC: how do special care baby units react to it? British Journal of Midwifery 3 (1): 8-10,12-15

Diakow P R, Gadsby T A, Gadsby J B et al 1991 Back pain during pregnancy and labour. Journal of Manipulative and Physiological Therapeutics 14 (2): 116-118

Doehring K M 1989 Relieving pain through touch. Advances in Clinical Care 4 (5): 32

Donnelly W J, Spykerboer J E, Thong Y H 1985 Are patients who use alternative medicine dissatisfied with orthodox medicine? Medical Journal of Australia 142: 439

Drevets W C et al 1995 Blood flow changes in human somatosensory cortex during anticipated stimulation. Nature 373 (6511): 249. Cited by Taylor A G 1999 Complementary/alternative therapies in the treatment of pain. In: Spencer J W, Jacobs J J Complementary/ alternative medicine – an evidence-based approach. Mosby, Edinburgh

Dryden S L, Holden S A, Mackereth P A 1999 'Just the ticket': the findings of a pilot complementary therapy service (part II). Complementary Therapies in Nursing and Midwifery 5: 15-18

Dunn C, Sleep J, Collett D 1995 Sensing an improvement: an experimental study to evaluate the use of aromatherapy, massage and periods of rest in an intensive care unit. Journal of Advanced Nursing 21: 34-40

Eichelberger G 1993 Study on foot reflex zone massage: alternative to tablets. Krankenpfledge-Soins Infirmiers 86 (5): 61-63

Engwquist A, Vibe-Hansen H 1977 Zone therapy and plasma cortisol during surgical stress. Ugeskrift for Laeger 139: 460-462

Enzer S 2000 Reflexology: a tool for midwives. Self-published, Australia

Eriksen L 1992 Zoneterapi mod knonisk forstoppelse [Zone therapy for chronic constipation]. Sygeplejersken 92 (26): 7

Ernst E 1999a Abdominal massage therapy for chronic constipation: a systematic review of controlled clinical trials. Forsch Komplementarmed 6: 149-151

Ernst E 1999b Massage therapy for low back pain: a systematic review. Journal of Pain and Symptom Management 17: 65-69

Ernst E, Koder K 1997 Reflexology: an overview. European Journal of General Practice 3: 52-57

Ernst E, Pittler M, Stevinson C et al 2001 The desktop guide to complementary and alternative medicine – an evidence-based approach. Mosby, Edinburgh

Fallon J M 1990 Chiropractic and pregnancy: a partnership for the future. International Chiropractors' Association International Review of Chiropractic 1: 39-42

Faustman W, Faull K, Whiteford H et al 1990 CSF-5-HIAA, serum cortisol, and age differentially predict vegetative and cognitive symptoms in depression. Biological Psychiatry 27: 311-318

Feder E, Liisberg G B, Lenstrup C et al 1993 Zone therapy in relation to birth. Proceedings of the International Confederation of Midwives 23rd International Congress 2: 651-656

Ferrell Torry A T, Glick O J 1993 The use of therapeutic massage as a nursing intervention to modify anxiety and the perception of pain. Cancer Nursing 16 (2): 93-101

Fibio R 1999 Manipulation of the cervical spine: risks and benefits. Physical Therapy 79: 50-65

Field T, Morrow C, Valdeon C et al 1992 Massage reduces anxiety in child and adolescent psychiatric patients. Journal of the American Academy of Child and Adolescent Psychiatry 31: 125-131

Field T, Grizzle N, Scafidi F et al 1996 Massage and relaxation therapies' effects on depressed adolescent mothers. Adolescence 31: 903-911

Field T, Ironson G, Pickens J et al 1996 Massage therapy reduces anxiety and enhances EEG pattern of alertness and math computations. International Journal of Neuroscience 86: 197-205

Fligg B 1986 Biomechanical and treatment considerations for the pregnant patient. Journal of the Canadian Chiropractic Association 30 (3): 145-147

Frankel B 1997 The effect of reflexology on baroreceptor reflex sensitivity, blood pressure and sinus arrhythmia. Complementary Therapies in Medicine 5: 80-84

Fraser J, Kerr J R 1993 Psychophysiological effects of back massage on elderly institutionalised patients. Nursing 18: 238-245

Friedman M H, Weisberg J 2000 The craniocervical connection: a retrospective analysis of 300 whiplash patients with cervical and temporomandibular disorders. Cranio 18 (3): 163-167

Golaszewski T, Frigo P, Mark H E et al 1995 Treatment of hyperemesis gravidarum by electrostimulation of the vestibular apparatus. Zeitschrift Geburtshilfe Neonatologie 199 (3): 107-110

Graham H 1999 Complementary therapies in context: the psychology of healing. Jessica Kingsley Publishers, London

Hansen A, Vendelbo Jensen D, Larsen E et al 1996 Relaxin is not related to symptom giving pelvic girdle relaxation in pregnant women. Acta Obstetrica et Gynecologica Scandinavia 75: 245-249

Harrison L L, Leeper J D, Yoon M 1990 Effects of early parent touch on preterm infants' heart rates and arterial oxygen saturation levels. Journal of Advanced Nursing 15 (8): 877-885

Hayes J, Cox C 2000 Immediate effects of a five-minute foot massage on patients in critical care. Complementary Therapies in Nursing and Midwifery 6 (1): 9-13

Heidt P R 1991 Helping patients to rest; clinical studies in Therapeutic Touch. Holistic Nursing Practice 5 (4): 57-66

Hernandez Rief M, Dieter J, Filed T et al 1999 Massage therapy effects on headache sufferers. International Journal of Neuroscience 96: 11

Hernandez Rief M, Martinez A, Field T et al 2000 Premenstrual symptoms are relieved by massage therapy. Journal of Psychosomatic Obstetrics and Gynecology 21: 9-15

Hertzman Miller R P, Morganstern H, Hurwitz E L et al 2002 Comparing the satisfaction of low back pain patients randomised to receive medical or chiropractic care: results from the UCLA low-back pain study. American Journal of Public Health 92 (10): 1628-1633

Hurwitz E L, Morganstern H, Harber P et al 2002 A randomised trial of chiropractic manipulation and mobilisation for patients with neck pain: outcomes from the UCLA neck pain study. American Journal of Public Health 92 (10): 1634-1641

Ironson G, Field T, Scafidi F et al 1996 Massage therapy is associated with enhancement of the immune system's cytotoxic capacity. International Journal of Neuroscience 84: 205-217

Jeffreys P 2000 Feng shui for the health sector: harmonious buildings, healthier people. Complementary Therapies in Nursing and Midwifery 6 (2): 61-65

Johanson R B, Spencer S A, Rolfe P et al 1992 Effect of post-delivery care on neonatal body temperature. Acta Paediatrica 81 (11): 859-863

Joyce M, Richardson J 1997 Reflexology can help MS. International Journal of Alternative and Complementary Medicine July: 10-12

Kaada B, Torsteinbo O 1989 Increase in plasma beta-endorphins in connective tissue massage. General Pharmacology 20 (4): 487

Kesselring A, Spichiger E, Muller M 1998 Foot reflexology - an intervention study. Pflege 11 (4): 213-218

King S W, Hosler B K, King M A 2002 Missed cervical spine fracture-dislocations: the importance of clinical and radiographic assessment. Journal of Manipulative and Physiological Therapeutics 25 (4): 263-269

Klougart N, Nilsson N, Jacobsen J 1989 Infantile colic treated by chiropractors: a prospective study of 316 cases. Journal of Manipulative and Physiological Therapeutics 12 (4): 281

Krieger D 1975 Therapeutic Touch: the imprimatur of nursing. American Journal of Nursing 5 (75): 784-787

Kristof O, Schlumpf M, Saller R 1997 Foot reflex zone massage – a review. Wiener Medizinische Wochenschrift 147 (18): 418-422

Kuhn C M, Schanberg S M, Field T et al 1991 Tactile-kinesthetic stimulation effects on sympathetic and adrenocorticol function in preterm infants. Journal of Pediatrics 119 (3): 434-440

Lafuente A, Noguera M, Puy C et al 1990 Effekt der Reflexzone behandlung am Fuss bezuglich der prophylaktischen behandlung mit Funarizin bei an Cephalea-kopfschmerzen leidenen Patienten. Erfarhungsheilkunde 39: 713-715

Langworthy J M, Breen A C, Vogel S 2002 Third-place chiropractic and the national health care system: a basis for partnership in the UK. Journal of Manipulative and Physiological Therapeutics 25 (1): 21-33

Launso Brendstrup E, Arnberg S 1999 An exploratory study of reflexological treatment for headache. Alternative Therapies 5 (3): 57-65

Leboeuf-Yde C, Hennius B, Rudberg E et al 1997 Side effects of chiropractic treatment: a prospective study. Journal of Manipulative and Physiological Therapeutics 20 (8): 511-515

Lett A 2000 Reflex zone therapy for health professionals. Churchill Livingstone, Edinburgh

Leylek O A, Toyaksi M, Erselcan T et al 1999 Immunologic

and biochemical factors in hyperemesis gravidarum with or without hyperthyroxinaemia. Gynecologic and Obstetric Investigation 47 (4): 229-234

Licciardone J, Gamber R, Cardarelli K 2002 Patient satisfaction and clinical outcomes associated with osteopathic manipulative treatment. Journal of the American Osteopathic Association 102 (1): 13-20

Loo M 1999 Complementary/alternative therapies in select populations: children. In: Spencer J W, Jacobs J J (eds) Complementary/alternative medicine: an evidence-based approach. Mosby, St Louis

Mackereth P 2001 'Reflexology techniques are not an effective tool for symptom recognition of the diagnosis of medical conditions': The case against. Complementary Therapies in Nursing and Midwifery 71: 45-49

Maier E 1999 Knowledge and effectiveness of so-called foot sole reflex massage. Versicherungsmedizin 51 (2): 75-79

Marcus D A 1993 Serotonin and its role in headache pathogenesis and treatment. Clinical Journal of Pain 9 (3): 159-167

Marieb E N 2001 Human anatomy and physiology, 5th edn. Addison Wesley Longman, San Francisco

Marquardt H 2000 Reflexotherapy of the feet. Thieme, Stuttgart

McKechnie B et al 1983 Anxiety states: a preliminary report on the value of connective tissue massage. Journal of Psychosomatic Research 27 (2): 125

Melzack R, Wall P D 1965 Pain mechanisms: a new theory. Science 150: 971-979

Motha G, McGrath J 1993 The effects of reflexology on labour outcomes. Reflexions: Journal of the Association of Reflexologists November: 2-4

Mueller S, Sahs A L 1976 Brain stem dysfunction related to cervical manipulation. Neurology 26: 547

Mur E, Schmidseder J, Egger I et al 2001 Influence of reflex zone therapy of the feet on intestinal blood flow measured by color Doppler sonography. Forsch Komplementarmed Klass Naturheilkd 8 (2): 86-89

Nilsson N 1985 Infantile colic and chiropractic. European Journal of Chiropractic 33: 264

Ohm J 2001 Chiropractors and midwives – a look at the Webster technique. Midwifery Today International Summer: 38-42

Oleson T, Flocco W 1993 Randomised controlled study of premenstrual symptoms treated with ear, hand and foot reflexology. Obstetrics and Gynaecology 82 (6): 906-911

O'Neill A 1994 Danger and safety in medicines. Social Sciences and Medicines 38 (4): 497-507

Oschman J L 2000 Energy medicine – the scientific basis. Churchill Livingstone, Edinburgh

Ostgaard H C, Zetherstrom G, Roos-Hansson E et al 1994 Reduction of back and posterior pelvic pain in pregnancy. Spine 19 (8): 804-900

Penna M 1989 Pregnancy and chiropractic care. American Chiropractic Association Journal of Chiropractic 1: 31-33

Petersen K L, Hvidman L, Uldbjerg N 1994 Normal serum relaxin in women with disabling pelvic pain during pregnancy. Gynecological and Obstetric Investigations 38: 21-23

Petersen L N, Faurschou P, Olsen O T 1992 Foot zone therapy and bronchial asthma: a controlled clinical trial. Ugeskrift for Laeger 154 (30): 2065-2068

Pistolese R A 2002 The Webster technique: a chiropractic technique with obstetric implications. Journal of Manipulative and Physiological Therapeutics 25 (6): E1-9

Pittler M H 2000 Osteopathy: a glaring lack of rigorous clinical trials from Europe. Focus on Alternative and Complementary Therapies 5 (2): 132-133

Plaugher G, Long C R, Alcantara J et al 2002 Practice-based randomised controlled-comparison clinical trial of chiropractic adjustments and brief massage treatment at sites of subluxation in subjects with essential hypertension ; a pilot study. Journal of Manipulative and Physiological Therapeutics 25 (4): 221-239

Plotkin B J, Rodos J J, Kappler R et al 2001 Adjunctive osteopathic manipulative treatment in women with depression: a pilot study. Journal of the American Osteopathic Association 101 (9): 517-523

Poole H M, Murphy P, Glenn S 2001 Evaluating the efficacy of reflexology for the management of chronic low back pain. Journal of Pain 2 (2): 47

Proctor M L, Hing W, Johnson T C et al 2001 Spinal manipulation for primary and secondary dysmenorrhoea (Cochrane Review) Cochrane Database Systematic Review 4: CD 002119 2.6.02

Quinn J F 1989 Therapeutic Touch as energy exchange: replication and extension. Nursing Science Quarterly 2 (2): 79-87

Rooney B, Fiocco G, Hughes P et al 2001 Provider attitudes and use of alternative medicine in a Midwestern medical practice in 2001. Wisconsin Medical Journal 100 (7): 27-31

Savarimuthu D, Bunnell T 2002 The effects of music on clients with learning disabilities: a literature review. Complementary Therapies in Nursing and Midwifery 8 (3): 160-165

Scafidi F, Field T, Wheedon A et al 1996 Behavioural and hormonal differences in preterm neonates exposed to cocaine in vitro. Pediatrics 97: 851-855

Schauberger C W, Rooney B L, Goldsmith L et al 1996 Peripheral joint laxity increase in pregnancy but does not correlate with serum relaxin levels. American Journal of Obstetrics and Gynecology 174 (2): 667-671

Schwerla F, Hass-Degg K, Schwerla B 1999 Evaluierng und kritische Bewertung von in der europaischen Literatur veroffentlichten, osteopathischen Studien im klinischen Bereich und im Bereich der Grundlagenforschung Forsch Komplementarmed 6: 302-310. Cited by Pittler M H 2000 Osteopathy: a glaring lack of rigorous clinical trials from Europe. Focus on Alternative and Complementary Medicine 5 (2): 132-133

Senstad O, Leboeuf-Y de C, Borchgrevink C 1997 Frequency and characteristics of side effects of spinal manipulative therapy. Spine 22: 435-441

Shvartzman P, Abelson A 1988 Complications of chiropractic treatment for back pain. Postgraduate Medicine 83 (7): 57-8

Siev-Ner I, Gamus D, Lerner-Geva L et al 1997 Reflexology treatment relieves symptoms of multiple sclerosis: a randomised controlled study. FACT 2: 196

Skargren E, Oberg B E 1998 Predictive factors for 1-year outcome of low-back and neck pain in patients treated in primary care: comparison between the treatment strategies chiropractic and physiotherapy. Pain 77: 201-207

Stano M, Haas M, Goldberg B et al 2002 Chiropractic and medical costs of low back care: results from a practice-based observational study. American Journal of Managed Care 8(9): 802-809

Stevenson C 1994 The psychophysiological effects of aromatherapy massage following cardiac surgery. Complementary Therapies in Medicine 2 (1): 27-35

Suen L K P, Thomas K, Wong S et al 2001 Is there a place for auricular acupuncture in the realm of nursing? Complementary Therapies in Nursing and Midwifery 7 (3): 132-139

Sunshine W, Field T, Schanberg S et al 1996 Massage therapy and transcutaneous electrical stimulation effects on fibromyalgia. Journal of Clinical Rheumatology 2: 18-22

Thomas M 1989 Fancy footwork. Nursing Times 85 (41): 42-44

Tiran D 2002 Supporting women during pregnancy and childbirth. In: Mackereth P, Tiran D (eds) Clinical reflexology: a guide for health professionals. Elsevier Science, London

Tovey P 2002 A single-blind trial of reflexology for irritable bowel syndrome. British Journal of General Practice 52 (474): 19-23

Trousdell P 1996 Reflexology meets emotional needs. International Journal of Alternative and Complementary Therapy November 9-12

Turgeon M 1994 Right brain, left brain reflexology [Translated by Guoin M A from the original Turgeon M 1988 La reflexologie du cerveau pour auditifs et vissels. Editions de Montagne, Quebec) Healing Arts Press, Vermont

Turgut M 2002 Ischaemic stroke secondary to vertebral and carotid artery dissection following chiropractic manipulation of the cervical spine. Neurosurgical Review 25 (4): 267

Vernon H, McDermaid C S, Hagino C 1997 Systematic review of randomised clinical trials of complementary/alternative therapies in the treatment of tension-type and cervicogenic headache. Complementary Therapies in Medicine 7: 142-155

Vernon H 2000 Qualitative review of studies of manipulation-induced hypoalgesia. Journal of Manipulative and Physiological Therapeutics 23: 134-138

Wagner F 1987 Reflex zone massage. Thorsons, London

Watkins A D 1994 The role of alternative therapies in the treatment of allergic diseases. Clinical and Experimental Allergy 24 (9): 813

Weinrich S P, Weinrich M C 1990 The effect of massage on pain in cancer patients. Applied Nursing Research 3 (4): 140

Williamson J, White A, Hart A et al 2002 Randomised controlled trial of reflexology for menopausal symptoms. British Journal of Obstetrics and Gynaecology 109 (9): 1050-1055

Yates R G, Lamping D L, Abram N L et al 1998 Effects of chiropractic treatment on blood pressure and anxiety: a randomised controlled trial. Journal of Manipulative and Physiological Therapeutics 11: 484-488

Yongsheng Xu Xiaolian S 1995 Hypertension of pregnancy treated with foot reflexology – a case report. Reflexology Symposium Report. Foot Reflexology Service Centre, Ankang City Shaanxi

8

The psychological approach

This chapter examines some of the psychological issues related to the causes, predisposing factors and care of women with gestational sickness. A short discussion on the concept of mind-body medicine sets in context the physiological impact of psychological stress. A range of complementary therapies is explored which may be of use in relieving nausea and vomiting in pregnancy, particularly when exacerbated by psychological factors.

INTRODUCTION

Diagnosis of pregnancy is frequently confirmed as a result of a suspicion triggered by nausea and vomiting, in the absence of any other aetiology. The discovery of impending parenthood produces conflicting emotions, including joy and anticipation, anxiety about the health of both mother and baby and concerns regarding work and finances or the relationship with the father. Often there is a feeling of ambivalence towards the pregnancy and the baby, and in some women this may be to the extent that they grieve for the approaching loss of independence. There may be a distorted perception of reality, disbelief regarding the conception and a real fear of increasing responsibilities.

A couple's conscious decision to conceive may, in part, be due to a desire to continue the human race and in particular, the family line, a factor which Raphael-Leff (1992) terms 'genetic immortality', but may also be an element of 'growing up', of becoming an adult, or may even subconsciously be an opportunity to prove that they can be better parents than their own. There is an element of control, of being able to make a choice about whether, when and how to become pregnant, although societal and family pressures to start a family can add to the trauma of infertility in some. Many women revel in the pregnancy itself, others view it as a means to an end, yet experience immense guilt that they do not conform to the socially expected image of the 'blooming' expectant mother (Raphael-Leff 1992). Lack of understanding about what is happening, coupled with fear of hospitals and reluctance to confide in maternity care staff, particularly male medical staff, increases overall anxiety.

Psychological issues in pregnancy are, today, often more significant than physical factors, with so many improvements in the safety of childbirth in the last century, although ironically, concerns may actually be due to those very developments and technological advances, the so-called 'medicalisation' of pregnancy and childbirth, resulting in women feeling they have lost control. For example, Clement, Wilson and Sikorski (1998) explore the positive and negative psychological aspects of women's experiences of ultrasound scanning and highlight the dilemmas presented to some women by either knowing too much or knowing too little. Safety is naturally paramount, for all women want to deliver a live healthy baby (Walton & Hamilton 1995), but the reality of pregnancy and childbirth does not always fulfill their emotional expectations. The apparent focus on childbirth as a normal life event does not seem to equate with the predominance of hospital-based care. Some attention is given to the mother's psychological wellbeing, but the emphasis continues to be on physical health and recognition of deviations from the norm, in a routine 'conveyor belt' fashion (Reid & Garcia 1989) which has essentially changed very little in the last decade, although Hirst et al (1998) doubt whether all women wish to receive this uniform care. Much of the attention is focused on the fetus rather than on the mother and she may think that she

is simply a 'carrier' for her baby, potentially causing feelings of resentment to arise. However, fears about physical changes which the woman may not understand, or concerns based on experience in a previous pregnancy, will lead most women to submit to conventional maternity care for the psychological security it brings about their physiopathological condition.

Pregnancy is one of the greatest and most rapid transitions in a woman's life, as identified by Holmes and Rahe (1967), and brings major social, economic and emotional changes, as well as a new identity. Role conflict and identity crisis can be a significant problem for some women, especially with the contemporary trend for professional women to have children later in life. Partners' reactions can also be variable, with some experiencing feelings of jealousy and resentment towards the baby, and a sense of loss for the changing nature of the relationship. Libido is affected by endocrine changes and by altered body image, and couples need to find other ways of expressing their feelings for each other, but sexual activity most commonly declines during the antenatal period. Thus pregnancy may either strengthen the emotional relationship between the couple, or, perhaps as a result of emotional immaturity and pre-existing difficulties, weaken it still further. Unplanned, unwanted pregnancies, especially in fragile relationships or where the mother is unsupported, will have an even more profound effect, especially if she has to make decisions about the future of the pregnancy and the baby.

Financial pressures when the mother stops working, even if only temporarily, put an increased reliance on the partner to provide, and may affect the mother's sense of independence. The current UK system of maternity leave and pay places the emphasis on financial wellbeing, at the expense of physical wellbeing, with some women insisting on working almost up to their due date, often to the detriment of their health. Social contact also changes as the woman progresses through the pregnancy, and after the birth of the baby, and in some may lead to feelings of isolation and loneliness.

The current political focus on 'family values'

may also have a detrimental effect, especially on women who are not in a conventional heterosexual, monogamous, two-parent family. The media's preoccupation with parenthood, particularly in advertisements, highlights the joys without acknowledging the demands, and the high profile exposure of celebrity pregnancies adds to feelings of inadequacy amongst women in the general antenatal population. To this may be added a sense of guilt about not enjoying the pregnancy, an emotion which may be much more widespread than is given credence.

Previous experiences of pregnancy and childbirth elicit powerful and vivid memories (Simkin 1992), sometimes leading to long-term distress which seriously impacts on subsequent pregnancies (Kitzinger 1992) and which may, indeed, be permanent (Moorhead 1996). A few women feel so traumatised by the childbirth experience that they suffer post-traumatic stress disorder resulting in prolonged nightmares and a fear of future pregnancies (Menage 1993), psychosexual difficulties and compromised relationships with their infants (Ballard et al 1995). Excessive stress during pregnancy, whether pregnancy-specific or not, is known to impair the immune system (Jabaaij 1993), which may be the aetiological stimulus to the development of symptoms such as nausea and vomiting (Minagawa et al 1999; Leylek et al 1999) or initiate complications such as preterm labour (Hedegaard et al 1993), or indeed, postmaturity (Sharma et al 1993). However, Buckwalter and Simpson (2002) dispute the traditional theory that pregnancy sickness is a conversion disorder in which psychological distress manifests as physical symptoms, although they do debate the suggestion that the psychological effect of the physiological symptom is a conditioned response, a theory supported by the successful use of psychological treatments such as hypnotherapy.

Emotions vary during pregnancy, both individually and between women, and may be influenced by many of the factors discussed above. Tearfulness is experienced by as many as 21% of primigravidae, although the incidence may decline with increasing parity (NCT/NOP 2002), suggesting that lack of knowledge and

uncertainty may play a part in affecting many women. Other negative emotions include fear and anxiety, mood swings, worry and depression, but these are usually balanced with feelings of happiness and anticipation.

Much has been written regarding the psychosomatic factors involved in gestational nausea and vomiting, and it is acknowledged that psycho-emotional and psychosocial issues can exacerbate the problem, particularly stress, inadequate information about the progress of pregnancy and relationship difficulties. Leeners et al (2000) also postulate that psychosocial factors impact on both the duration and intensity of symptoms and on the resistance towards conventional pharmacological approaches to resolving the problem. Work by Murray (1997) suggests that increasing age may adversely affect the degree of nausea suffered by people when traveling by air, sea, rail, road or in space. It is known that older expectant mothers experience many more physiopathological problems than younger women, so increased frequency, duration or severity of sickness is understandable. The influence of the family, especially the pregnant woman's own mother or her mother-in-law, may also impact on her attitude towards gestational sickness, as may her personality and approach to pregnancy. While a genetic predisposition to gestational sickness may forewarn a woman of the likelihood of its occurrence in her own pregnancies, the woman with no family history may be made to feel uncomfortable by relatives, friends or colleagues who fail to appreciate her distress. Embarrassment may be another issue related specifically to uncontrolled and inopportune vomiting, and the fear of spontaneous emesis in a public place may prevent the mother from feeling able to leave home, adding to her sense of isolation. Other physical changes occurring in early pregnancy may contribute to more severe sickness, particularly tiredness, an increase in which has been shown to be positively correlated with increasing nausea (van Lier et al 1993), and although it is impossible to determine whether the sickness leads to more tiredness or vice versa, it is evident that recumbent rest vastly improves

---

Practice point

Midwives, obstetricians, GPs and other members of the maternity care team must acknowledge the woman's interpretation of the severity of her symptoms, and take sensitive steps towards determining the possible psychological causes and predisposing factors, as well as the physiopathological causes.

---

women's perceptions of their condition (O'Brien & Naber 1992).

Mack (2000) discusses the effects of a previous concealed termination of pregnancy on the emotional state of a woman in a subsequent planned pregnancy, in which she attributed the severe sickness she was experiencing to a form of retribution for killing her first baby. Frequently women view the impact of their sickness on the baby as their own 'fault', even when no such significant reason may be present. This can add to their distress, and in the event of pregnancy loss or more severe complications, to immense feelings of guilt.

Measurement of specific variables such as duration of nausea and number of episodes of both nausea and vomiting can assist in identifying the need for hospitalisation (see Chapter 1), but scoring systems such as those from the Motherisk Programme (Koren et al 2002; 2001), the Rhodes scoring system (Rhodes & McDaniel 1999) or the McGill system (Lacroix et al 2000) fail to take into account any accompanying psychophysical factors. It has been shown that the need for hospital care increases with greater severity and duration of vomiting (Atanackovic et al 2001), notably in primigravidae. However, little could be found in the research literature on the psychological impact of hospitalisation itself on the course of the hyperemesis gravidarum, taking into account the inclination of hospital staff to concentrate on the reason for admission, i.e. the condition, rather than on the person and all the components which contribute to the woman's daily life. In certain instances, this can lead to a misplaced dependence of the woman on her caregivers. In others, exacerbation of symptoms may occur, despite medical interventions, as a result of the enforced admission and the inability to attend to the rest of the family or to fulfill work commitments.

An interesting phenomenon appears to be more prevalent today than hitherto, in that women seem inclined to expect maternity care professionals to resolve *all* their symptoms, without a conscious understanding that pregnancy is naturally a time which brings with it a whole range of physical changes, some less pleasant than others. Perhaps the increase in the amount of disposable income of many people, with the option to pay for services and solutions to a whole variety of daily problems, leads them to expect a totally problem-free pregnancy, which, when it is not, triggers disillusionment and discontentment. The severity of nausea and vomiting may be one example of this, but if health professionals can assist women to acknowledge that the symptoms are a normal part of early pregnancy, it may contribute to improved coping skills. Added to the physical discomforts of the sickness are anxiety and worry about what could happen to the baby, but facilitating a positive outlook, such as recognising the nausea as a response to sufficiently high hormone levels to sustain the pregnancy may also help the woman to cope better.

Communication is vital to the mother's attainment of a safe and satisfying pregnancy and childbirth experience (Tennant & Butler 1999) and is in keeping with the woman-centred philosophy of the Department of Health's strategy for the 21st century (SNMAC 1998). Sjogren (1998) acknowledges that women with severe anxiety about the impending birth need special individualised antenatal support, including psychotherapy or counselling. Antenatal classes, whether National Health Service or private, such as those offered by the National Childbirth Trust (NCT), provide a forum for discussion, mutual support and reassurance. The survey for the NCT conducted by NOP Research (2002) found that 50% of women who attended antenatal classes did so in order to receive evidence-based information or professional advice (31%), while 36% benefited from the opportunity to meet other expectant mothers, especially within the local area. The use of group sessions can be especially beneficial in helping women to realise that they are not alone, and the establishment of a 'natural remedies for morning sickness' group at a south London hospital has been reported by Tiran (2003).

MIND-BODY MEDICINE

One of the fundamental aspects of complementary medicine is the focus on the interaction between the body, mind and spirit, taking account of the whole person. Considerable research has been undertaken in recent years to demonstrate a link between the mind (psychology), the brain (neurology) and the body's natural defences (immunology) and to identify the pathways connecting the body and mind. Thus there is an emerging body of knowledge on psycho-neuro-immunology (PNI), refuting the original assumptions that the immune system is autonomous and independent of other systems and providing evidence of the role of the central nervous system in the defence of the body via neurochemicals, and vice versa.

Stress elicits a range of chemical responses in the body. For example, it is known that human chorionic gonadotrophin (hCG), amongst other hormones, is capable of affecting the immune system (Blalock 1994; Reichlin 1993) and that endorphins and other opiates have a variety of effects on its cells (Bateman et al 1989), whilst the ability of the hypothalamus to synthesise catecholamines suggests an inter-regulatory function (Terao et al 1993). Autonomic flow to different target tissues and neurohormone and neuropeptide production are influenced by the different stressors affecting the individual, interacting at either a tissue or cellular level to trigger or inhibit an immune response. Stressful situations activate central autonomic nuclei and the sympathetic-adreno-medullary (SAM) axis, as well as the hypothalamic-adreno-corticol (HPAC) axis. The SAM pathway is responsible for the 'fight or flight' response, and the feelings of anger and anxiety, involving noradrenaline and the central nucleus of the amygdala, or adrenaline and the basal nuclei of the amygdala

respectively, whereas the HPAC pathway triggers submission, despair and defeat, probably through the septohippocampal system (Henry 1986).When stress is chronic the individual vascillates between anger and fighting to gain control over the situation, and despair and feelings of loss of control, prompting them to 'give up'. This cycle stimulates the production of certain destructive catabolic hormones which eventually affect not only the immune system but also other body systems. Examples of this include the incidence of the development of the common cold in stressed individuals compared to those who are not stressed (Cohen et al 1991), and the reduction of leucocyte cytokine mRNA expression which can affect wound healing in stressed patients (Kielcolt-Glaser et al 1995).

Conversely, acute stress activates other immune responses such as a depression in humoral and cellular immunity for students under examination stress (Kielcolt-Glaser et al 1986), or the inhibition of neutrophil phagocytosis for someone who is deprived of sleep (Palmblad et al 1976). However, since these early studies, it is now believed that chronic, mild to moderate stress is overall more harmful to the immune system than single major life events such as bereavement.

Neurological factors may influence the individual's response to stressful events, including the emotional centres in the brainstem, particularly the amygdala, which is involved in emotional memory. The emotional impact of an event is stored in the memory together with all the associated contextual and environmental cues, with the increased adrenergic input potentiating the memory of the event. Thus, in a woman with a negative emotional memory of a previous pregnancy, a subsequent pregnancy could initiate psychosomatic symptoms, such as severe sickness.

The issue of somatisation is debated by Sharpe and Wessely (1997:170-1), a term implying the conversion of psychological distress into physical symptoms, in which organic disease may not be identified. They prefer the term 'functional somatic symptoms', indicating physical symptoms for which no pathological cause

---

Case 8.1

A 31-year-old multigravida attended the hospital antenatal booking clinic at 12 weeks' gestation. Whilst waiting to be called in to the midwife for her history to be taken, she proceeded to sit on the floor of the clinic waiting area, back against the wall, legs splayed wide and a bucket placed between them. She attracted much attention from other expectant mothers by groaning, sighing and audibly retching into the bucket, although she was not seen to vomit.

It was unfortunate that when she was eventually called in to see the midwife, the clinic was running extremely late and the midwife was unable to spend as much time with the woman as she would have liked but suggested that she might attend the next available 'walk in' pregnancy sickness group.

The woman attended the group, thankfully minus her bucket, and was able to talk over her feelings towards the sickness, her pregnancy and the problems she had experienced in her last pregnancy. She was also able to hear the fears and concerns of other expectant mothers, reducing her impression that she alone was suffering. She seemed grateful for suggestions for self-help strategies and departed without having once complained of nausea or shown the need to retch or vomit. Although she was given the opportunity to return, she did not reappear and it was later confirmed that her sickness had, almost immediately, improved significantly to the point where she was able to cope.

Box 8.1 Psychological approaches to care of women with pregnancy sickness

Validate the symptoms – they are what the mother says they are
Establish a collaborative partnership with the mother
Provide adequate explanations for the symptoms and of the treatment

Avoid unnecessary investigations and treatment
Negotiate a plan of action which gives the mother a sense of empowerment
Treat the whole person – body, mind and spirit

Box 8.2 Complementary therapies which may alleviate pregnancy sickness exacerbated by psychological factors

Hypnotherapy, autogenic training
Biofeedback
Counselling, psychotherapy
Bach flower remedies

Exercise therapies eg Tai Chi, Qi Gong, yoga
Relaxation therapies e.g. Therapeutic Touch, music, visualisation

---

can be determined, yet avoiding the possible stigma attached to psychiatric origins. Common functional somatic disorders in the general population include back, joint, chest or abdominal pain, headache, fatigue or dizziness. Bridges and Goldberg (1985) found that 20% of GP consultations are for somatic symptoms, with many of these patients being referred for secondary consultations, particularly in gastroenterology, neurology and cardiology clinics, although the majority receive no treatment since no organic disease can be detected despite the time and expense of a range of investigations. Patients remain dissatisfied and frequently turn to com-plementary and alternative medicine for answers. Sharpe and Wessely (1997:177) argue that it is the time taken by complementary practitioners to listen to and to validate the patient's symptoms which result in a measure of success in caring for these people, even when the symptoms are not fully resolved. Providing adequate information and education about the causes, effects and management of the symptoms can contribute to a more successful outcome, and the use of group settings can help to counter psychosocial and emotional isolation which may accompany the condition (Easton 1997:199).

HYPNOTHERAPY, AUTOGENIC TRAINING, BIOFEEDBACK

Hypnotherapy is the therapeutic use of the hypnotic condition, an altered state of consciousness or awareness, which may be indistinguishable from simple mental relaxation or 'day dreaming'. During hypnotherapy, the client in the hypnotic state is treated with a variety of therapeutic tools, ranging from simple suggestion to psychoanalysis. These tools may be employed either by the therapist (facilitator) or by the client, in the form of 'self-hypnosis'. Synonymous terms include imagery, meditation, relaxation or autogenic training (Ernst et al 2001).

Hypnosis has been used since ancient times but became a therapeutic practice in the late 18th century when Anton Mesmer devised a treatment based on magnetism. Despite the investigations of a Royal Commission concluding that its effects were due to imagination, the therapy was revised in the mid 19th century when it was used successfully as a replacement for anaesthesia. By the 1950s, both the British and American Medical Associations recognised hypnotherapy as an acceptable medical tool (Simon & James 1999). Although the vast majority of hypnotherapists are lay practitioners, many doctors, dentists and psychotherapists utilise hypnotherapeutic techniques in their practice.

Autogenic training (AT) is related to the principles of hypnotherapy but emphasises the empowerment of the client by reducing the passivity and dependence on the practitioner which is a feature of hypnosis. It involves specific mental exercises, relaxation and auto – or self – suggestion which aim to work on an increased awareness of the origins of physical and mental disorders to help individuals to self-treat the conditions. Original work by Schultz focused on teaching clients to consider the warmth and heaviness experienced when in an hypnotic state, and to extend these feelings to the whole body, followed by a conscious awareness of heart rate, respiration, warmth in the stomach and coolness of the forehead. The cardiac physician, Luthe, developed AT further by adding individualised 'intentional' exercises involving repeated therapeutic suggestions. Meditative exercises are also now a feature of the technique.

Biofeedback involves the use of apparatus to monitor, amplify and feed back information to the patient about physiological responses to stimuli, in order that the person can learn to self-regulate those responses. It originated in the 1960s when researchers studying electroencephalograms (EEGs) found that volunteers' attempts to produce alpha waves also produced deep relaxation and meditative clarity. The commonest physiological responses on which treatment is focused are skin temperature, muscle tension, blood pressure, respiratory rate, blood flow and cerebral activity (via EEG), with information presented to the client as a continuous signal, either visual or auditory. Treatment aims to assist the person to establish mastery over the response, independent of the biofeedback apparatus.

It is difficult to determine exactly how hypnotherapy or AT work, or indeed, *if* they work purely as a result of the practitioner's intervention, since other factors, such as the placebo effect, susceptibility to suggestion or even the environment may have an effect on improving the client's wellbeing. Some authorities challenge hypnotherapy as being extremely subjective and affected by factors such as patient compliance or their attitude towards role playing (Heap 1996; Coe & Sarbin 1991). Hypnosis is certainly associated with deep relaxation which, in itself, may act as the therapeutic trigger, since years of debate have concluded that analgesia and other responses may be achieved with suggestion, rather than specifically with hypnosis. However, formal induction of the hypnotic state by a practitioner is not always needed, for highly susceptible people may be able to self-hypnotise and, under hypnosis, deliberately control involuntary physiological processes such as heart rate, skin temperature and intestinal secretions, which is the basis for AT. Biofeedback works on the mind-body interaction, presumably on the limbic system, thereby affecting the hypothalamo-pituitary axis and autonomic control.

Hypnotherapy is normally used to treat anxiety, stress, psychosomatic conditions, pain, addictive behaviours and phobia. Many conditions require a course of six to ten treatments under the facilitation of the therapist although the client can be taught how to induce the hypnotic state in themselves for home use. Group sessions can be useful in certain circumstances including smoking cessation groups and antenatal preparation for childbirth classes. Where short-term goals are required, hypnotherapy is often used as a tool for cognitive behavioural therapy (Kirsch et al 1995; Schoenberger 2000). It may also be used in combination with other therapeutic strategies such as music (Nilsson et al 2001).

Like hypnotherapy, autogenic training is used to assist people with stress-related disorders, anxiety and depression and the medical conditions which arise as a result of these, such as sleep disturbances, headaches, premenstrual syndrome, chronic pain, asthma, hypertension, angina and functional bowel and bladder disorders. Commonly, treatment is initially given in small groups of about three, teaching the recommended exercises, which participants then practise daily and record their personal responses. Intentional exercises are then taught individually, with a course of treatment normally being between eight and ten sessions, with no need for further attendance.

Biofeedback is useful for alleviating conditions associated with muscular tension and spasm, such as headache and chronic pain, and those improved by psychological relaxation, including stress and anxiety-related problems, attention deficit, asthma, substance abuse and sleep disorders. Other conditions which have been treated successfully include enuresis, encopresis, Raynaud's phenomenon and irritable bowel syndrome.

Safety of hypnotherapy and autogenic training

Hypnotherapy is generally considered to be a safe therapeutic tool, although professional theory identifies certain contraindications to treatment such as psychosis, personality disorders, epilepsy and children younger than five years of age. Psychological problems may potentially be exacerbated especially when the hypnotic process is used to reveal repressed memories. One study of adolescent teenagers treated with hypnotherapy for resistant obesity elicited several adverse reactions in some of the subjects, including anxiety, fears, dissociation and depersonalisation. Those in whom deep trance could not be induced also perceived this as a failure of the process (Haber et al 1979).

Many people worry that hypnosis can be used to elicit embarrassing or degrading behaviour, and the trend for communal hypnosis for entertainment has done little to reassure them that this is not the case. Those people who choose to submit themselves to hypnosis for the purpose of entertainment have already expressed a conscious or subconscious willingness to be encouraged to perform certain feats in public, such as incessantly running up and down steps or barking like a dog. Another potential problem of uncontrolled sessions is that there are likely to be some highly suggestible people in whom group hypnosis induces a deep trance, from which it may be difficult to ensure they have recovered. It is this type of scenario which is occasionally sensationalised in the press when someone fails to emerge from a deep trance then proceeds to walk out into traffic, or a similar potentially fatal action. However, a professional hypnotherapist, trained to practise *clinical* hypnotherapy, works in partnership with the client, to facilitate only the desired behavioural changes.

Little could be found in the literature about the potential hazards of AT or biofeedback, but contraindications and precautions are similar to those for hypnotherapy. They should be used only to *complement* conventional treatment, as there is a theoretical potential for interaction with orthodox therapy, so that any medication, e.g. antihypertensives or insulin, should be monitored carefully. Adverse effects occasionally occur with biofeedback, such as dizziness, anxiety and disorientation.

Practice point

Hypnotherapy and autogenic training are contraindicated in women with a history of psychological or personality disorders, those who have epilepsy and those on medication for pre-existing medical conditions.

General research into hypnotherapy, autogenic training and biofeedback

Addictive behaviour is one of the most common problems associated with hypnosis, and its use in smoking cessation has been studied in several trials, although not all of these have proved successful (Green & Lynn 2000; Abbott et al 1998; Valbo & Eide 1996). People with substance abuse have had variable responses, with positive outcomes to biofeedback produced by Taub et al (1994), Denney et al (1991) and Peniston and Kulkosky (1990), but negative or inconclusive results in hypnotherapy studies by others (Katz 1980; Jacobson & Silfverskiold 1973). Work by Somer (1995) on patients with intractable phobic anxiety has used a combination of hypnotherapy and biofeedback, with some success.

Symptoms and side-effects of major medical conditions may be helped by any of the relaxation therapies. Relief of anxiety, depression and fears associated with chemotherapy treatment has been demonstrated by Kaye and Schindler (1990), who found total or almost total symptom relief in 68% of cancer patients, and by Curtis (2001) with a reported 82% success rate. Combined relaxation and biofeedback has similar effects (Burish & Jenkins 1992). The use of hypnosis in trauma has been studied (Cardena 2000; Brom et al 1989) and perception of both acute and chronic pain can be altered positively (NIH Technology Assessment Statement 1997; Kiefer & Hospodarsky 1980). Headache and migraine appear to improve when biofeedback is used (Herman et al 1995; Bogaards & ter Kuile 1994; Holroyd & Penzien 1990), which appears to be more effective than relaxation techniques alone, although there seems to be a synergistic effect when both are used together (Rokicki et al 1997). There are also reports of victims of cerebrovascular accident and other neurological disorders showing improvement following a course of hypnotherapy (Manganiello 1986; Crasilneck & Hall 1970) or with biofeedback (Basmajian 1998).

The psychological impact on asthma may also be affected by hypnotherapy, with Morrison (1988) finding a 62% improvement in symptoms and a corresponding reduction in the need for hospital admission. Children with asthma appear to respond especially well to hypnotherapy (Kohen & Wynne 1997; Watkins 1994), although this may be either because children are more susceptible to hypnosis, or because pre-adolescent asthma has a more reversible disease process.

Other medical conditions with psycho-emotional factors have been shown to be positively affected when patients are given a course of hypnotherapy. Irritable bowel syndrome, for example, has been researched extensively (Camilleri 1999; Camilleri & Choi 1997; Houghton et al 1996; Elkins & Wall 1996; Talley et al 1996). Gonsalkorale et al (2002) report on the first unit in the UK in which a team of hypnotherapists provide a clinical service for people with irritable bowel syndrome, with early audits showing it to be successful in the majority of patients. Hypnotherapy was also used for people suffering irritable bowel syndrome by Forbes et al (2000), with treatment administered via audio-tape as a less time-consuming – and therefore more cost-effective – means of reducing anxiety and consequent physiopathological symptoms. Patients with gastric motility disorders have also responded well to autogenic training with guided imagery (Rashed et al 2002).

Within maternity care, hypnotherapy may have a contribution to make in the care of women with infertility when combined with other therapies (Poehl et al 1999), although it is difficult to extrapolate precisely the role of the therapy in such a complex aetiological phenomenon.

Jenkins and Pritchard (1993) conducted a study of 126 primigravid and 136 multigravid women, each with 300 age-matched controls, to assess the effects of antenatal hypnotherapy on the first and second stages of labour. There was a reduction in the requirement for analgesia in the first stage for primigravid and multigravid women who received hypnotherapy compared to controls. There was also an interesting reduction in the mean length of labour of primigravidae in the hypnotherapy group compared to their controls, which caused the researchers to reflect on the psychological components involved in the length of the first stage of labour.

In Harmon et al's study (1990), 60 women were divided into high and low susceptibility groups and then given six sessions of childbirth preparation and skill mastery, with half of each group receiving hypnotic suggestion before the sessions and the other half being taught conventional relaxation and breathing exercises. All women who had received hypnotherapy had shorter labours culminating in normal deliveries, required less analgesia and the babies had higher Apgar scores, while the highly susceptible, hypnotically treated women also had lower postnatal depression scores.

Pain control in labour is perhaps one of the commonest indications for the use of hypnotherapy. Antenatal preparation for labour assists in reducing maternal stress, anxiety and pain (Bernat et al 1992), which Oster (1994) claims is superior to the Lamaze method of psychoprophylaxis. Zimmer et al (1988) demonstrated an increase in fetal movements in response to maternal relaxation, particularly when the hypnotic state was induced by a physician rather than self-induced. Schauble et al (1998) use hypnosis as a 'conditioned reflex' to produce a positive outcome for labour by enhancing the mother's sense of readiness and control, which they call the 'hypnoreflexogenous' method, while Guthrie et al (1984) suggested that partners could be taught to induce hypnosis in labouring women to reduce the time required by staff to do so. Biofeedback has been found to be helpful for the relaxation of early first stage labour, but in a study by St James-Roberts et al (1983), did not result in the

prevention or management of severe pain in more established labour.

Problems occurring in pregnancy have been treated with hypnosis including correction of breech presentation (Mehl 1994). Antenatal blood pressure may be kept within manageable limits for women at risk of pre-eclampsia (Somers et al 1989). However, although a study of hypertensive expectant mothers found a reduced incidence of hospital admission and lower blood pressure readings in groups given biofeedback and/or relaxation compared to a control group, there was no more significant improvement in the biofeedback/relaxation group than in those who used relaxation alone (Little et al 1984). Skin-cooling biofeedback with health education information was also found to be less effective than combined non-pharmacological treatments for headaches during pregnancy (Marcus et al 1995).

However, Omer and Sirkovitz (1987) dispute the value of hypnotherapy in inducing labour in post-dates pregnancy, and indeed, Omer et al (1986) found it effective in *prolonging* pregnancy and increasing infant birth weight in women admitted to hospital for preterm labour.

Postnatally, faecal incontinence following traumatic or operative delivery has been treated with biofeedback. Fynes et al (1999) compared sensory biofeedback with augmented biofeedback, and found improved continence scores in both groups, but significantly better anal resting and squeeze pressures in the group of women who had used biofeedback augmented with relaxation.

In another study, however, only limited success was achieved with biofeedback and electrostimulation as an adjunct to pelvic floor exercises, reducing urinary, but not faecal, stress incontinence, nor intravaginal or intra-anal pressures or bladder neck integrity (Meyer et al 2001).

It may be possible that hypnosis could be used to increase prolactin levels in breastfeeding mothers (Cepicky et al 1995) and may positively influence the duration of breastfeeding (Brann & Guzvica 1987).

Hypnotherapy, autogenic training and biofeedback for nausea and vomiting

The value of hypnosis in the treatment of iatrogenic nausea and vomiting associated with cancer treatments has been reported for many years (Keller 1995; Genuis 1995; Stoudemire et al 1984; LaClave & Blix 1989; Fortuin 1988; Blum 1988). Hypnotherapeutic techniques seem to be especially helpful in children with nausea after cancer treatments (Hawkins et al 1995; Jacknow et al 1994; Zeltzer et al 1991). An investigation of 16 patients undergoing chemotherapy demonstrated complete cessation of *anticipatory* nausea and vomiting and significant reduction in the intensity of drug-induced vomiting (Marchioro et al 2000), although Burish and Tope (1992) advocate that patients should learn the techniques before chemotherapy commences. The issue of anticipatory nausea and vomiting is explored also by Montgomery et al (2002) for women due to undergo excisional breast biopsy for suspected malignancy. It was found that postoperative pain and distress were significantly reduced following hypnotherapy, possibly resulting from a change in the women's preoperative expectations. The use of hypnotic suggestion combined with music *during* surgery also appears to have significant effects on postoperative recovery, as with Nilsson et al's study (2001) of women undergoing hysterectomy, and the specific reaction of post-surgical nausea and vomiting has been shown to be reduced by approximately half in patients receiving hypnotherapeutic suggestion during thyroidectomy (Eberhart et al 1998). A case report of a nine-year-old boy with intractable post-prandial reflex vomiting claimed cessation of symptoms within four weeks using self-hypnotherapeutic suggestion, relaxation and imagery, and no recurrence of the condition after a 12 month review (Sokel et al 1990). Marchand et al (2002) report on the case of a 76-year-old woman with a three month history of uncontrollable vomiting which was unresponsive to pharmacological treatment but was successfully resolved with hypnosis.

The psychological aetiology of hyperemesis gravidarum has been acknowledged by Schouenborg et al (1992) and by Goldman (1990), who claim hypnotherapy to be one of the most effective forms of treatment, together with psychotherapy, environment change, ginger and relevant pharmaceutical medications. Henker (1976) also examined encouraging results of combining hypnotherapy with psychotherapy and behaviour modification for ten women with gestational sickness, and Bartholomew and Klapp (1992) similarly found psychotherapy to be helpful. Interestingly, Apfel et al (1986) suggest that women with hyperemesis gravidarum appear to be more susceptible to hypnosis and that hypnotisability may contribute to the aetiology of the condition.

Simon and Schwartz (1999) reviewed the empirical studies of hypnosis to treat women with hyperemesis gravidarum, stressing the need for differential diagnosis and appropriate referral. They suggest that more widespread use of medical hypnosis in the large numbers of pregnant women suffering moderate sickness may assist in reducing the incidence of hyperemesis gravidarum, while Poliakov (1989) regards it as a safer option for the fetus than conventional drug management, but postulates that patient doubt and prejudice may contribute to its failure. Case reports of women with hyperemesis gravidarum, successfully treated with hypnotherapy, are also found in the literature (Torem 1994; Stanford 1994; Smith 1982; Long et al 1986), although it is difficult to determine whether improvement occurred as a direct result of the therapy, an indirect impact of extraneous factors, or spontaneously with the passage of time. Adaptive biofeedback has also been shown to reduce the severity of motion sickness symptoms in susceptible individuals (Smirnov et al 1988).

Very few papers on the subject of AT for nausea and vomiting could be found, and all referred to motion sickness. A comparative study on aviators of the efficacy of AT, 'sham' training using an alternative cognitive task and a control group (Toscano & Cowings 1982) showed that the AT group could withstand significantly longer periods of excessive motion by regulating their own autonomic responses, although a replication of this study by Jozsvai and Pigeau (1996) failed to demonstrate a clear distinction between the three groups. However, further work by the original team (Cowings & Toscano 2000) in a randomised, matched study showed that AT is superior to pharmacological promethazine in reducing symptoms of severe motion sickness, despite high rotational velocity.

BACH FLOWER REMEDIES

Bach flower remedies (BFRs) are liquid preparations containing plant essences which have been specially prepared and which are thought to have a positive effect on the emotions. The founder of the BFR system was Dr Edward Bach, a medical practitioner and homeopath in the early 20th century, who became disillusioned with the reductionist, physical approach to treating illness and devised a range of remedies claimed to balance the whole person by working on the emotional elements of illness. A range of 38 remedies plus the Rescue remedy, a universal first aid/stress reliever, is available in health stores, and although CAM practitioners may advise the use of these remedies in conjunction with other therapies, they are most commonly self-administered by patients. However, it is important to remember that Bach flower remedies can have an 'onion peeling' effect on the emotions, gradually revealing concealed feelings, and for some women careful psychological counselling may be required.

The remedies are prepared by placing freshly picked flowers from the relevant plants into spring water, with brandy added to preserve the energy. It is not known how they work, although there are some similarities with homeopathy, but there is no acknowledged pharmacological action. Although there are no known contraindications, the fact that the remedies contain alcohol must be taken into account, either on moral or physical grounds. However, as very few drops are used and the remedy is already diluted at the point of administration, their use in pregnancy is acceptable.

Practice point

Bach flower remedies are preserved in brandy; while the amount used is safe in pregnancy, it is wise to refrain from recommending BFRs to women with a history of hepatic disease or alcohol abuse.

Bach flower remedy research

There appears to be very little rationale for the effectiveness of BFRs and any positive results are largely attributed to a placebo effect. Few scientific studies have been conducted on this therapy, and of those available, most are inconclusive. Rescue remedy seems to be the most popular and well known of the remedies and has been assessed as to its usefulness in relieving examination stress in students. One hundred students were given either rescue remedy or placebo in a double-blind placebo-controlled trial prior to examinations, but no significant differences were demonstrated between the two groups (Armstrong & Ernst 1999). Similar results were achieved in a smaller study by Walach et al (2000).

Only one small obstetric study of BFRs has been found (Ruhle 1996, unpublished). A controlled trial of 24 women with post-dates pregnancy was undertaken, in which one group received individually prescribed BFRs, dependent on the emotional state of the women, one group received counselling and a control group received no psychological care except the conventional obstetric care given to all three groups. The researcher ambitiously assessed factors such as the date of onset of labour, intrapartum drug use, mode of delivery, anxiety state and psychological wellbeing, but was forced later to acknowledge the confounding variables which could have affected these factors in any of the groups. A conclusion was drawn that the women in the BFR group went into spontaneous labour sooner, had more normal labours and deliveries with less medication and were emotionally more positive about the event than those in the other two groups. However, it was

---

Box 8.3 Examples of Bach flower remedies to ease negative emotions

(Dosage: 2 drops of each remedy in water 3 times daily)
Anger with self for weakness – Centaury, oak
Concealing feelings behind a 'brave face' – Agrimony
Constantly needing reassurance – Cerato
Difficulty in adapting to changing situation – Walnut
Fear and anxiety due to known factors – Mimulus
Fear and anxiety due to unknown factors – Aspen
Frustration – inability to continue as normal – Vervain, oak
Irritability – Impatiens
Intolerance for physical condition – Beech
Over-concern for the health of the baby – Red chestnut

Overwhelmed – memories of previous pregnancy
Honeysuckle
Overwhelmed with responsibilities – Elm
Refusal to give in, carries on as normal – Oak
Resentment towards the baby or pregnancy – Willow
Self-obsession – Heather
Self-pity – Chicory
Tearfulness – Scleranthus, sweet chestnut
Terror (perhaps due to previous history) – Rock rose
Tiredness, weariness – Olive
Uncleanliness (after vomiting) – Crab apple

Case 8.2

A multigravida of 28 weeks' gestation attended the complementary therapy clinic for persistent nausea although her reports of very frequent vomiting did not correlate with her appearance, since she looked hydrated and generally well, if a little tired, dispirited and feeling sorry for herself. On meeting with the CT midwife, she revealed marital difficulties, as well as the need to care for a disabled child, and admitted that this pregnancy was unplanned. She seemed to have tried every possible natural remedy and alternative strategy with little effect on her nausea and vomiting, but it was obvious that she needed to talk over her psychosocial problems. Rather than deal with the physical symptoms,

the CT midwife advised her to try BFR elm, to overcome her sense of being overburdened by responsibility, olive for lethargy, walnut for adaptation to change and chicory for self-pity. The following week the mother telephoned to cancel her appointment, saying she felt better than she had done for weeks, with no vomiting and little nausea. Whether this success resulted from the use of the BFRs, the placebo effect, being listened to, or spontaneous resolution is difficult to determine, but since the BFRs were not considered harmful, it was worth attempting to help this woman with natural remedies, rather than admit her to hospital for 'hyperemesis gravidarum'.

---

recognised that the numbers (n=8 per group) were too small for statistical significance.

Although there is a lack of data to support the claimed effects of BFRs, experience suggests, at the very least, a strong placebo effect. Pregnant women suffering sickness seem to grasp at anything which may help to relieve their symptoms and rarely do they question the safety of the remedies, even when informed of the alcohol content. Whether women view the remedies as a 'prop' onto which they can cling, or as a means of empowerment, since they can choose whether, when and how they take them, is unclear, but they usually welcome the suggestion of an inexpensive, readily available and self-administered remedy.

There are various publications accompanying supplies of the remedies which women can obtain from healthfood stores and which guide

them to the most appropriate remedy. Suitable remedies for some of the emotions which can accompany gestational sickness are given in Box 8.3.

OTHER RELAXATION THERAPIES

Music has been used as a therapeutic intervention on many occasions, perhaps hitherto without any scientific acknowledgement of its benefits. Increasingly, the focused use of music is proving to have psychophysiological effects on patients undergoing a range of treatments. For example, postoperative recovery may be easier and quicker when music is used prior to, during or after surgery, sometimes in conjunction with guided imagery. Nilsson et al (2001) exposed women about to undergo hysterectomy to music on the day of operation and demonstrated reduced pain, nausea, vomiting, fatigue and improved sense of wellbeing. Post-operative music and relaxation exercises in gynaecological patients from five different hospitals in Cleveland, USA, showed similar recuperative effects (Good et al 2002). Ezzone et al (1998) demonstrated the value of music as a means of decreasing antiemetic requirements in oncology patients. Guided imagery, via audio-tape, was used by Troesch et al (1993) to reduce chemotherapy-related nausea and vomiting and improve patients' coping strategies, and progressive muscle relaxation techniques have had similar effects (Molassiotis et al 2002; Luebbert et al 2001; Arakawa 1997).

Music is universally acceptable, although care should be exercised when selecting pieces for therapeutic use, particularly in group settings, as memories can be evoked which can be emotionally upsetting to some individuals. Similarly, the use of relaxation tapes in which the sound of water is incorporated could, theoretically, produce feelings of anxiety or panic in someone who is afraid of water or who has had a near-drowning experience.

Standley (2002) carried out a meta-analysis of the use of music therapy on preterm infants and found a consistent and statistically significant benefit to progress and prognosis in babies in the intensive care unit. Investigations by Benzaquen et al (1990) suggest that the fetus is acoustically receptive to the intrauterine environment, and, indeed, medical resonance music could contribute to a reduction in the incidence of preterm labour in women at risk (Sidorenko 2000).

Relaxation exercises may also prevent the onset of preterm labour (Janke 1999). It is known that various relaxation techniques can help to alleviate women's fears about birth (Sjogren 1998), and the effects of music on pain levels in labouring women has long been investigated (Durham & Collins 1986; Robinson 2002). Relaxation exercises which encourage the patient to focus inwards on themselves could potentially exacerbate depression, so care must be taken in identifying anyone at risk. Therapeutic Touch (TT), a specific therapy akin to the laying on of hands or Reiki, has been used with good psycho-emotional effects on newly-delivered women, but the study by Kiernan (2002) was too small to be statistically significant.

Tai Chi, originally devised as an ancient Chinese martial art, is of increasing interest in the west, not only as a form of sport and exercise but also for its therapeutic and relaxation effects. Its philosophy is to promote health in individuals and population groups, helping people to achieve and maintain optimum health and wellbeing through a sequence of formulated movements which stimulate internal energy flow (see also Chapter 4) and have been shown to be aerobic in nature and of moderate intensity (Lan et al 2001). Tai Chi is claimed to affect the inter-related and inseparable physical, psychological, spiritual and energy levels of the individual, with emphasis on physical and mental relaxation, focus through meditation and balance between all elements of the person's life and health (Lewis 2002). In recent years Tai Chi has become the subject of several clinical trials exploring its potential as a therapeutic tool for specific conditions. It is known, for example, that it has a significant impact on the cardiovascular system (Wang et al 2002; Vaarnanen et al 2002), reducing blood pressure (Selvamurthy et al 1998; Young et al 1999; Lai et al 1995) and improving cardiorespiratory function (Lan et al 1999). It has also been suggested that, as it is a mild, non-strenuous form of exercise, it may contribute to the care of patients with rheumatoid arthritis (Kirsteins et al 1991), and to a reduction in the incidence of osteoporosis in postmenopausal women (Qin et al 2002; Lane & Nydick 1999; Henderson et al 1998; Lan et al 1998; Forrest 1997; Schaller 1996; Wolfson et al 1996; Wolf et al 1996).

Similarly, yoga is beneficial for maintaining relaxation and improving cardiovascular functioning (Raju et al 1997; Stachenfeld et al 1998; Schmidt et al 1997; Peng et al 1999) and can be used to treat a range of other conditions including carpal tunnel syndrome (Garfinkel et al 1998) and obsessive compulsive disorders (Shannahoff-Khalsa & Beckett 1996). However, some yoga positions are contraindicated during pregnancy and any expectant mother who

<table>
<tr><td>

Practice point

Relaxation therapies can be recommended to women with a history of sickness in previous pregnancies, as a preventative measure, or as a means of giving 'me time' to those currently suffering mild to moderate nausea and vomiting.

</td></tr>
</table>

wishes to practice yoga should ensure her teacher is aware of the pregnancy.

Although these latter studies were not specific to the care of patients with nausea and vomiting, the relaxation effects can be applied to pregnant women in whom stress, anxiety and depression appear to exacerbate their physical symptoms. However, in practical terms, it is unlikely that women suffering anything more than mild to moderate nausea would feel able to participate in activity-based therapies, although they may have some value as preventative interventions.

CONCLUSION

Pregnancy is a time of immense physical and psychosocial upheaval, and stress can compound any hormonally-induced sickness. A range of complementary strategies can be employed to relieve symptoms associated with psychological and emotional distress, including hypnotherapy and the related therapies of autogenic training and biofeedback, Bach flower remedies and general relaxation therapies. Symptoms may be perceived as improving when the expectant mother feels that her feelings are acknowledged, or when an associated emotional symptom is alleviated, enabling her to cope better with the continuing physical symptoms. Midwives, obstetricians and GPs should endeavour always to identify related psychological problems as early as possible, in order that steps can be taken to seek the most appropriate care and treatment of the individual.

REFERENCES

Abbott N C, Stead L F, White A R et al 2000 Hypnotherapy for smoking cessation. Cochrane Database Systematic Review (2): CD 001008

Apfel R J, Kelley S F, Frankel F H 1986 The role of hypnotizability in the pathogenesis and treatment of nausea and vomiting of pregnancy. Journal of Psychosomatic Obstetrics and Gynaecology 5: 179-186

Arakawa S 1997 Relaxation to reduce nausea, vomiting and anxiety induced by chemotherapy in Japanese patients. Cancer Nursing 20 (5): 342-349

Armstrong N C, Ernst E 1999 A randomized double-blind placebo-controlled trial of Bach flower remedy. Perfusion 11: 440-446

Ballard C G, Stanley A K, Brockington I F 1995. Post traumatic stress disorder (PTSD) after childbirth. British Journal of Psychiatry 165 (3): 525-528

Bartholomew A, Klapp B F 1992 Inpatient psychotherapy of hyperemesis gravidarum – a case report. Zeitschrift Geburtshilfe Perinatologie 196 (3): 134-139

Basmajian J V 1998 Biofeedback in physical medicine rehabilitation. In: DeLisa J A, Gans B M (eds) 1998 Rehabilitation medicine: principles and practice, 3rd edn. Lippincott-Raven, Philadelphia

Bateman A, Singh A, Kral T et al 1989 The immune-hypothalamic-pituitary-adrenal axis. Endocrine Review 10 (1): 92-112

Bernat S H, Wooldridge P J, Marecki M et al 1992 Biofeedback-assisted relaxation to reduce stress in labour. Journal of Obstetric Gynecological and Neonatal Nursing 21 (4): 295-303

Benzaquen S, Gagnon R, Hunse C et al 1990 The intrauterine sound environment of the human fetus during labour. American Journal of Obstetrics and Gynecology 163 (2): 484-490

Blalock J E 1994 The immune system: our sixth sense. Immunologist 2: 8-15

Blum R H 1988 Hypothesis: a new basis for sensory-behavioral pretreatmens to ameliorate radiation therapy-induced nausea and vomiting? Cancer Treatment Reviews 15 (3): 211-227

Bogaards M C D, ter Kuile M M 1994 Treatment of recurrent tension headache: a meta-analytical review Clinical Journal of Pain 10: 174-190

Brann L R, Guzvica S A, 1987 Comparison of hypnosis with conventional relaxation for antenatal and intrapartum use: a feasibility study. Journal of the Royal College of General Practitioners 37 (303): 437-440

Bridges K W, Goldberg D P 1985 Somatic presentation of DSM III psychiatric disorders in primary care. Journal of Psychosomatic Research 29: 563-569

Brom D, Kleber R J, Defares P B 1989 Brief psychotherapy for post traumatic stress disorders. Journal of Consultations in Clinical Psychology 57: 607-612

Buckwalter J G, Simpson S W 2002 Psychological factors in the etiology and treatment of severe nausea and vomiting in pregnancy. American Journal of Obstetrics and Gynecology 185 (5 Suppl Understanding): S210-214

Burish T G, Jenkins R A 1992 Effectiveness of biofeedback

and relaxation training in reducing the side-effects of cancer chemotherapy. Health Psychology 11 (1): 17-23

Burish T G, Tope D M 1992 Psychological techniques for controlling the adverse side effects of cancer chemotherapy: findings from a decade of research. Journal of Pain and Symptom Management 7: 287-301

Camilleri M 1999 Review article: clinical evidence to support current therapies of irritable bowel syndrome. Alimentary Pharmacology and Therapeutics 13 (suppl 2): 48-53

Camilleri M, Choi M C 1997 Review article: irritable bowel syndrome. Alimentary Pharmacology and Therapeutics 11 (1): 3-15

Cardena E 2000 Hypnosis in the treatment of trauma: a promising, but not fully supported, efficacious intervention. International Journal of Clinical and Experimental Hypnosis 48: 125-138

Crasilneck H B. Hall J A 1970 The use of hypnosis in the rehabilitation of complicated vascular and post-traumatic neurological patients. International Journal of Clinical and Experimental Hypnosis 18 (3): 145

Cepicky P, Pecena M, Roth Z et al 1995 A successful inducement of prolactin secretion and an unsuccessful attempt to influence the luteinizing hormone secretion by a hypnotic suggestion of breastfeeding. International Journal of Prenatal and Perinatal Psychology and Medicine 7 (3): 303-307

Clement S, Wilson J, Sikorski J 1998 Women's experiences of antenatal ultrasound scans. In: Clement S (ed) Psychological perspectives on pregnancy and childbirth. Churchill Livingstone, London

Coe W, Sarbin T 1991 Role theory. Hypnosis from a dramaturgical and narrational perspective. In: Lynn S, Rhue J (eds) Theories of hypnosis, general models and perspectives. Guildford Press, New York

Cohen S, Tyrell D A, Smith A P 1991 Psychological stress and susceptibility to the common cold. New England Journal of Medicine 325: 606-612

Cowings P S, Toscano W B 2000 Autogenic-feedback training exercise is superior to promethazine for control of motion sickness symptoms. Journal of Clinical Pharmacology 40 (10): 1154-1156

Curtis C 2001 Hypnotherapy in a specialist palliative care unit: evaluation of a pilot service. International Journal of Palliative Care Nursing 7(12): 604-605

Durham L, Collins M 1986 The effect of music as a conditioning aid in prepared childbirth education. Journal of Obstetric Gynecological and Neonatal Nursing 15 (3): 268-270

Easton S 1997 Psychological health: helping people in stress and distress. In: Watkins A (ed) Mind body medicine: a clinician's guide to psychoneuroimmunology. Churchill Livingstone, New York

Eberhart L H, Doring H J, Holzrichter P et al 1998 Therapeutic suggestions given during neurolept-anaesthesia decrease post-operative nausea and vomiting. European Journal of Anaesthesiology 15 (4): 446-452

Elkins G R, Wall V J 1996 Medical referrals for hypnotherapy: opinions of physicians, residents, family practice outpatients and psychiatry outpatients. American Journal of Clinical Hypnosis 38 (4): 254-262

Ernst E, Pittler M H, Stevinson C et al 2001 The desktop guide to complementary and alternative medicine: an evidence-based approach. Mosby, Edinburgh

Ezzone S, Baker C, Rosselet R et al 1998 Music as an adjunct to antiemetic therapy. Oncology Nurses' Forum 25 (9): 1551-1556

Forbes A, MacAuley S, Chiotakakou-Faliakou E 2000 Hypnotherapy and therapeutic audiotape: effective in previously unsuccessfully treated irritable bowel syndrome? International Journal of Colorectal Disease 15 (5-6): 328-334

Forrest W R 1997 Anticipatory postural adjustment and Tai chi chuan. Biomedical Sciences Instrumentation 33: 65-70

Fortuin A A 1988 Hypnotherapy as antiemetic treatment in cancer chemotherapy. Recent Results in Cancer Research 108: 112-116

Fynes M M, Marshall K, Cassidy M et al 1999 A prospective randomized study comparing the effect of augmented biofeedback with sensory feedback alone on fecal incontinence after obstetric trauma. Diseases of the Colon and Rectum 42 (6): 753-758

Garfinkel M S, Singhal A, Katz W A et al 1998 Yoga-based intervention for carpal tunnel syndrome: a randomized trial. Journal of the American Medical Association 280 (18): 1601-1603

Genuis M L 1995 The use of hypnosis in helping cancer patients control anxiety, pain and emesis: a review of recent empirical studies. American Journal of Clinical Hypnosis 37 (4): 316

Goldman L 1990 Control of hyperemesis. In: Hammond D (ed) Handbook of hypnotic suggestions and metaphors. Norton, New York

Gonsalkorale W M, Houghton L A, Whorwell P J 2002 Hypnotherapy in irritable bowel syndrome: a large-scale audit of a clinical service with examination of factors influencing responsiveness. American Journal of Gastroenterology 97 (4): 954-961

Good M, Anderson G C, Stanton-Hicks M et al 2002 Relaxation and music to reduce pain after gynecologic surgery. Pain Management in Nursing 3 (2): 61-70

Green J P, Lynn S J 2000 Hypnosis and suggestion-based approaches to smoking cessation: an examination of the evidence. International Journal of Clinical and Experimental Hypnosis 48: 195-224

Guthrie K, Taylor D J, Defriend D 1984 Maternal hypnosis induced by husbands during childbirth. Journal of Obstetrics and Gynaecology 5 (2): 93-95

Haber C H, Nitkin R, Shenker I R 1979 Adverse reactions to hypnotherapy in obese adolescents: a developmental viewpoint. Psychiatric Questions 51 (1): 55-63

Harmon T M, Hynan M T, Tyre T E 1990 Improved obstetric outcome using hypnotic analgesia and skill mastery combined with childbirth education. Journal of Consultations in Clinical Psychology 58 (5): 525-530

Hawkins P J, Liossi C, Ewart B W et al 1995 Hypnotherapy for control of anticipatory nausea and vomiting in children with cancer: preliminary findings. Psycho-oncology 4: 101-106

Heap M 1996 Special hypnosis supplement. The Psychologist 9 (11): 498

Hedegaard M, Henrikson T B, Sabroe S et al 1993 Psychological distress in pregnancy and preterm delivery. British Medical Journal 307: 234-239

Henderson N K, White C P, Eisman J A 1998 The roles of exercise and fall risk reduction in the prevention of osteoporosis. Endocrinology and Metabolism Clinics of North America 27 (2): 369-387

Henker F O 1976 Psychotherapy as adjunct in treatment of vomiting during pregnancy. Southern Medical Journal 69 (12): 1585-1587

Henry J P 1986 Mechanisms by which stress can lead to coronary heart disease. Postgraduate Medical Journal 62: 687-693

Hermann C, Kim M, Blanchard E B 1995 Behavioural and prophylactic pharmacological intervention studies of pediatric migraine: an exploratory meta-analysis. Pain 60: 239-256

Hirst J, Hewison J, Dowswell T et al 1998 Antenatal care: what do women want? In: Clement S (ed) 1998 Psychological perspectives on pregnancy and childbirth. Churchill Livingstone, London

Holmes T H, Rahe R H 1967 Social readjustment rating scale. Journal of Psychosomatic Research 11: 219

Holroyd K A, Penzien D B 1990 Pharmacological versus non-pharmacological prophylaxis of recurrent migraine headache: a meta-analytic review of clinical trials. Pain 42: 1-13

Houghton L A, Heyman D J, Whorwell P J 1996 Symptomatology, quality of life and economic factors of irritable bowel syndrome – the effect of hypnotherapy. Alimentary Pharmacology and Therapeutics 10 (1): 91-95

Jabaaij L 1993 Stress and the immune system. Journal of Psychosomatic Research 37: 361-369

Jacknow D S, Tschann J M, Link M P et al 1994 Hypnosis in the prevention of chemotherapy-related nausea and vomiting in children: a prospective study. Journal of Developmental and Behavioural Pediatrics 15: 258-264

Janke J 1999 Effect of relaxation therapy on preterm labour outcomes. Journal of Obstetric, Gynecologic and Neonatal Nursing 28 (3): 255-263

Jenkins M W, Pritchard M H 1993 Hypnosis: practical applications and theoretical considerations in normal labour. British Journal of Obstetrics and Gynaecology 100 (3): 221-226

Jozsvai E E, Pigeau R A 1996 The effect of autogenic training and biofeedback on motion sickness tolerance. Aviation Space and Environmental Medicine 67 (10): 963-968

Kaye J M, Schindler B A 1990 Hypnosis on a consultant-liaison service. General Hospital Psychiatry 12 (6): 379-383

Keller V E 1995 Management of nausea and vomiting in children. Journal of Pediatric Nursing 10 (5): 280

Kiernan J 2002 The experience of Therapeutic Touch in the lives of five postpartum women. American Journal of Maternal and Child Nursing 27 (1): 47-53

Kiefer R C, Hospodarsky J 1980 The use of hypnotic techniques in anesthesia to decrease postoperative meperidine requirements. American Journal of the Osteopathic Association 79: 693

Kielcolt-Glaser J K, Glaser R, Strain E et al 1986 Modulation of cellular immunity in medical students. Journal of Behavioural Medicine 9: 5-21

Kilecolt-Glaser J K, Marucha P T, Malarkey W B et al 1995 Slowing of wound healing by psychological stress. Lancet 346: 1194-1196

Kirsch I, Montgomery G, Sapirstein G 1995 Hypnosis as an adjunct to cognitive behavioural psychotherapy: a meta-analysis. Journal of Consultations in Clinical Psychology 63: 214-220

Kirsteins A E, Dietz F, Hwang SM 1991 Evaluating the safety and potential use of a weight-bearing exercise, Tai-Chi Chuan, for rheumatoid arthritis patients. American Journal of Medical Rehabilitation 70 (3): 136-141

Kitzinger S 1992 Birth and violence against women: generating hypotheses from women's accounts of unhappiness after childbirth. In: Roberts H (ed) Women's health matters. Routledge, London

Kohen D P, Wynne E 1997 Applying hypnosis in a preschool family asthma education program: uses of storytelling, imagery and relaxation. American Journal of Clinical Hypnosis 39 (3): 169

Koren G, Boskovic R, Hard M et al 2002 Motherisk – PUQE (pregnancy-unique quantification of emesis and nausea) scoring system for nausea and vomiting of pregnancy. American Journal of Obstetrics and Gynecology 186 (5suppl): S228-231

Koren G, Magee L, Attard C et al 2001 A novel method for the evaluation of the severity of nausea and vomiting of pregnancy. European Journal of Obstetrics, Gynecology and Reproductive Biology 94 (1): 31-36

La Clave L J, Blix S 1989 Hypnosis in the management of symptoms in a young girl with malignant astrocytoma: a challenge to the therapist. International Journal of Clinical and Experimental Hypnosis 37 (1): 6-14

Lacroix R, Eason E, Melzack R 2000 Nausea and vomiting during pregnancy: a prospective study of its frequency, intensity and patterns of change. American Journal of Obstetrics and Gynecology 182 (4): 931-937

Lai J S, Lan C, Wong M K et al 1995 Two year trends in cardiorespiratory function among older Tai Chi Ch'uan practitioners and sedentary sunjects. Journal of the American Geriatrics Society 43 (11): 1222-1227

Lan C, Chen S Y, Lai J S et al 1999 The effect of tai ch'i on cardiorespiratory function in patients with coronary artery bypass surgery. Medicine and Science in Sports and Exercise 30 (3): 345-351

Lane J M, Nydick M 1999 Osteoporosis: current modes of prevention and treatment. Journal of the American Academy of Orthopaedic Surgeons 7 (1): 19-31

Leeners B, Sauer I, Rath W 2000 Nausea and vomiting in early pregnancy/hyperemesis gravidarum. Current status of psychosomatic factors. Zeitschrift Geburtshilfe Neonatologie 204 (4): 128-134

Lewis D E 2002 T'ai chi ch'uan. Complementary Therapies in Nursing and Midwifery 6 (4): 204-206

Leylek O A, Toyaksi M, Erselcan T et al 1999 Immunologic and biochemical factors in hyperemesis gravidarum with or without hyperthyroxinaemia. Gynecologic and Obstetric Investigation 47 (4): 229-234

Little B C, Hayworth J, Benson P et al 1984 Treatment of hypertension in pregnancy by relaxation and biofeedback. Lancet 1 (8382): 865-867

Long M A D, Simone S S, Tucher J J 1986 Outpatient treatment of hyperemesis gravidarum with stimulus control and imagery procedures. Journal of Behavioural and Therapeutic Experimental Psychiatry 17: 105

Luebbert K, Dahme B, Hasenbring M 2001 The effectiveness of relaxation training in reducing treatment-related symptoms and improving emotional adjustment in acute non-surgical cancer treatment: a meta-analytical review. Psycho-oncology 10 (6): 490-502

Mack S 2000 Therapies for the relief of physical and emotional stress In: Tiran D, Mack S (eds) Complementary therapies for pregnancy and childbirth, 2nd edn. Bailliere Tindall, London

Manganiello A J 1986 Hypnotherapy in the rehabilitation of a stroke victim: a case study. American Journal of Clinical Hypnosis 29 (1): 64

Manjunath N K, Telles S 1999 Factors influencing changes in tweezer dexterity scores following yoga training. Indian Journal of Physiology and Pharmacology 43 (2): 225-229

Marchand P, Moulin J L, Merle J C 2002 Hypnosis for the treatment of nausea and vomiting: it works! Revue Medicale de Liege 57 (6): 382-384

Marchioro G, Azzarello G, Vivifani F et al 2000 Hypnosis in the treatment of anticipatory nausea and vomiting in patients receiving cancer chemotherapy. Oncology 59 (2): 100-104

Marcus D A, Scharff L, Turk D C 1995 Nonpharmacological management of headaches during pregnancy. Psychosomatic Medicine 57 (6): 527-535

Mehl L E 1994 Hypnosis and conversion of the breech to the vertex presentation. Archives of Family Medicine 3: 881-887

Menage J 1993 Post-traumatic stress disorder in women who have undergone obstetric and/or gynaecological procedures. Journal of Reproductive and Infant Psychology 11 (2): 221-228

Meyer S, Hohlfeld P, Achtari C et al 2001 Pelvic floor education after vaginal delivery. Obstetrics and Gynecology 97 (5 Pt 1): 673-677

Minagawa M, Narita J, Tada T et al 1999 Mechanisms underlying immunologic states during pregnancy: possible association of the sympathetic nervous system. Cellular Immunology 196 (1): 1-13

Molassiotis A, Yung H P, Yam B M et al 2002 The effectiveness of progressive muscle relaxation training in managing chemotherapy-induced nausea and vomiting in Chinese breast cancer patients: a randomised controlled trial. Support Care Cancer 10 (3): 237-246

Montgomery G H, Weltz C R, Seltz M et al 2002 Brief presurgery hypnosis reduces distress and pain in excisional breast biopsy patients. International Journal of Clinical and Experimental Hypnosis 50 (1): 17-32

Moorhead J 1996 New generations: 40 years of birth in Britain. National Childbirth Publishing Trust, HMSO London

Morrison J B 1988 Chronic asthma and improvement with relaxation induced by hypnotherapy. Journal of Royal Society of Medicine 81 (12): 701-704

Murray J B 1997 Psychophysiological aspects of motion sickness. Perception and Motor Skills 85 (3 Pt 2): 1163-1167

National Childbirth Trust 2002 NCT/Calpol Survey: Report of Key Findings. NOP World, London

NIH Technology Assessment Statement 1995 Integration of behavioral and relaxation approaches into the treatment of chronic pain and insomnia. NIH Technology Assessment Statement 16-18: 1-34

Nilsson U, Rawal N, Unestahl L E et al 2001 Improved recovery after music and therapeutic suggestions during general anaesthesia: a double-blind randomized controlled trial. Acta Anaesthesiology Scandinavia 45 (7): 812-817

O'Brien B, Naber S 1992 Nausea and vomiting during pregnancy: effects on the quality of women's lives. Birth 19 (3): 138-143

Omer H, Friedlander D, Paltzi Z 1986 Hypnotic relaxation in the treatment of premature labour. Psychosomatic Medicine 48 (5): 351-361

Omer H, Sirkovitz A 1987 Failure of hypnotic suggestion in inducing postterm pregnancies. Psychosomatic Medicine 49 (6): 606-609

Oster M I 1994 Psychological preparation for labour and delivery using hypnosis. American Journal of Clinical Hypnosis 37 (1): 12-21

Palmblad J, Cantell K, Strandler H et al 1976 Stressor exposure and immunological response in man: Interferon producing capacity and phagocytosis. Journal of Psychosomatic Research 20: 193-199

Peng C K, Mietus J E, Liu Y et al 1999 Exaggerated heart rate oscillations during two meditation techniques. International Journal of Cardiology 70 (2): 101-107

Poehl M, Bichler K, Wicke V et al 1999 Psychotherapeutic counselling and pregnancy rates in in vitro fertilization. Journal of Assisted Reproduction and Genetics 16 (6): 302-305

Poliakov V V 1989 Treatment of hyperemesis gravidarum by hypnosis. Akush Ginekol (Mosk) 5: 57-7 [article in Russian] cited on www.nccam.nih.gov (accessed 29.8.02)

Qin L, Au S, Choy W et al 2002 Regular Tai Chi Chuan exercise may retard bone loss in postmenoausal women: a case control study. Archives of Physical Medicine and Rehabilitation 83 (10): 1355-1359

Raghuraj P, Telles S 1997 Muscle power, dexterity skill and visual perception in community home girls trained in yoga or sports and in regular schoolgirls. Indian Journal of Physiology and Pharmacology 41(4): 409-415

Raju P S, Prasad K V, Venkata R Y et al 1997 Influence of intensive yoga training on physiological changes in 6 women: a case report. Journal of Alternative and Complementary Medicine 3 (3): 291-295

Raphael-Leff J 1992 Psychological processes of childbearing. Chapman & Hall, London

Rashed H, Cutts T, Abell T et al 2002 Predictors of response to a behavioural treatment in patients with chronic gastric motility disorders. Digestive Diseases and Science 47 (5): 1020-1026

Reichlin S 1993 Neuroendocrine-immune interactions. New England Journal of Medicine 327 (10): 1246-1253

Reid M, Garcia J 1989 Women's views of care during pregnancy and childbirth. In: Chalmers I, Enkin M, Keirse M J N C (eds) Effective care in pregnancy and childbirth. Oxford University Press, Oxford

Rhodes V A, McDaniel R W 1999 The index of nausea, vomiting and retching: a new format of the index of nausea and vomiting. Oncology Nursing Forum, 26 (5): 889-894

Robinson A 2002 Music therapy and the effects on laboring women. Kentucky Nurse 50 (2): 7

Rokicki L A, Holroyd K A, France C R et al 1997 Change mechanisms associated with combined relaxation/EMG biofeedback training for chronic tension headache. Applied Psychophysiological Biofeedback 22: 21-41

Ruhle G 1996 Pilot study on the use of Bach flower essences in primiparae with postdate pregnancy [unpublished dissertation]. Heidelberg University Hospital for Women, Heidelberg

Schaller K J 1996 Tai Ch'i chuan: an exercise option for older adults. Journal of Gerontological Nursing 22 (10): 12-17

Schauble P G, Werner W E, Rai S H et al 1998 Childbirth preparation through hypnosis: the hypnoreflexogenous protocol. American Journal of Clinical Hypnosis 40 (4):

273-283

Schmidt T, Wijga A, Von Zur Muhlen A et al 1997 Changes in cardiovascular risk factors and hormones during a comprehensive residential three month kriya yoga training and vegetarian nutrition. Acta Physiologica Scandinavia Supplementum 640: 158-162

Schoenberger N E 2000 Research on hypnosis as an adjunct to cognitive behavioural psychotherapy. International Journal of Clinical and Experimental Hypnosis 48: 154-169

Schouneborg L O, Honnens de Lichtenberg M, Djursing H et al 1992 Hyperemesis gravidarum. Ugeskr Laeger 154 (15): 1015-1019

Selvamurthy W, Sridharan K, Ray U S et al 1998 A new physiological approach to control essential hypertension. Indian Journal of Physiology and Pharmacology 42 (2): 205-213

Shannahoff-Khalsa D S, Beckett L R 1996 Clinical case report: efficacy of yogic techniques in the treatment of obsessive compulsive disorders. International Journal of Neuroscience 85 (1-2): 1-17

Sharpe M, Wessely S 1997 Non-specific ill health: a mind-body approach to functional somatic symptoms. In: Watkins A (ed) Mind body medicine: a physician's guide to psychoneuroimmunology. Churchill Livingstone, New York

Sharma J B, Smith R J, Wilkin D J 1993 Induction of labour at term. British Medical Journal 306: 1413

Sidorenko V N 2000 Clinical application of medical resonance therapy music in high-risk pregnancies. Integr Physiol Behav Sci 35 (3): 199-207

Simon E P, Schwartz J 1999 Medical hypnosis for hyperemesis gravidarum Birth 26 (4): 248-254

Simon E P, James L C 1999 Clinical applications of hypnotherapy in a medical setting. Hawaii Medical Journal 58 (12): 344-347

Simkin P 1992 Just another day in a woman's life? Part 2: nature and consistence of women's longterm memories of their first birth experiences. Birth 19 (2): 64-81

Sjogren B 1998 Fear of childbirth and psychosomatic support. A follow up of 72 women. Acta Obstetrica Gynecologica Scandinavia 778: 819-825

Smirnov S A, Aizikov G S, Kozlovskaia I B 1988 Effect of adaptive biofeedback on the severity of vestibule-autonomic symptoms of experimental motion sickness. Kosm Biol Aviakosm 22 (4): 35-39 [article in Russian] cited at www.nccam.nih.gov (accessed 29.08.02)

Smith B J 1982 Management of the patient with hyperemesis gravidarum in family therapy with hypnotherapy as an adjunct. Journal of New York State Nurses' Association 13: 17

Sokel B S, Devane S P, Bentovim A et al 1990 Self hypnotherapeutic treatment of habitual reflex vomiting. Archives of Diseases in Children 65 (6): 626-627

Somer E 1995 Biofeedback-aided hypnotherapy for intractable phobic anxiety. American Journal of Clinical Hypnosis 37 (3): 54-64

Somers P J, Gevirtz R N, Jasin S E et al 1989 The efficacy of biobehavioral and compliance intervention in the adjunctive treatment of mild pregnancy-induced hypertension. Biofeedback and Self-Regulation 14 (4): 309-318

Stachenfeld N S, Maack G W, Di Pietro L et al 1998 Regulation of blood volume during training in postmenopausal women. Medicine and Science in Sports and Exercise 30 (1): 92-98

Standing Nursing and Midwifery Advisory Committee 1998 Midwifery: delivering our future. HMSO, London.

Standley J M 2002 A meta-analysis of the efficacy of music therapy for premature infants. Journal of Pediatric Nursing 17 (2): 107-113

Stanford J B 1994 Hypnosis for nausea and vomiting in pregnancy. American Family Physician 49 (8): 1733-1736

St James-Roberts I, Hutchinson C M P A, Haran F J et al 1983 Can biofeedback-based relaxation training be used to help women with childbirth? Journal of Reproductive and Infant Psychology 1 (1): 5-10

Stoudemire A, Cotanch P, Laszlo J 1984 Recent advances in the pharmacologic and behavioral management of chemotherapy-induced emesis. Archives of Internal Medicine 144 (5): 1029-1033

Talley N J, Owen B K, Boyce P et al 1996 Psychological treatments for irritable bowel syndrome: a critique of controlled treatment trials. American Journal of Gastroenterology 91(2): 277-283

Tennant J, Butler M 1999 Communication: issues for change. British Journal of Midwifery 7 (6): 359-362

Terao O, Oikawa M, Saito M 1993 Cytokine induced changes in the hypothalamic norepinephrine turnover: involvement of corticotrophin-releasing hormone and prostaglandins. Brain Research 622: 257-261

Tiran D 2003 CTNM report on CTs innovations. Complementary Therapies in Nursing and Midwifery

Tiran D 2002 Supporting women during pregnancy and childbirth. In: Mackereth P, Tiran D (eds) Clinical reflexology: a guide for health professionals. Elsevier Science, London

Torem M S 1994 Hypnotherapeutic techniques in the treatment of hyperemesis gravidarum. American Journal of Clinical Hypnosis 37 (1): 1-11

Toscano W B, Cowings P S 1982 Reducing motion sickness: a comparison of autogenic -feedback training and an alternative cognitive task. Aviation Space and Environmental Medicine 53 (5): 449-453

Troesch L M, Rodehaver C B, Delaney E A et al 1993 The influence of guided imagery on chemotherapy-related nausea and vomiting. Oncology Nurses' Forum 20 (8): 1179-1185

Vaananen S, Laitinen T, Pekkarinen H et al 2002 Tai chiquan acutely increases heart rate variability. Clinical Physiology and Functional Imaging 22 (1): 2-3

Valbo A, Eide T 1996 Smoking cessation in pregnancy: the effect of hypnosis in a randomised study. Addictive Behaviors 21 (1): 29-35

Van Lier D, Manteuffel B, Dilorio C et al 1993 Nausea and fatigue during early pregnancy. Birth 20 (4): 193-197

Walach H, Rilling C, Engelke U 2000 Bach flower remedies are ineffective for test anxiety: results of a blinded, placebo-controlled randomized trial. Forsch Komplementarmed Klass Naturheilkd 7: 55

Walton I, Hamilton M 1995 Midwives and changing childbirth. Books for Midwives Press, Hale

Wang J S, Lan C, Chen S Y et al 2002 Tai Chi Chuan training is associated with enhanced endothelium-dependent dilation in skin vasculature of healthy older men. Journal of the American Geriatric Society 50 (6): 1024-1030

Watkins A D 1994 The role of alternative therapies in the treatment of allergic diseases. Clinical Experimental Allergy 24 (9): 813

Wolf S L, Barnhart H X, Kutner N G et al 1996 Reducing frailty and falls in older persons: an investigation of Tai chi and computerized balance training. Journal of the American Geriatrics Society 44 (5): 489-497

Wolfson L, Whipple R, Derby C et al 1996 Balance and strength training in older adults: intervention gains and Tai chi maintenance. Journal of the American Geriatrics Society 44 (5): 498-506

Young D R, Appel L J, Jee S et al 1999 The effects of aerobic exercise and Tai chi on blood pressure in older people: results of a randomized trial. Journal of the American Geriatrics Society 47 (3): 277-284

Zeltzer L K, Dolgin M J, LeBaron S et al 1991 A randomized controlled study of behavioral intervention for chemotherapy distress in children with cancer. Pediatrics 88: 34-42

Zimmer E Z, Peretz B A, Eyal E et al 1988 The influence of maternal hypnosis on fetal movements in anxious pregnant women. European Journal of Gynecology and Reproductive Biology 27 (2): 133-137

9

The Tiran integrated approach

This chapter draws together the themes which have emerged from the preceding chapters and applies them to practice for healthcare professionals caring for pregnant and childbearing women, namely obstetricians, GPs and midwives. The concept of holistic maternity care, with particular reference to the impact of nausea and vomiting on pregnant women, is explored and the advantages of integrated maternity care are considered. Finally, a new tool for a combined approach to the care of expectant mothers suffering nausea and vomiting, the Tiran Integrated Approach, is proposed.

INTRODUCTION

Pregnancy and childbirth are normal life events, arguably the most significant in the lives of most people and, increasingly, a single episode for many couples. Obviously there is a universal desire for women to produce live, healthy infants and to maintain their own health and wellbeing. Thankfully, maternal mortality and morbidity rates in the western world are minimal, neonatal deaths are infrequent and professionals and parents welcome the relative safety of the childbearing event, yet there remains a fundamental emphasis of the conventional maternity services on the presence of *physical* health, or rather, on the *absence* of pathological complications.

Nowhere is this more apparent than in the care of women suffering the *symptoms* of pregnancy, which are given scant attention by obstetricians and by some GPs, and although midwives often express sympathy and offer advice, they may feel powerless to deal with the woman's concerns at anything more than a superficial level. The implication is that, as these symptoms are normal, expected and not usually pathological in either cause or effect, there is no real need to do anything to resolve them, and in any case, symptoms such as nausea and vomiting have often resolved spontaneously by the time the expectant mother first meets her midwife. Furthermore, it is considered that, as prescribed medication is contraindicated for all but those with the most severe sickness, there is very little that can be offered to help the woman other than 'reassurance' that it is normal and will resolve spontaneously after the first trimester.

Conversely, there is an inherent professional obligation to detect early and treat promptly any possible pathological conditions which arise, in order to prevent further complications developing. This results in standardised routine observations and investigations being performed, often unthinkingly, more as a defensive attempt to avoid litigation than with any real acknowledgement of their value, which Tiran (1999) refers to as the 'just-in-case' syndrome. Indeed, it is this very 'routineness' which may lead to reduced vigilance in identifying nuances in the appearance, behaviour or overall condition of a single woman amongst many, which could ironically cause professionals to fail to recognise deviations from the norm. On the other hand, repetitive technological monitoring may reveal biophysical changes, of which we are not yet cognisant as being normal, with a premature diagnosis of 'complications' requiring medical action. Over-reliance on technological replacements for human care has fuelled the medical *management* of pregnancy and childbirth which is standard in most of the western world. The paternalism of conventional obstetrics encourages doctors to want to 'take charge' of the woman's condition, while she becomes a 'patient', a passive recipient of care. Emotional blackmail is unwittingly used by many providers of conventional maternity care to persuade women to submit to procedures such as induction of labour or Caesarean section, in which control is handed very firmly to the expert. In addition, obstetric progress has led to a range of specialisms within the specialism, such as fetal medicine and the highly technical management of infertility, which are more adventurous, more exciting and more newsworthy than uncomplicated pregnancies and births.

The aims of maternity care are, surely, to provide the means for women to achieve as safe *and satisfying* a childbirth experience as possible, within the constraints of their personal biophysical and psycho-social circumstances. Unfortunately, whilst obstetricians and, to a certain extent, midwives, focus on physiopathological *safety*, mothers are often more concerned with psycho-emotional and social *satisfaction*, although, of course, none would wish for a problematic pregnancy or labour. The principles of UK Maternity Service policy (Department of Health 1998), namely continuity of care and carer, informed choice, responsiveness and accessibility, patient involvement and clinical effectiveness, should facilitate individualised care, thereby avoiding routine procedures and investigations for the sake of them. The *Changing Childbirth* report (Department of Health 1993) also advocated, amongst other suggestions for quality care, that maternity professionals should facilitate the empowerment of pregnant women and their families, yet, ten years on, it appears that this concept continues to be paid 'lip service' without actually being fully achieved. Anderson (2002) challenges the 'misleading myth of choice' offered to expectant mothers, suggesting that there is 'continuing oppression' of women, even when choices appear to be available. She goes so far as to question whether newly-introduced options will eventually become compulsions, and expresses concern about the impact of restricted choice and its implicit overtones of control on both mothers and midwives. Waldenstrom (1996) suggests that the emphasis on safety should not be at the expense of maternal satisfaction, both of which are elements of high quality care, and

Johanson et al (2002) add to the debate by questioning whether the medicalisation of childbirth has gone too far as a result of medicolegal pressures leading to defensive practice (by midwives as well as obstetricians), thus contributing to reduced choices for women.

Providing women with sufficient information to be involved in the decision-making process regarding their pregnancies adds to their sense of *empowerment*, increasing their cooperation to comply with professional advice. However, whilst acknowledging that the healthcare professional is merely a facilitator in the healing process, providing people with education requires individuals to take responsibility for their own health, something which not all are prepared to do. Also, offering a full choice of options for women is dependent on their availability and *accessibility*, which may be limited due to socioeconomic factors, either locally, nationally or internationally – an example of the latter being the reluctance to budget routinely for any potentially pre-eclamptic mother to receive magnesium sulphate, despite overwhelming evidence as to its benefits (Sheth & Chalmers 2002). Another example of 'choices' being presented in a biased way is that of breech presentation, in which the mother may be offered external cephalic version or Caesarean section, with no comprehensive explanation of the benefits *and* risks of either, nor of any other options, at the very least, that of vaginal breech delivery. (In the majority of centres, alternative suggestions to encourage version, such as moxibustion, yoga positions or homeopathy are not even mentioned.)

This can hardly be considered to be 'informed choice', neither is it ethically acceptable, even leaving aside the non-conventional approaches. All healthcare professionals are bound by the ethical duties of beneficence (benefiting) and non-maleficence (not harming), yet it could be argued that there is a very fine distinction between these two concepts in numerous procedures and techniques of orthodox care. Stone (2002) suggests that the notion of what constitutes 'benefiting' is much wider in complementary than in conventional medicine.

Conventional medical benefit focuses on the *outcome* of treatment, namely the removal of symptoms or 'curing', whilst complementary medicine may either prevent the development or exacerbation of ill health, or improve psychological wellbeing through the relaxation effects of many therapies, and is therefore equally concerned with the *process*. Additionally, there is a legal duty of care towards patients, which could be called into question if healthcare professionals fail to disclose comprehensively the risks, as well as the benefits, of treatment, thereby potentially exposing themselves to accusations of negligence.

Thus, there appears to be a difference of opinion about what constitutes *effectiveness* in maternity care. Medical effectiveness is concerned with intermittent antenatal (and continuous intrapartum) monitoring to achieve a positive outcome in the delivery of a live, healthy baby from a live, healthy mother. The mechanistic and increasingly technological approach to biomedicine reflects also a materialistic orientation towards healthcare (Engebretson 2002). The 'institutionalisation' of childbirth (Campbell & Macfarlane 1987) has persisted into the 21st century, producing a 'snapshot' approach to care which does not reflect fully the nine months of pregnancy and the period of adaptation to parenthood which mothers, and their families, experience. Maternal effectiveness more often involves 'making it through' the nine months of waiting, enduring unpleasant symptoms and, sometimes, challenging health professionals in order to achieve an experience which is in keeping with their personal philosophy.

'Effectiveness' is also concerned with undertaking procedures or treatment strategies which achieve that *which is expected*, but treatment aims are generally determined by health professionals without any recourse to the mother's needs other than her immediate physiopathological ones, or those of the fetus. Psychosocial needs must, at best, take second place and at worst, are disregarded, this attitude often being disguised in a language which demonstrates the paternalistic bias of care, and does not allow for anything other than conventional (medical) treatment (Stan 2002). More fundamentally, effectiveness should be about achieving that *which the mother desires* for herself and her baby, involving her in the decision making, leading to a greater sense of empowerment and therefore greater collaboration, which will ultimately result in a safer childbearing experience for all concerned.

Engebretson (2002) debates the dualistic nature of healthcare in which there is a division between general medicine and psychiatry and a marginalisation of spiritual aspects of health. This orthodox division is compounded by the traditional sense of superior status of physicians over psychiatrists and of surgeons over physicians. Gynaecology/obstetrics is a specialism which has the uniquely fortunate status of being both medicine and surgery, with some psychological care, yet the same attitude prevails in the covert implication of superiority of men (i.e. doctors) over women (i.e. mothers and midwives). Much still has to be done within the conventional health system in general to encourage attitudinal changes in all parties involved, to reflect better a more balanced weighting of choices and responsibilities which have a direct effect on those requiring care.

To a certain extent, attitudes of scepticism, and occasionally downright antagonism, continue to prevail amongst conventional healthcare professionals about CAM, although thankfully this is declining as more evidence becomes available to demonstrate its safety and efficacy. However, until CAM therapies are more widely integrated into mainstream healthcare provision, it will continue to be regarded more as an alternative by the vast majority of doctors, nurses and other practitioners, as they have only limited experience of seeing CAM in practice. The complementary approach could be better incorporated into conventional healthcare by its inclusion in the curricula of medical, nursing and pharmacy schools, enabling future practitioners to appreciate the different perspective which it brings (Konefal 2002; Kreitzer et al 2002). Education and training of both conventional and complementary practitioners is essential, particularly in maternity care. It is of

concern that some complementary therapists are attracted to the pleasant, fashionable and lucrative specialism of pregnancy and childbirth, yet they have little appreciation of the possible complications which may arise, nor or their legal position in the maternity services, one which was set in statute in the UK in order to protect mothers and babies (see Case 9.1). Similarly, conventional professionals may reject CAM or remain sceptical through lack of knowledge, yet they owe it to their patients to have at least a modicum of awareness, as the general public is increasingly turning to the alternatives. Trust and cooperation of colleagues in orthodox healthcare can be achieved through greater education and more opportunities for research so that the benefits of the individual therapies can be demonstrated (Peace 2002). Additionally, clear guidelines need to be identified to ensure 'best practice' when a complementary therapy, such as homeopathy, is incorporated into the orthodox health services, including assessment and referral processes and audit and evaluation systems (Peters et al 2000). Policies and protocols will not only protect the mothers but also the staff and can be a positive and constructive means of integrating the two systems (Tiran 2000).

The common argument against trying anything different or new, especially complementary strategies, is that they are untested as to either effectiveness or safety, yet numerous techniques have been introduced in conventional healthcare without any prior evidence of either. An obstetric example is that of ultrasound scans, the safety of which was only called into question many years after its inception as a diagnostic tool, and which today is used at considerably higher levels of power than previously, with a greater possibility of thermal and non-thermal insults to patients (Miller et al 1998). Conversely, there is a growing body of evidence for some areas of complementary medicine, notably acupuncture and herbal medicine (see Chapters 4 and 5), as well as other therapies, although the conventional scientific community is at pains to challenge the research methodology, advocating the credibility of randomised blinded controlled

---

Case 9.1

A student of aromatherapy, who was already a qualified reflexologist, attended the antenatal clinic to work under the supervision of the CT midwife, providing aromatherapy massages for relaxation of pregnant women. She saw one expectant mother and, unbeknown to the midwife, decided to perform reflexology on her own initiative to treat the mother's constipation, although the midwife had discussed the use of suitable essential oils and massage techniques. The following week the mother returned and complained of having suffered headaches, immense fatigue and vomiting in the 24 hours after the treatment. This was undoubtedly more than a mere healing crisis and had probably arisen as a result of over-zealous and inappropriate reflexology. The CT midwife discussed this with the student and asked her to refrain from using reflexology with future clients. However, a few weeks later, a member of staff produced a small bottle of nutmeg essential oil belonging to the CT midwife. Nutmeg is an oil which should never be used in pregnancy and only in labour under controlled circumstances. The midwife reported that the student had asked her to return it to the CT midwife, although on questioning she denied this. It was obvious however that she had 'borrowed' the oil without the knowledge of the CT midwife and, as she had not been in the labour ward, must have used it for one of the pregnant women without permission. She was, of course, counselled and informed that she was excluded from the clinic as her reliability and professionalism were suspect.

---

studies over any other methods. One of the problems of standardising methodology is the disparity between the two philosophies. The biomedical approach is disease-orientated, facilitating examination of specific treatments for specific conditions, with hypothesis testing and linear reasoning being the fundamental components of scientific study. The more comprehensive multidimensional approach of CAM therapies requires investigations in which care and management is focused not on whether or not a specific treatment is effective but rather on the sense of wellbeing obtained by the person (Spencer 1999). Another criticism of CAM research is the small numbers of subjects tested in any one study, although greater integration into mainstream healthcare might partially resolve this problem. Randomisation between those who do and those who do not receive the test treatment is more difficult with small numbers, a factor which also increases variability. Blinding of studies is also more difficult with therapies such as manual techniques (acupuncture, reflexology, massage) as the practitioner and often the recipient will be aware of whether or not they are exposed to the test treatment. There is also an element of subjectivity which is less easy to eliminate from CAM investigations – not the subjectivity of the practitioners/researchers but that of the clients, whose improved 'wellness' may result from psychological and emotional factors even in the absence of

'cure' for the pathological condition. Spencer (1999) suggests that, irrespective of whether it is conventional or CAM, medical research requires a range of evidence for results to be valid, including experimental and clinical evidence of safety, efficacy and comparability with existing treatments, as well as evidence that there is a demand for, satisfaction with and cost-effectiveness of the strategies being studied.

Much has been postulated about the efficacy of complementary medicine being due to the 'placebo effect', although the word is frequently used in the restrictive sense of an intervention which has no intention of having a therapeutic effect, but is simply a sham treatment used 'to please' (from the Latin). However, physiological changes resulting from placebo conventional treatment have been shown to affect between 30 and 70% of patients, including pharmacokinetics, dose-related responses, endorphin release and long-term effects (Beecher 1955; Pogge 1963; Levine et al 1978; Oh 1994). A broader definition of placebo is that in which therapeutic strategies are shown to work in isolation from, or despite, the impact of the extraneous factors such as the environment, the time availability or the personal interaction between client and therapist. White (2000) identifies other elements which can have a positive or negative impact on the effectiveness of treatments, including the gender, reputation and charisma of the caregiver, aspects of interaction

Figure 9.1 Safety and satisfaction in maternity care

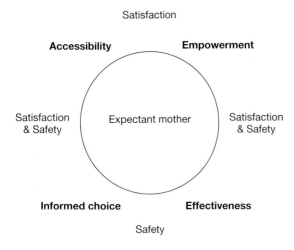

such as empathy and touch, as well as the therapeutic environment. Placebos may work solely as a means of reducing anxiety or through a conditioning response in the form of 'remembered wellness' (Shapiro & Shapiro 1984; Benson 1996; Vincent & Furnham 1997). However, conventional medicine can also be criticised for failing to acknowledge its own placebo effect, including attention and compassionate care, patient anxiety or awareness and patient and doctor expectation of outcomes of treatment (Kaptchuk 2002; Moyad 2002), or, indeed, the locus of control by 'powerful others' (So 2002). Much of the work of midwives actually involves giving expectant mothers the time to ask questions about issues of concern and worry to them and to gain information about the progress of their pregnancies. The 'expected *outcome*' of a live healthy baby is almost taken for granted in modern obstetrics and more emphasis is put by women on the *process* of the pregnancy.

INTEGRATED MATERNITY CARE

The concept of '*holism*' within healthcare implies that the person is viewed as a single entity comprised of many individual facets, but with the whole being more than the sum of its parts. Unfortunately, however, contemporary use of the term 'holism' appears to have deflected understanding away from its true meaning, with the word becoming a synonym for 'complementary' (Buckle 1993), although Vincent and Furnham (1997) do not believe that complementary therapies, *per se*, are intrinsically holistic, and Todd (1990) maintains that common usage has led to the trend of defining holism as a treatment modality. Health professionals should aim to work towards 'whole person' care (Benor 1996), in keeping with the original meaning of the word as defined by Jan Smuts in 1926 (cited by Pietroni 1997), and within which there is an emphasis on the integration and inter-relationship between body, mind and spirit. Integral to this relationship are the concepts of energy and balance, spirituality and empowerment (Hebert et al 2001).

'Energy' is a difficult concept to comprehend for many practitioners of conventional healthcare, who may see it as a 'new age' element without foundation. However, many traditional and contemporary systems of healthcare, acknowledge the existence of a fundamental life force, referred to by numerous terms. For example, Traditional Chinese Medicine (TCM, see Chapter 4) refers to the energy as 'chi' or 'Qi', distributed via channels called meridians which have been shown to exist as electrically-charged points throughout the body (Bensoussan 1991). Indian Ayurvedic medicine uses the term 'Prana', with energy distributed via a series of seven wheel-like or funnel-shaped chakras. Miccozzi (1996) refers to the 'vitalism' or vital force, a term used also in homeopathic theory, in which it is believed that there is an inherent internal force within each of us which facilitates the promotion of self-healing. Even within conventional healthcare, the concept of energy fields, which were formerly inexplicable, is now a component of some clinical specialities, as with the use of oscillatory magnetic fields to 'jump start' the healing process (Oschman 2000:122), although Basford (2001) laments the continuing scepticism of conventional medical practitioners about these techniques. Within complementary medicine, many therapies have evolved from a belief in a therapeutic energy between the client and the therapist, as in Reiki, reflexology or Therapeutic Touch, or as a conceptual component of the therapeutic medium, as in acupuncture or homeopathy. However, in simple, western terms, this rather nebulous 'energy' may be as basic as the interaction which occurs between the patient and her carer, or even, simply, an applied use of intuition on the part of the healthcare professional (see Case 9.2).

'Spirituality' is also a little-understood phenomenon in conventional healthcare. Sulmasy (2002) postulates that people are 'beings-in-relationship', a balanced interaction of all biopsychosocial and spiritual facets of life, and that illness should be considered a biological disruption which has a direct or indirect effect on their psychosocial and spiritual components. He presents a framework for understanding the four domains of spirituality, namely religion, religious coping and support, spiritual wellbeing and spiritual need. Religion and spirituality are a source of comfort for many people and can have a profound effect on health, particularly mental wellbeing (Larson & Milano 1996), and healthcare professionals should enquire about patients' coping and support mechanisms and respect their values (Hebert et al 2001). Boudreaux et al (2002) explore further the nature of spirituality, which is associated with an enhanced sense of wellbeing, improved ability to cope ('resiliency') and decreased adverse physiological and psychological symptoms. Guinn (2001) argues that there is a need to adopt a new subset of ethical principles in order to accommodate the increased integration of complementary practices into conventional care, which includes not only the spirituality, naturalistic and relational approaches, but also the concepts of humanity and ecological integrity. Therapeutic strategies which impact on spiritual wellbeing may include prayer, music, dance or relaxation therapies, and have been studied in respect of chronic illness such as diabetes mellitus (Johns 2001; Landis 1996), but apply equally well to short-term, acute phases of adaptations in health status, such as pregnancy, or the life-changing events of parenthood. It is, however, interesting to note that some people are averse to receiving complementary therapies because of their personal religious views, deeming them 'new age' or irreligious.

Most importantly, there is a need for *balance*, whether this is defined in terms of Yin and Yang as in Traditional Chinese Medicine, biochemically as in conventional physiopathology, or a sociological balance between caregivers and recipients. The function of the 'life force' (Qi, prana, etc.) is to maintain the balance between all parts of the body, mind and spirit, with each having an impact, either negative or positive, upon the others. Conventional medicine more frequently employs a reductionist approach to care, which views the body as a series of relatively independent systems, each of which can be treated by separate specialists. There remains an apparent lack of understanding amongst medical practitioners, in particular those in hospital-based specialisms, of the multifactorial nature of health changes. The focus of obstetricians is overtly on the patient's reproductive tract so that they appear to become partially blinded to any other factors affecting the woman, such as the potential exacerbation of her condition by worry over social, financial or relationship issues. Also, within general medicine, there is a need to recognise the biological influences of female hormones on non-gynaecological systems, (and of male hormones on other systems), as well as the gender differences in health and illness (Autry et al 2002).

Reductionism tends to be based on medical pathophysiological treatment provided by 'experts', paternalistic information giving, with a mechanistic, routine and institutionalised approach. Requirements for healthcare are viewed as one-off 'episodes' in which the patient is a passive recipient and treatment is determined on deduction and analysis. Conversely, holistic, or 'naturalistic' (Whitehead 2000) care focuses on the individual human experience; the client is an active partner in the process, their empowerment is facilitated by healthcare professionals and the ongoing client-identified needs are taken into consideration through socially or environmentally-based care.

The intention of *all* professionals involved in the care of pregnant and childbearing women is to aid the process of 'healing', which, in maternity care can be taken to mean facilitating the acquisition of optimum health and wellbeing during pregnancy, labour and the puerperium. The aim may be the same for both conventional and complementary care providers, but its implementation may vary according to the inherent philosophical origins. Duggan debates the 'false dichotomy' of the technique-focused approach of orthodox medical care and the relationship-centred care of complementary medicine, and identifies the need for a 'coming together', or an integration, of practitioners from both directions, a process which Tiran (1999) has termed the 'evolution' of healthcare. Within holistic maternity care, the fundamental aim of the therapeutic interaction should be to assist the mother to achieve optimum health and wellbeing through empowerment. This may be helped by the natural warmth, sensitivity and empathy of the care-giver, or could be hindered by the pressures of time, venue and cost-effectiveness of the system, in essence, the placebo response. Fahy (2002) debates the inseparability of power and knowledge, with medical power being dependent on the cooperation of the midwife and the submission of the mother, only becoming overt when resistance from either of these is encountered. It is suggested that, in order for mothers to become more empowered, women should not only be able to acquire knowledge about physiopathological benefits *and* risks, but also socio-legal information to equip them to deal with varying circumstances.

Using research evidence may also increase compliance from the mother to meet the needs of the healthcare professional. An example would be a reduction to weekly, rather than daily, iron supplementation to avoid gastrointestinal disturbance, in women who have borderline haemoglobin levels, as no real benefit has been found by administering the more frequent dosage (Hyder et al 2002). The provision of a situation in which the mother can determine her own needs will contribute towards a more productive relationship and a more successful outcome in the therapeutic interaction (Liossi & Mystakidou 1997), which should be a partnership between the mother and the doctor/midwife and other members of the maternity care team. Mitchell and Cormack (1998) suggest that good practice (in complementary medicine, but equally in conventional healthcare) is built on the principles of an open, facilitative environment, a contract devised with informed consent or the opportunity to decline treatment if desired, contemporary evidence and an individualised approach. Care should be effective, safe, provided within the personal professional boundaries of the caregiver and constantly evolving as a result of high quality initial and continuing education. Wright and Sayre-Adams (2000) debate the provision of a 'sacred space', a therapeutically positive environment, in which the patient can be autonomous but guided by the expertise of professionals. Cumbie (2001) suggests that there is also a need for healthcare professionals to develop the art of the 'therapeutic use of self' as an essential component of a therapeutic relationship, in which each individual professional strives to achieve a personal sense of harmony

---

Case 9.2

A 28-year-old mother of three small children in the 32nd week of pregnancy was referred to the complementary therapy (CT) midwife for reflexology treatment to reduce her blood pressure. On her first visit, the midwife commenced a visual and manual examination of the mother's feet (see Chapter 7) and identified a possible change in physiology related to her eyes. Taking an educated guess she asked the mother if she had experienced any visual disturbance, at which the mother burst into tears and asked how the midwife knew. On being questioned the day before by her own midwife, the mother had denied any symptoms of pre-eclampsia because she did not want to leave her children if she was admitted to hospital. The CT midwife took the mother's blood pressure which was excessively high and accompanied by other symptoms of impending eclampsia, and the mother was transferred to the labour ward, for immediate delivery.

Figure 9.2 The integrated maternity care team

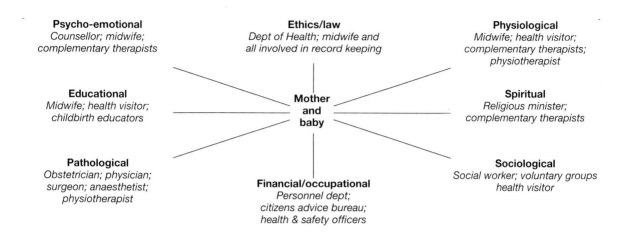

and balance, and an empathic sensitivity, as a means of actualising the potential for good in clients or patients.

This sense of harmony should, however, extend beyond the boundaries of individuals, to the *system* which provides care for pregnant and childbearing women. A multidisciplinary team approach to maternity care is essential, particularly as it is virtually impossible, given the resourcing and staffing shortages of contemporary services, to provide universally-available holistic continuity of *carer*, as advocated by the *Changing Childbirth* report (1993), although continuity of *care* can be achieved through good interdisciplinary communication. Modern western maternity care persists in a hierarchical structure which enforces the paternalism and engenders a culture in which medical expertise is seen as superior to that of other professionals such as midwives, physiotherapists, social workers or religious ministers. This reinforces the anticipation of pathological complications as being of most importance, with a 'birth is only normal in retrospect' attitude, which may inadvertently transmit itself to the woman, possibly affecting outcomes. For example, labour has been found to be prolonged in women being cared for by obstetricians rather than by midwives, which Heres et al (2000)

attribute to increased maternal stress levels caused by the emphasis on avoidance of complications rather than facilitating progress of normality. The hierarchy of the maternity services also places the passive 'patient' firmly at the bottom of the structure, dismissing her knowledge in the process of childbearing, although Tranmer (2000) challenges whether it is the professional or the patient who is actually the most knowledgeable about her condition. In order to achieve holistic care, an integrated *team* is required, with different professionals providing different elements of care, determined according to an holistic framework (Tiran 1999, see Figure 9.2). Viewing the mother as integral to the whole decision-making process, with a flatter structure for more effective teamwork, would enhance the experience, not only for women and their families but also for professionals.

It would be untrue, unrealistic and unfair to promote the idea that complementary approaches are entirely positive, while reductionist (i.e. conventional) approaches are only negative. In reality, many practitioners of conventional maternity care would wish to and, indeed, strive to provide individualised, yet evidence-based care *despite* the constraints of the system such as poor resources, lack of time and unsatisfactory venues. Conversely, some practitioners of complementary medicine could be accused of working in a mechanistic and disease-focused way, hidden under the guise of those trappings of the therapeutic environment which lead clients to depart satisfied, even if not 'cured'. More than this, however is the need to achieve a maternity care system in which the expectant mother, together with her baby and family, is the pivotal focus on which decision-making and care provision is determined. This philosophy should take priority over any other means of delivering maternity care, including both the condition-focused approach of conventional obstetrics, or the alternative and sometimes confrontational approach of complementary medicine. It is equally as inappropriate for practitioners of conventional midwifery, general practice or obstetrics to dismiss alternative options, as it is for complementary practitioners to denigrate orthodox care. It is vital also to consider what exactly is the aim of any treatment, care or management, and strive to achieve that purpose in the most effective and safest way possible.

Chapter 2 discussed the reasons for an increasing use of complementary and alternative medicine, including people's desires for greater satisfaction and effectiveness in healthcare. Furnham (1996) suggested a 'push-pull' effect, in which dissatisfaction with and rejection of the orthodox system, desperation and high costs of private conventional healthcare are pushing people away from the mainstream, while differing philosophies and client-therapist relationships, personal control, increased accessibility and the achievement of a greater sense of wellbeing are enticing people towards CAM therapies. In an ever-increasing climate of competition, even in state-run services, providers and managers of conventional healthcare services, too, are looking to ways to improve patient satisfaction, and may be persuaded to consider the incorporation of complementary therapies once they can be shown to be *cost* effective as well as therapeutically effective, often in lieu of conclusive evidence of their mechanism of action (Reilly 2001). One of the

issues of integrating CAM therapies into conventional healthcare is the cost of time, especially as the majority of therapies involve time-consuming interactions such as talking and touching. It has been shown that the general public would be in favour of complementary medicine being more available in nationally provided healthcare, especially as the personal costs of use can often be prohibitive (Lewis et al 2001). An example of this is the trend amongst peri-menopausal women to self-administer herbal alternatives, although the ultimate cost of long-term use is considerably higher than for medical prescriptions of hormone replacement therapy. From a service provision perspective the fundamental question is whether complementary medicine can be substituted for orthodox treatment, at less cost, or whether the enhancement of wellbeing and satisfaction is worth extra expenditure.

Conversely, the public is now, more than ever, prepared to spend money on their health and wellbeing, including beauty aids, speciality foods and diets, vitamins and minerals, fitness and exercise products, water and air filtration systems, smoking cessation aids, natural remedies such as herbal, homeopathic and aromatherapy substances and consultations with complementary and alternative practitioners. A 2000 survey in the UK by Ernst and White showed that approximately £1.6 billion is spent on CAM each year by the general public, representing about 4% of public expenditure on health, in addition to private medical insurance expenditure. Individuals are willing to search the Internet for health information and to purchase numerous books on health, self-development and other related topics. Furnham (1996) refers to this as 'shopping for health', in which people view CAM therapies as additions to the range of options available, enabling them to make their own choices, although its lack of universal availability on the NHS means that it is most likely to be accessed by those who are more affluent. (One US survey (Ernst 1999) found an interesting positive correlation between greater use of herbal medicines and purchasing of BMW cars!)

Fiigure 9.3 Advantages of integrated maternity care

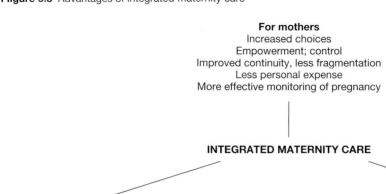

For mothers
Increased choices
Empowerment; control
Improved continuity, less fragmentation
Less personal expense
More effective monitoring of pregnancy

INTEGRATED MATERNITY CARE

For conventional maternity care staff
Maintenance of 'gatekeeper' role
Retention of legal responsibilities
Enhanced education re. CAM
Awareness of interactions
Early detection of abnormalities

For complementary practitioners
Advocacy of CAM therapies
Opportunities for audit and research
Greater credibility, respectability
Enhanced education re. maternity
physiopathology and services

However, more than just encouraging the increased use of complementary and alternative therapies, it is vital that these therapies should be more fully *integrated* into conventional healthcare in order to fulfil the demands of people who can now be seen as 'activist health consumers' rather than passive, dependent patients (Jacobs 1999). A survey in 1998 by Astin identified that 40% of people accessing health services also used CAM therapies, not because they were dissatisfied with conventional healthcare but because they were closer to their personal philosophies about health, although very few (less than 5%) used CAM therapies exclusively. Pregnant women often experience a period of reflection which causes them to challenge their personal (spiritual) beliefs about life, and will frequently be prepared to make lifestyle changes for the good of their offspring. Integration can be better achieved through improving the knowledge of both conventional and complementary practitioners, who need to appreciate each other's philosophies and methods of working. Eisenberg (1997) suggests the need to share information between healthcare professionals and consumers, including ensuring that the client understands his/her symptoms fully, documenting *all*

symptoms and assumptions made by the client as well as the professional, considering risks and benefits of *all* treatments, including the potential for interactions and follow-up of effectiveness of any CAM treatment used by the client.

Integrated maternity care, in which complementary therapies are incorporated as components of normal provision, facilitates the philosophy in which the mother is central to care planning and delivery, yet ensures that the requirements of maternity care are maintained, with the obstetrician, GP or midwife retaining responsibility for overseeing the health and wellbeing of pregnant and childbearing women. The woman can be involved in decision making, enabling her to feel more empowered and to take control of and responsibility for her own health. From a conventional professional perspective, monitoring of physiological progress will allow pathological complications to be detected and acted upon early, and any possible interactions between conventional and complementary strategies, especially pharmacological, can be avoided. Complementary practitioners will be able to work in partnership with colleagues in orthodox care, with increased collaboration and opportunities for research and

---

Box 9.1 Principles of integrated maternity care

Woman-focused, individualised	Safe and effective
Empowering and satisfying	Relationship-centred, not technique-focused
Trustful and respectful	Vitalistic, not mechanistic
Collaborative and facilitative	Assessment of needs
Available and accessible	Evaluation of efficacy
Based on informed choice	Analysis of risks *and* benefits of conventional *and*
Process-focused, not outcome-obsessed	complementary care

---

audit, ultimately contributing to a greater body of knowledge. Institutionally, a wider availability of treatment options could reduce the requirements for hospital admissions, thus decreasing overall service costs, notably for prescribed medications. Finally, it must be remembered that the only professionals legally permitted to take sole responsibility for the care of pregnant and childbearing women are those already working in the conventional maternity services, yet women are frequently self-administering, or consulting practitioners of, complementary medicine. Therefore, a combination of aspects of the two systems is eminently practical and cost effective, as well as legally and medically safer for the women (see Figure 9.3).

THE TIRAN INTEGRATED APPROACH TO GESTATIONAL SICKNESS

In Chapter one we examined a range of potential causes for pregnancy sickness, primarily physiopathological, but also psychosocial, occupational and other factors which may contribute towards a greater severity of symptoms. In later chapters, we debated the wide variety of manifestations and aetiological theories for gestational sickness and the approaches of different complementary therapies to treating women who are suffering from it. It is noticeable that practitioners of the different therapies utilise a common philosophy of holism, albeit interpreted in many different ways. There is a far deeper understanding of the interaction between body-mind-spirit of an individual, and no seemingly insignificant aspect of the person is disregarded in the practitioner's quest for the most appropriate treatment. Whilst conventional maternity care professionals attribute nausea and vomiting primarily to endocrine factors, different complementary practitioners view the condition as imbalances in nutritional (nutritional therapists), energy (TCM practitioners and homeopaths), structural (osteopaths, chiropractors) or psychological (hypnotherapists) factors, with a universal whole-person approach.

Before considering further the ways in which complementary medicine can be incorporated into conventional maternity care and to the care of expectant mothers with nausea and vomiting, it is necessary to explore the holistic *impact* of the condition on women and their families in order to appreciate better an integrated approach to its management. Utilising an holistic framework for care can assist in this process and may, indeed, facilitate reflective practice (Taylor 2002). Various authorities have explored the concept of 'comfort' in maternity care, including the use of a psycho-neuroimmunological framework to provide holistic care of women in preterm labour (Ruiz & Pearson 1999) and the impact of relaxation techniques to reduce stress hormones during childbirth (DePunzio et al 1994). In nursing practice, Kolcaba and Steiner (2000) suggested that total comfort is greater than the sum of its parts, with optimum comfort being not only the physical, but also psycho-emotional and spiritual. Kolcaba and Wilson (2002) revisit this theory of comfort and suggest that there are four elements, namely physical, psychospiritual, sociocultural and environmental. Koehn (2000) applies these principles to the use of complementary and alternative therapies as a means of providing holistic care for labouring women. Kolcaba and

Figure 9.4 An holistic approach to the causes, predisposing and exacerbating factors of nausea and vomiting in pregnancy

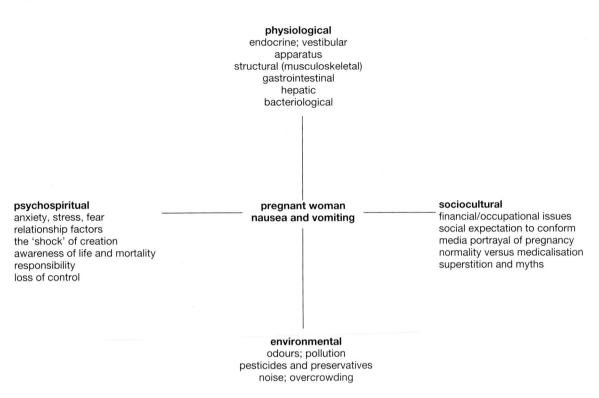

Adapted from Kolcaba and Wilson, 2002, with permission of American Society of PeriAnesthesia Nurses

Wilson's comfort model has been adapted here to consider the *causes* and predisposing factors to gestational nausea and vomiting (see Figure 9.4) and Tiran's holistic framework (1999) has been used to consider its *impact* on the woman and her family (Figure 9.5).

The *Tiran Integrated Approach* to gestational sickness is designed to focus on the *mother's experience* of nausea and vomiting, to identify the impact on each individual and to assist the mother in determining for herself the most appropriate means of coping with the condition in order that she can continue her daily life. Professional experience suggests that women are affected in many different ways and that the perception of 'severity' is dependent on a range of factors according to the mother's lifestyle, commitments, personality and personal philosophy. The existing models for assessing the severity of nausea and vomiting, such as the Rhodes Index (Rhodes & McDaniel 1999) are based solely on the biophysical impact and attempt to measure quantifiable elements such as duration of nausea, number of vomiting episodes or amount of weight loss. This artificially reduces the condition to one in which only the endocrine, gastrointestinal and fetal causes or effects are deemed to be of importance, signifying the need for various forms of biophysical management, such as medication, intravenous rehydration and hospitalisation. The onus of responsibility for this management

Figure 9.5 Using an holistic framework to identify the impact of pregnancy sickness on the woman, her family and society

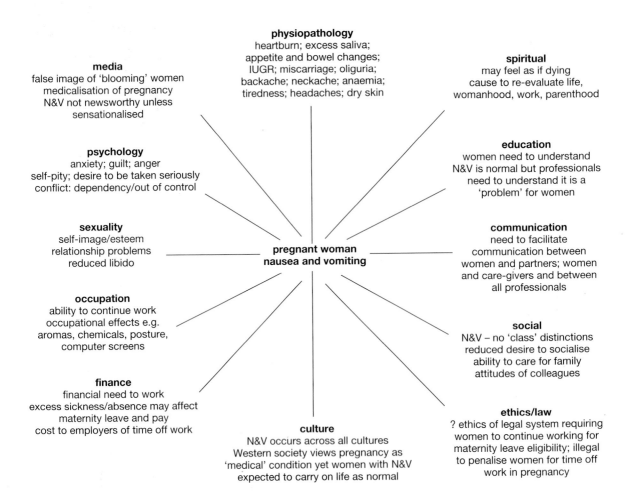

physiopathology
heartburn; excess saliva;
appetite and bowel changes;
IUGR; miscarriage; oliguria;
backache; neckache; anaemia;
tiredness; headaches; dry skin

spiritual
may feel as if dying
cause to re-evaluate life,
womanhood, work, parenthood

media
false image of 'blooming' women
medicalisation of pregnancy
N&V not newsworthy unless
sensationalised

education
women need to understand
N&V is normal but professionals
need to understand it is a
'problem' for women

psychology
anxiety; guilt; anger
self-pity; desire to be taken seriously
conflict: dependency/out of control

sexuality
self-image/esteem
relationship problems
reduced libido

**pregnant woman
nausea and vomiting**

communication
need to facilitate
communication between
women and partners; women
and care-givers and between
all professionals

occupation
ability to continue work
occupational effects e.g.
aromas, chemicals, posture,
computer screens

social
N&V – no 'class' distinctions
reduced desire to socialise
ability to care for family
attitudes of colleagues

finance
financial need to work
excess sickness/absence may affect
maternity leave and pay
cost to employers of time off work

ethics/law
? ethics of legal system requiring
women to continue working for
maternity leave eligibility; illegal
to penalise women for time off
work in pregnancy

culture
N&V occurs across all cultures
Western society views pregnancy as
'medical' condition yet women with N&V
expected to carry on life as normal

is passed to the experts rather than determined by the mother in a way which best suits her personal circumstances.

In Chapter 1 it was suggested that a simple Likert or visual analogue scale could be employed to assess the severity of each woman's nausea and vomiting. However, a more explicit method of assessment might be to use a system based on the Personal Construct Theory developed from the work of Kelly (1955) who suggested that each of us as individuals form ideas and opinions about the world around us which we test out against reality and adapt accordingly. Personal views of life are constantly evolving in response to experiences

and our ideas and beliefs become an integral component of the concept of ourselves. Using this model offers a practical tool since it is based on reality as perceived by the individual, yet encompasses the body, mind and spirit approach which is an essential facet of integrated healthcare. From a professional perspective it enables the midwife, doctor, therapist or other clinician to adapt care to each mother and facilitates continuing professional development by encouraging reflective practice. It allows for changes to be introduced in accordance with the personal interpretation of the severity of gestational sickness (or any other symptom or medical condition).

In practical terms, the mother can be invited to select three words or phrases which best describe how *she* feels about her pregnancy sickness, and these can assist in the process of selection of the most appropriate strategies to alleviate the problem. For example, choosing words which identify a psycho-emotional impact of the nausea (e.g. frightened, 'fed up' or miserable) may indicate the use of Bach flower remedies, hypnotherapy or autogenic training; focusing on the lifestyle impact (e.g. exhausting, inconvenient, stressful) may suggest relaxation therapies or homeopathy; and emphasising the physical symptoms (constant nausea, headaches, heartburn) could signify the need for prescribed medication. The most important aspect of care is to provide women with the information to make choices for themselves and to take responsibility for implementing those choices. Group settings can be useful in alerting women to the commonality yet variations in symptoms and in providing peer and professional support when it is most needed (Tiran 2003). There is no single solution to dealing with the multitude of biopsychosocial effects of nausea and vomiting in pregnancy, but women can be assisted to adapt their choices as their condition varies. Selection of appropriate strategies will be dependent on the nature and effect of the symptoms, and it is important to distinguish between those which women can self-administer, and those which require an expert practitioner, of either conventional or complementary medicine (see Box 9.2). In cases where a mother chooses natural remedies which can be purchased in a health store, for mild to moderate symptoms, she must have adequate evidence-based information for safe use. Additionally, in the event of hyperemesis gravidarum developing, while the mother has the option not to accept conventional medical treatment, her health and that of her baby may be seriously compromised if appropriate care is rejected, and treatment may need to be professionally led as objective rationalisation of thought may be difficult.

The *Tiran Integrated Approach* combines the full range of both conventional and complementary treatments and allows the mother to try whichever seems most suited to her personal circumstances, altering those choices if the first is unsuccessful or unacceptable. For example, a woman may decide to try homeopathic remedies as she has no time to receive any physical or manual treatments, but then finds the healing crisis and consequent exacerbation of symptoms too unbearable. This will require a reassessment and she may opt for an appropriate herbal remedy, for example, cooling peppermint, combined with the vestibular apparatus audiotape. As her condition improves she could omit the peppermint but continue with the audiotape and adapt her diet to include cooling foods such as cucumber. A woman admitted to hospital for hyperemesis gravidarum will initially require intravenous rehydration and possibly pharmacological medication, but could benefit from in-patient relaxation therapies such as reflexology or aromatherapy. Once transferred home, she may use acupressure wristbands or acumagnets but return on an outpatient basis for therapy and monitoring of her condition by the midwife. It can be seen from Figure 9.6 that there is a far wider choice available to women than is generally appreciated within the conventional maternity services and a combined approach facilitates a more effective and safe management of the problem. It must also be acknowledged that there may be specific medical or personal reasons why a woman may not wish to use some of the suggested strategies, and these can be taken into account without overly limiting her options (see Box 9.3).

Ongoing professional support for the woman is important and could be offered face-to-face in a group or individual setting, or via a telephone helpline, as with the Motherisk programme in Toronto, Canada (Magee et al 2002). Auditing of the several thousands of calls to this helpline has provided data from which to consider further investigation into the condition and currently ongoing studies include an exploration of the economic cost such as medication, and the time and cost of absence from work of women in Canada (Motherisk website 26.11.02).

Figure 9.6 An integrated approach to the care of women with pregnancy sickness

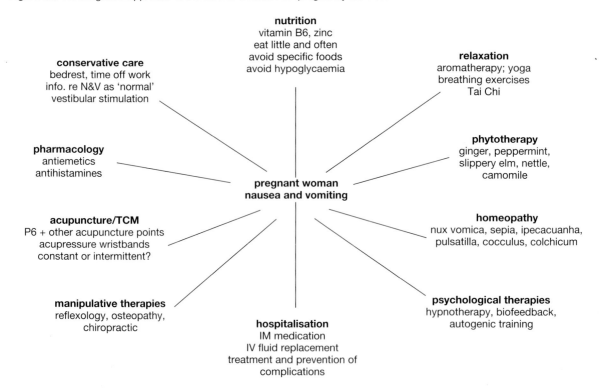

Box 9.2 Summary of modes of treatment for pregnancy sickness

Degree of nausea and vomiting	Conventional treatment	Complementary self-administered treatment	Complementary treatment requiring expert practitioner
Mild	Rest and relaxation Small, frequent meals Avoid certain foods Avoid hypoglycaemia	Nutrition – vitamin B6, zinc or multivitamin supplement Aromatherapy – ginger, lime, lavender, camomile Herbal medicine – ginger, peppermint, slippery elm Bach flower remedies	Aromatherapy/massage Hypnotherapy Biofeedback/autogenic training Alexander technique
Moderate	Maintain hydration Avoid anaemia Oral antiemetics or antihistamines Advise time off work	P6 acupressure wristbands or acumagnets Vestibular audiotape Homeopathy	Acupuncture, shiatsu Reflexology Homeopathy Hypnotherapy
Severe	Hospitalisation IM antiemetics IV fluid replacement Total parenteral nutrition	P6 acupressure wristbands or acumagnets Vestibular audiotape *In conjunction with conventional treatment*	Osteopathy/chiropractic if structural misalignment or relaxation therapies *In conjunction with conventional treatment*

Box 9.3 Reasons why women may not wish to use certain strategies to treat their nausea and vomiting

STRATEGY	REASON	STRATEGY	REASON
Dietary changes	Dislike of advised foods	Acupuncture	Fear of needles
	Unable to retain any food		Eastern philosophy
	Expense of specific foods		conflicts with religious
	Practicalities of cooking		beliefs
Multivitamin supplements	Expense unless		May be contraindicated
	prescribed		Expense, availability
	Regarded as drugs		Credibility of practitioner
	Unable to swallow/retain	Reflexology	Dislike feet being touched
	May exacerbate		Seen as 'new age'
	symptoms		Credibility of practitioner
	May be contraindicated		Disbelief in effectiveness
	with other drugs	Homeopathic remedies	Profound healing crisis –
Relaxation techniques	No time or motivation		exacerbates symptoms
	Feeling too unwell		Tablets regarded as drugs
	Cost of private therapists		Expense, availability
Aromatherapy oils	Odour exacerbates n&v		Difficult to select most
	Dislike of smell		appropriate remedy
	Rejection of massage	Hypnotherapy	Fear of 'mind control'
	Fear of safety (chemicals)		Refuse to acknowledge
Herbal medicines	Regarded as drugs		psychological cause/effect
	May be contraindicated		Accessibility, expense
	Expense, accessibility	Osteopathy, chiropractic	Embarrassed by close contact
	Preparation (tinctures)		with practitioner
Bach flower remedies	Alcohol content		Expense, availability
	Seen as 'new age'		Credibility of practitioner
	Refuse to acknowledge	Alexander technique	Time, expense
	psychological		Not viewed as appropriate
	cause/effect		Availability of classes
Vestibular audiotape	No personal headphones	Prescribed drugs	Fear of effects on baby
	Difficult to use when		Forget to take medication
	working		Don't consult doctor
	N&V not triggered by	Hospitalisation	Family and work commitments
	motion		Emphasis on abnormality
	Lack of availability		May exacerbate stress
P6 acupressure	Uncomfortable to wear		Dislike of institutionalisation
wristbands	Forget to put on before		
	rising		
	Don't understand		
	instructions		
	Expense, availability		

CONCLUSION

Nausea and vomiting is more than simply a transient insignificant symptom of pregnancy. It is an extremely common condition of complex and varied aetiology which affects women in many different ways and impacts to varying degrees on their lives and those of their partners, families and colleagues. Left untended, it may resolve spontaneously, leaving the woman with nothing more than an unpleasant memory, or it may progress to a pathological problem requiring concentrated professional care and management and with the risk of complications which could, in extreme cases, lead to long-term morbidity or even death.

Most women will seek help from their midwives, obstetricians or general practitioners, who

Box 9.2 Tool: Tiran integrated approach to gestational sickness page 1

Tool Page 1	Vitamin B6 & zinc	Ginger (herb/EO)	Peppermint (herb/EO)	Acupressure/ puncture at P6 point
Nausea/vomiting	Constant nausea, frequent vomiting	Constant nausea, better after vomiting – vomits food soon after eating	AM nausea & intermittent, worse after vomiting – watery vomit later after eating	Constant or intermittent nausea, frequent vomiting
Notable characterstics	Insomnia Bitter taste in mouth (zinc) May have recently been on Pill	Thirsty for cold drinks, feels hot, red tongue, severe abdo pain	Craves hot drinks but no thirst, feels cold, pale tongue, dull abdo pain	P6 point dips & feels tender, located 3 fingers up from inner wrist crease
Mood/BFRs	Depressed BFR walnut, gorse, sweet chestnut	Anger BFR holly, cherry, plum, rock water, impatiens	Worry BFR heather, white chestnut, agrimony	Variable according to excess or deficiency
Contraindications Precautions	Avoid coffee, tea, bran, iron supps, soya & with low serum copper B6 50mg/day in vit. B complex Zinc 50mg/day	Anticoagulants, antihypertensives Use grated root ginger for tea, not biscuits or beer	Cardiac disease, epilepsy, G6PD Do not use with homeopathy	Coagulation disorders; needle phobia

Box 9.3 Tool: Tiran integrated approach to gestational sickness page 2

Tool page 2	Reflexology Osteopathy Chiropractic	Bach flower remedies	Hypnotherapy Autogenic training	Vestibular stimulation (audiotape)
Nausea/vomiting	Nausea variable, frequent vomiting	Nausea variable, hyperemesis gravidarum	Constant nausea, frequent vomiting	Constant nausea and vomiting
Notable characteristics	H/O neck, back injury or condition; heartburn; N & V unresponsive to other treatments	Variable	Variable	Worse with any motion, normally prone to travel sickness
Mood/BFRs	Miserable BFR walnut, gorse	Variable	Changeable but intense according to specific emotion	Variable
Contraindications Precautions	Epilepsy, APH, diabetes, renal or gall stones, thyroid disease, pacemaker, anticoagulants	Alcoholics, cirrhosis, moral objection to alcohol; dose 2 drops in water, Rescue remedy 4 drops neat prn	Clinical depression, schizophrenia, mania	None known; must be used with personal headphones

Box 9.4 Tool: Tiran integrated approach to gestational sickness page 3

Tool page 3	Homeopathic Nux Vomica	Homeopathic Ipecacuanha	Homeopathic Sepia	Homeopathic Pulsatilla
Nausea/vomiting	Nausea AM, & after eating, initially better after vomiting – vomit bile, mucus, bitter	Nausea constant, especially on waking, vomits ++ after food, + saliva, no effect on nausea	Intermittent, AM & after 1700 till sleep; vomits bile soon after eating	Constant nausea especially late afternoon/evening, worse after eating
Notable characteristics	Ravenous, craves coffee, tea, alcohol Averse to noise Constipation with backache	No appetite or thirst but craves cold drinks, averse to tobacco Heartburn, headaches	Nausea worse when hungry, better after eating, craves sour foods, vinegar, averse to food enjoyed previously Dark haired, tall, angular women	No thirst, bitter taste in mouth, non-specific cravings, averse to rich, spicy food, sensitive to over-eating. Heart-burn, flatulence, needs reminding to drink. Fair haired feminine women
Mood **NB Bach flower remedy unnecessary**	Angry, violent, workaholic	Frustrated, anxious, irritable	Indifferent, wants to be alone, regrets pregnancy, fear of miscarriage	Tearful, changeable, needs comfort, fears mothering abilities
Contraindications Precautions	No food, drink, smoking or cleaning the teeth for 15 minutes *before and after* taking each remedy. Contraindicated with coffee, mint toothpaste, analgesics, antacids, antibiotics, antifungals, anticoagulants. Dosage 30C potency, 1 tablet 2-3 hourly, not to be handled or dispensed on metal spoon.			

Box 9.5 Tool: Tiran integrated approach to gestational sickness page 4

Tool page 4	Homeopathic Cocculus	Homeopathic Colchicum	Other homeopathic remedies	Conventional treatment
Nausea/vomiting	Nausea afternoon, better with food, worse when tired and with motion	Nausea constant especially AM & evening, better if curled in fetal position, gagging & retching +++	Nausea evening, night & after vomits, craves acid fruits, apples = *antim tart* Nausea from 10am, worse later, hungry but loses weight = *natrum mur*	Constant nausea, frequent vomiting; unresponsive to other treatments NB Consider differential diagnosis
Notable characteristics	Hunger but no appetite, thirsty, metallic taste in mouth, craves cold drinks, averse to odours, first treatment for *motion sickness*	Thirsty for fizzy drinks, cravings intense but unable to satisfy them, averse to *any odours* especially food e.g. fish, eggs. Diarrhoea, sensitive to cold	Vomiting like food poisoning = *arsenicum* Excessive saliva = *kreosotum* Averse to water, even washing = *phosphorus*	Weight loss; no appetite; signs/symptoms of dehydration; hospitalisation if weight loss more than 3kg or 5%; nutrient deficiency, electrolyte imbalance
Mood **NB Bach flower remedy unnecessary with homeopathic remedies**	Emotional excitement, worry, insomnia, sensitive to loss of sleep	Want to be totally motionless & uninterrupted, variable energy levels	Bilious, right shoulder pain, constipation, nausea better with hot drinks = *chelidonium*	Psychologically unable to cope, distressed, anxious, tearful
Contraindications, precautions	No food, drink, smoking or cleaning the teeth for 15 minutes *before and after* taking each remedy. Contraindicated with coffee, mint toothpaste, analgesics, antacids, antibiotics, antifungals, anticoagulants. Dosage 30C potency, 1 tablet 2-3 hourly, not to be handled or dispensed on metal spoon.			? evidence on teratogenicity; monitor thiamin & clotting status in severe cases

will advise conservative rest, dietary and lifestyle adaptations and, in the event of an apparently more severe situation, may prescribe one of several medications available, or resort to admitting the woman to hospital. Many conventional healthcare professionals feel impotent to do more, and are reluctant even to consider pharmacological preparations unless the woman is showing signs of impending dehydration and weight loss, when outpatient medication is given in an attempt to prevent hospitalisation.

In cases where the mother self-selects alternatives to conventional care, she may opt for natural remedies which she can administer to herself, or may consult a practitioner of a complementary therapy. However, unless she has received adequate evidence-based information she may choose inappropriate or incorrect herbal medicines, essential oils or dietary supplements or try to use strategies such as acupressure wristbands which she finds ineffective as a result of inaccurate use through lack of knowledge. Consulting a practitioner of complementary medicine may be impractical due to lack of availability, geographical or economic factors and has the potential for problems if the therapist is not registered, underinsured, or inadequately qualified or experienced to treat pregnant women. Where reputable expert professional complementary practitioners are accessed, the women may need to commit to a course of treatment in order to gain maximum benefit, which will require her to find the time and finances to do so. The initial healing crisis which may occur with many therapies may cause an undesired exacerbation of symptoms with which the woman feels unable to cope, possibly causing her to discontinue treatment, but potentially leaving her in a worse condition than previously. Although many complementary practitioners utilise elements of several therapies in their work, the mother will need to make a decision about her preferred form of treatment which she is ill-equipped to do, and may choose those which are less effective for her personal condition than others.

The *Tiran Integrated Approach* to gestational sickness focuses on the mother as central to the decision-making process, and places the professional in the role of educator, supporter and facilitator, rather than in the 'parent-child' scenario of managing the woman's care. The use of a personal construct theory applied to the assessment and evaluation process enables adaptations to be made to the mother's choices as her condition alters, allows her to be the determinant of effectiveness and facilitates a 'seamless integration' of different systems of care (Mantle 2001). Acknowledgement, by both mothers and professionals, of a variety of causes, manifestations and effects ensures a more comprehensive mind-body-spirit overview of this aspect of pregnancy, whilst the use of a range of both conventional and complementary treatment strategies in combination with one another ensures 'best practice' for each individual and maintains the legal responsibility of midwives and obstetricians without compromise. Encouraging the mother to view her sickness in a more positive light and assisting her to cope with it for its duration improves her sense of satisfaction and involvement, adding to her feeling of empowerment and consequently enhancing efficacy. Furthermore, increased ability of doctors and midwives to help women will improve their professional sense of satisfaction and may initiate reflection on practice which ultimately reduces demand on the services.

Nausea and vomiting is probably the commonest and most well known of all symptoms of pregnancy yet there has not, hitherto, been a concerted nor a comprehensive means of relieving it. It is hoped that the *Tiran Integrated Approach* will expand the range of effective, safe and satisfying options which can be offered by maternity professionals for the benefit of mothers and their families.

REFERENCES

Anderson T 2002 The misleading myth of choice: the continuing oppression of women in childbirth. MIDIRS Midwifery Digest 12 (3): 405-407

Astin J A 1998 Why patients use alternative medicine: results of a national study. Journal of the American Medical Association 279 (19): 1548

Autry A M, Meurer L N, Barnabei V M et al 2002 A longitudinal women's health curriculum: a multi-method multiperspective needs assessment. American Journal of Obstetrics and Gynecology 187 (3 Suppl): S12-14

Basford J R 2001 Medical electromagnetism: 3000 years of history. Focus on Alternative and Complementary Therapies 6 (1): 70

Beecher H K 1955 The powerful placebo. Journal of the American Medical Association 159: 1602

Benor D 1996 Reaching towards wholeness. European Nurse 4: 240-249

Benson H 1996 Timeless healing: the power of biology and belief. Scribner, New York

Bensoussan A 1991 The vital meridian. Churchill Livingstone, Edinburgh

Boudreaux E D, O'Hea E, Chasuk R 2002 Spiritual role in healing. An alternative way of thinking. Primary Care 29 (2): 439-454 , viii

Buckle J 1993 When is holism not complementary? British Journal of Nursing 2 (15): 744-745

Campbell R, Macfarlane A 1987 Where to be born: the debate and the evidence. National Perinatal Epidemiology Unit Oxford

Cumbie S A 2001 The integration of mind-body-soul and the practice of humanistic nursing. Holistic Nurse Practitioner 15 (3): 56-62

Department of Health 1993 Changing Childbirth: Report of the Expert Committee. HMSO, London

Department of Health 1998 Midwifery: delivering our future: report of the standing nursing, midwifery and health visiting committee. HMSO, London

De Punzio C, Neri E, Metelli P et al 1994 The relationship between maternal relaxation and plasma beta-endorphin levels during parturition. Journal of Pyschosomatic Obstetrics and Gynaecology 15 (4): 205-210

Duggan R M 2001 Diverse practitioners join at the heart of healing. Complementary Therapies in Nursing and Midwifery 7 (1): 1-3

Eisenberg D M 1997 Advising patients who seek alternative medical therapies. Annals of Internal Medicine 127: 61

Engebretson J 2002 Culture and complementary therapies. Complementary Therapies in Nursing and Midwifery 8 (4): 177-184

Ernst E 1999 Alternative views of alternative medicine. Ann Intern Med 131: 230

Ernst E, White A 2000 The BBC survey of complementary use in the United Kingdom. Complementary Therapies in Medicine 8: 32-36

Fahy K 2002 Reflecting on practice to theorise empowerment for women: using Foucault's concepts. Australian Journal of Midwifery 15 (1): 5-13

Furnham A 1996 Why do people choose and use complementary therapies? In: Ernst E (ed) 1996 Complementary medicine: an objective appraisal. Butterworth-Heinemann, Oxford

Guinn D E 2001 Ethics and integrative medicine: moving beyond the biomedical model. Alternative Therapies in Health and Medicine 7 (6): 68-72

Hebert R S, Kenckes M W, Ford D E et al 2001 Patient perspectives on spirituality and the patient-physician relationship. Journal of General Internal Medicine 16 (10): 685-692

Heres M H, Pel M, Borkent-Polet M et al 2000 The hour of birth: comparisons of circadian pattern between women cared for by midwives and obstetricians. Midwifery 16 (3): 173-176

Hyder S M, Person L A Chowdhury A M et al 2002 Do side-effects reduce compliance to iron supplements? A study of daily- and weekly-dose regimens in pregnancy. Journal of Health Population and Nutrition 20 (2): 175-179

Jacobs J J 1999 Complementary/alternative medicine in the 21st century. In: Spencer J W, Jacobs J J (eds) 1999 Complementary/alternative medicine: an evidence-based approach. Mosby, St Louis

Johanson R, Newburn M, Macfarlane A 2002 Has the medicalisation of childbirth gone too far? British Medical Journal 324 (7342): 892-895

Johns C 2001 The caring dance. Complementary Therapies in Nursing and Midwifery 7 (1): 8-12

Kaptchuk T J 2002 The placebo effect in alternative medicine: can the performance of a healing ritual have clinical significance? Annals of Internal Medicine 136 (11): 817-825

Kelly G 1955 The psychology of personal constructs Vol 1. Norton, New York

Koehn M L 2000 Alternative and complementary therapies for labor and birth: an application of Kolcaba's theory of holistic comfort. Holistic Nursing Practice 15 (1): 66-77

Kolcaba K, Steiner K 2000. Empirical evidence for the nature of comfort. Journal of Holistic Nursing 18 (1): 46-62

Kolcaba K, Wilson L 2002 Comfort care: a framework for perianaesthesia nursing. Journal of Perianaesthesia Nursing 17 (2): 102-111

Konefal J 2002 The challenge of educating physicians about complementary and alternative medicine. Academic Medicine 77 (9): 847-850

Kreitzer M J, Mitten D, Harris I 2002 Attitudes toward CAM among medical, nursing and pharmacy faculty and students: a comparative analysis. Alternative Therapies in Health and Medicine 8 (6): 44-47; 50-53

Landis B J 1996 Uncertainty, spiritual wellbeing and psychosocial adjustment to chronic illness. Issues in Mental Health Nursing 17 (3): 217

Larson D, Milano M 1996 Religion and mental health: should they work together? Alternative and Complementary Therapies March/April: 91

Levine J K D, Gordon N C, Fields H L 1978 The mechanism of placebo analgesia. Lancet 2: 654

Lewis D, Paterson M, Beckerman S et al 2001 Attitudes toward integration of complementary and alternative medicine with hospital-based care. Journal of Alternative and Complementary Medicine 7 (6): 681-688

Liossi C, Mystakidou K 1997 Heron's theory of human needs in palliative care. European Journal of Palliative Care 4 (1): 32-35

Magee L A, Chandra K, Mazzotta P et al 2002 Development

of a health-related quality of life instrument for nausea and vomiting of pregnancy. American Journal of Obstetrics and Gynecology 186 (5 suppl): S232-238

Mantle F 2001 Complementary therapies and nursing models. In: Rankin Box D (ed) The nurses' handbook of complementary therapies, 2nd edn. Bailliere Tindall/RCN, London

Miccozzi M S 1996 Fundamentals of complementary and alternative medicine. Churchill Livingstone, Edinburgh

Miller M W, Brayman A A, Abramowicz J S 1998 Obstetric ultrasonography: a biophysical consideration of patient safety – the 'rules' have changed. American Journal of Obstetrics and Gynecology 179 (1): 241-254

Mitchell A, Cormack M 1998 The therapeutic relationship in complementary health care. Churchill Livingstone, Edinburgh

Moyad M A 2002 The placebo effect and randomised trials: analysis of alternative medicine. Urological Clinics of North America 29 (1): 135-155

Oh V M 1994 The placebo effect – how can we use it better? British Medical Journal 309: 69

Oschman J L 2000 Energy medicine: the scientific basis. Churchill Livingstone, London

Peace G 2002 Integrated cancer care: linking medicine and therapies. Nursing Times 98 (34): 35-37

Pietroni P 1997 Is complementary medicine holistic? Complementary Therapies in Nursing and Midwifery 3: 9-11

Peters D, Pinto G J, Harris G 2000 Using a computer-based clinical management system to improve effectiveness of a homeopathic service in a fundholding general practice. British Homeopathic Journal 89 (Suppl 1): S14-19

Pogge R C 1963 The toxic placebo 1. Side and toxic effects reported during the administration of placebo medicine. Medical Times 91: 1

Reilly D 2001 Comments on complementary and alternative medicine in Europe. Journal of Alternative and Complementary Medicine 7 (Suppl 1): S23-31

Rhodes V A, McDaniel R W 1999 The index of nausea, vomiting and retching: a new format of the index of nausea and vomiting. Oncology Nursing Forum 26 (5): 889-894

Ruiz R K, Pearson A J 1999 Psychoneuroimmunology and preterm birth. A holistic model for obstetrical nursing practice and research. American Journal of Maternal and Child Nursing 24 (5): 230-235

Shapiro A K, Shapiro E 1984 Patient-provider relationships and the placebo effect. In: Matarazzo J D et al (eds) Behavioral health: a handbook of health enhancement and disease prevention. Wiley-Interscience, New York

Sheth S S, Chalmers I 2002 Magnesium for preventing and treating pre-eclampsia: time for international action. The Lancet 359 (9321): 1872-1873

So D W 2002 Acupuncture outcomes, expectations, patient-provider relationship and the placebo effect: implications for health promotion. American Journal of Public Health 92 (10): 1662-1667

Stan N H 2002 Deconstructing paternalism – what serves the patient best? Singapore Medical Journal 43 (3): 148-151

Stone J 2002 Ethicolegal and professional principles. In: Mackereth P, Tiran D (eds) Clinical reflexology: a guide for health professionals. Elsevier Science, London

Sulmasy D P 2002 A biopsychosocial-spiritual model for the care of patients at the end of life. Gerontologist 42 (3): 24-33

Taylor B 2002 Becoming a reflective nurse or midwife: using complementary therapies while practising holistically. Complementary Therapies in Nursing and Midwifery 8 (2): 62-68

Tiran D 1999 A holistic framework for maternity care. Complementary Therapies in Nursing and Midwifery 5: 127-135

Tiran D 2000 Incorporation of complementary therapies into maternity care. In: Tiran D, Mack S (eds) Complementary therapies for pregnancy and childbirth, 2nd edn

Tiran D 2003 Implementing complementary therapies into midwifery practice. Complementary Therapies in Nursing and Midwifery 9

Todd B 1990 Holistic nursing: a new paradigm for practice. NSNA/Imprint Sept/Oct: 75-80

Tranmer J E 2000 Who knows best: the patient or the provider? A nursing perspective. Hospital Quarterly 3 (4): 25-29

Vincent C, Furnham A 1997 Complementary medicine: a research perspective. John Wiley & Sons, Chichester

Waldenstrom U 1996 Modern maternity care: does safety have to take the meaning out of birth? Midwifery 12 (4): 165-173

White A 2000 Integration ... beyond placebo? Complementary Therapies in Medicine 8 (4): 225

Whitehead D 2000 Naturalistic vs reductionistic approaches to health-related practice: opposing dichotomy or symbiotic partnership? Complementary Therapies in Nursing and Midwifery 6 (3): 149-154

Wright S G, Sayre-Adams J 2000 Sacred space: right relationships and spirituality in healthcare. Churchill Livingstone, London

Glossary, Appendix & Index

Glossary

Acupressure: similar to acupuncture, but without the use of needles to stimulate the tsubos; see *acupuncture*.

Acupuncture: based on the principle that the body has energy lines, called meridians, which run through major organs, after which they take their names. There are 12 major meridians and 365 minor meridians. Focus points, called *tsubos*, occur periodically along the meridians and can be treated by the insertion of needles to stimulate or sedate energy levels and so rebalance the person, improving and maintaining their health.

Alexander technique: devised by Frederick Alexander, an actor, who discovered that his recurring loss of voice could be corrected by improving his posture. Involves a re-education to improve postural balance and coordination so that the body is able to maximise its potential with minimal strain.

Anthroposophical medicine: a combined approach to treatment, incorporating both conventional and complementary medicine as well as an exploration of the individual's inner feelings and concept of illness and health.

Aromatherapy: the therapeutic use of concentrated plant essences and essential oils which act pharmacologically, aesthetically and psychologically. Oils can be applied via the skin, the respiratory tract, the mucus membranes and, occasionally, gastrointestinally.

Autogenic training: an adapted hypno-therapeutic technique using relaxation, mental imagery and auto-suggestion.

Ayurvedic medicine: a traditional form of healing originating from India and involving the use of indigenous plants, manual therapeutic techniques and energy medicine.

Bach flower remedies: a system of using homeopathic (minute) doses of specific plant infusions, usually in liquid preparations, to treat the psycho-emotional aspects of health. There are 38 remedies plus the Rescue remedy.

Biofeedback: a form of psychophysiological programming, using apparatus to monitor and feed back physiological responses in order to effect changes; a form of psychophysiological re-education.

Carbon dioxide extraction: a method of using compressed carbon dioxide as a solvent to extract essential oils from plants; although expensive, it has the advantage of using lower temperatures than steam distillation, thus ensuring less damage to the essential oils.

Chinese herbal medicine: see *Traditional Chinese Medicine*.

Chiropractic: similar to *osteopathy*, chiropractic is based on the principle that the neuromusculoskeletal system is fundamental to health determination and that spinal misalignment predisposes people to disease which can be treated by spinal manipulation.

Cold expression: a method of extracting essences from citrus fruits, either by crushing the fruit and separating the juice from the peel, or by abrading the rind and using centrifugal force to separate the oil from the debris.

Craniosacral therapy: a gentle form of osteopathy in which the cranium and sacrum are balanced by minute manipulations to correct a range of disorders; sometimes termed cranial osteopathy.

Crystal healing: the use of various crystals believed to possess energies which can be channeled into or absorbed by the recipient in order to effect healing and maintenance of optimum health and wellbeing.

Decoction: similar to infusion but used for hard, woody parts of plants, left to simmer, then strained; should be used within 24 hours.

Emmenagoguic: an agent with the potential to cause uterine bleeding, but not necessarily an abortifacient.

Energy medicine: any form of therapeutic intervention involving an assumed transfer of energy from an identified source (the practitioner (as in *Reiki)* or a substance (as in *homeopathy*) and the client.

Essential oils: highly concentrated substances extracted by various means from plants for their therapeutic properties, used in *aromatherapy*.

Feldenkrais: a system involving re-education of the ways in which dysfunctional habits of movement of the body lead to impaired health and wellbeing; awareness through movement and 'functional integration' of the body aim to restore the individual to optimum health.

Foundation for Integrated Medicine (FIM): a charitable organisation founded in 1996 which is committed to greater integration of complementary and alternative medicine within conventional healthcare. Renamed, in 2002, the Prince of Wales' Foundation for Integrated Health.

Healing: see *spiritual healing.*

Herbal medicine: the medicinal use of plants. Generically includes all types of botanical medicine from around the world but is used primarily to indicate western herbal medicine, or phytotherapy.

Homeopathy: a discrete system of healthcare in which minute doses of vegetable, mineral or animal substances are used to treat conditions which, in larger doses, would actually cause the symptoms being treated; also explained as 'like treating like'.

Hypnotherapy: the medical use of the hypnotic or trance-like state to induce deep relaxation and make use of enhanced suggestibility to treat psychological conditions and effect behavioural changes.

Infusion (tea): soft parts of the dried plant (leaves, stems, seeds) are added to boiling water, left to infuse, strained and drunk, hot or cold.

Infused oil: plant material is covered with cold pressed oil and heated, either in sunlight or artificial heat: used as the basis for creams, pessaries, ointments, suppositories.

Iridology: a diagnostic system which uses the irises of the eyes to represent a map of the rest of the body and so enables the practitioner to determine areas of changing physiology and potential or actual pathology.

Massage: a generic term to describe the manipulation of soft tissues of the body, using pressure, traction and movement to treat physiological and emotional conditions; there are many types of massage around the world, including Swedish, lymphatic, aromatherapy, rolfing, Feldenkrais, lomi-lomi and others.

Medical herbalism: see *herbal medicine*.

Moxibustion: a technique in *Traditional Chinese Medicine* in which a stick of dried, compressed mugwort herb is used as a heat source above specific tsubos; in maternity care, this is used to turn breech presentations to cephalic.

Naturopathy: an all-encompassing system of healthcare incorporating both conventional and complementary medicine, including diet and nutrition, internal and external hydrotherapy, exercise, relaxation, spinal manipulation and other techniques to initiate the body's innate self-healing powers.

Osteopathy: a discrete manual system of healthcare in which massage, spinal manipulation and mobilisation are used to rebalance misalignments in the musculoskeletal system which are predisposed to deviations from health and cause illness and disease.

Phytotherapy: a generic term to describe the medicinal use of plants; see *herbal medicine*; also incorporates *aromatherapy* and Traditional Chinese herbal medicine.

Proving: in homeopathy, the process of determining the exact nature of symptoms which can be treated by a particular remedy; usually achieved by testing reactions of healthy volunteers to an overdose of the test substance.

Qi gong: a Chinese system of movements and postures similar to *Tai Chi*.

Reflexology: based on the principle that a small area of the body, normally the feet or hands, reflects in miniature the whole body, so that treatment can be applied distally via manual manipulation; can also be performed on the face, ear or back. Also termed reflex zone therapy or reflexotherapy.

Reiki: a form of energy medicine in which there is a direct intervention between the practitioner and the client intended to enhance health and wellbeing; it is believed that therapeutic effects occur as a result of a channeling of energy between the practitioner and client. Also called *spiritual healing*, distant healing, faith or psychic healing, 'laying on of hands', Therapeutic Touch.

Relaxation therapies: a range of different therapies aimed at triggering the relaxation response of the autonomic nervous system; includes *autogenic training, biofeedback, hypnotherapy, meditation* and others

Reverse proving: process which can occur in the event of a patient being given an incorrect homeopathic remedy, which leads to the development of symptoms which the remedy is intended (when used correctly) to relieve.

Rolfing: a deep, intense form of soft tissue massage, intended to release tensions in the fascia, thus improving body structure; also termed structural integration.

Shiatsu: a modern, Japanese system similar to *acupressure*, using the meridians and tsubos of *acupuncture* but in the form of complete body pressure massage; 'shiatsu' literally means 'thumb pressure'.

Solvent extraction: a method of obtaining essential oils from delicate flowers such as jasmine, rose or orange blossom, using hydrocarbons to extract aromatic material from the resins of the plants; the hydrocarbons are then filtered off by distillation.

Spiritual healing: a direct interaction, in the form of a channeling of energy, between therapist and patient to promote or facilitate self-healing; also referred to as faith healing, psychic healing or distant healing.

Steam distillation: the oldest and commonest method of extracting essential oils from plants, using steam to soften the plant tissues, allowing the oils to escape, and vaporise on cooling; the mixture of oil and water is then separated by centrifugal force.

Succussion: the process of vigorously shaking diluted substances in the preparation of homeopathic remedies; it is thought that this releases the active energies from the original substances into the water in which they have been diluted, thus making the remedy more powerful.

Tai Chi: a Chinese approach incorporating gentle movements and postures derived from martial arts to enhance mental and physical health and wellbeing.

Tibetan medicine: ancient traditional style of natural medicine from Tibet, using plants, exercise and meditation techniques.

Therapeutic Touch (TT): a formalised type of 'laying on of hands', adapted by the American nursing professor, Dolores Krieger, and used by nurses throughout America. It is not, however, performed within a religious context. Contact with the physical body does not occur; rather the practitioner uses the hands about 2 to 3 inches above the patient's body in order to detect energy flow and unblock energy deficits.

Tincture: dried or fresh plant material macerated in alcohol or glycerine for 2 to 3 weeks, then pressed; commonest form of administration.

Traditional Chinese Medicine (TCM): ancient traditional natural medicine from China, involving herbal medicine, acupuncture and acupressure, moxibustion, bone-setting and other techniques.

Tuina: a component of Traditional Chinese Medicine; a form of massage using pulling and rubbing movements to stimulate pressure points.

Vibrational medicine: alternative name for energy medicine, in which energy principles are thought to vibrate; *homeopathy* is sometimes referred to as vibrational medicine.

Yoga: involves gentle stretching, breathing exercises, meditation and a range of postures and positions for mental and physical wellbeing. There are several different styles of yoga, some more physical, others more spiritual.

Appendix: Useful addresses and resources

British Complementary Medicine Association
A general CAM organisation, providing registers of practitioners, information on educational programmes and insurance cover for registrants.
Kensington House, 33 Imperial Square,
Cheltenham, Gloucs GL50 1QZ

Complementary Maternity Forum
An independent, multidisciplinary professional networking and support organisation for those providing or interested in specialising in integrating complementary medicine into conventional maternity care. Members are midwives, complementary practitioners, GPs, obstetricians, obstetric physiotherapists, NCT teachers and journalists from pregnancy consumer publications and websites. Meetings are held three times a year, non-members welcome. Membership for individuals or groups; regular newsletters. Register of Complementary Maternity Services being developed for access by professionals and consumers.
Contact: Denise Tiran (Chair), University of
Greenwich, School of Health and Social Care,
Mansion Site, Avery Hill Campus, Eltham,
London SE9 2PQ
Tel: 07956 235456
www.c-m-f.co.uk

Complementary Therapies in Medicine
Complementary Therapies in Nursing and Midwifery
Professional research-based quarterly journals.
www.harcourt-international.com/journals

Daval Ltd
Produces Morningwell auditory tapes to relieve pregnancy sickness (see Chapter 7).
Victoria House, 23 Winchester Road, Andover,
Hants SP10 2EQ
Tel: 01264 364 474
www.morningwell.co.uk

Expectancy Ltd
Expectant Parents' Complementary Therapies Consultancy.
www.expectancy.co.uk

HerbMed
Herbal medicine database of related evidence.
www.herbmed.org

Hom-Inform information service
References from Glasgow Faculty of Homeopathy's comprehensive research database.
www.hominform.soutron.com/homqbel.asp

National Center for Complementary and Alternative Medicine
US database of CAM research and high quality review papers.
www.nccam.nih.gov/research

Prince of Wales' Foundation for Integrated Health (formerly the Foundation for Integrated Medicine)
12 Chillingworth Road, London N7 8QJ
Tel: 020 7688 1881
email: enquiries@fimed.org
www.fimed.org.uk

Research Council for Complementary Medicine
email: info@rccm.org.uk
www.rccm.org.uk

Royal College of Obstetricians and Gynaecologists
27 Sussex Place, London NW1
Tel: 0207 772 6200

Royal College of Midwives
15 Mansfield Street, London W1M 0BE
Tel: 020 7312 3535

Society of Homeopaths
Principal organisation for non-medical homeopaths.
www.homoeopathy-soh.org

Zita West Pregnancy Products
Natural remedies for pregnancy, including acu-magnets and herbal remedies for nausea.
www.zitawest.com

Index